The Faber Book of Seductions

The Faber Book of
SEDUCTIONS

Edited by
Jenny Newman

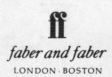

faber and faber
LONDON · BOSTON

First published in 1988
by Faber and Faber Limited
3 Queen Square London WC1N 3AU

This paperback edition first published in 1990

Photoset by Wilmaset Birkenhead Wirral
Printed in Great Britain by
Cox and Wyman Ltd Reading Berkshire

A CIP record for this book is
available from the British Library
ISBN 0-571-13751-2

Contents

Introduction ix

The Whole Artillery of Love

from Love for Love *William Congreve*	3
Going to Bed *John Donne*	6
Chagrin in Three Parts *Graham Greene*	8
from The White Devil *John Webster*	15
from Tom Jones *Henry Fielding*	19
Delight in Disorder *Robert Herrick*	21
from Rates of Exchange *Malcolm Bradbury*	22
from Hero and Leander *Christopher Marlowe*	32
from Sanditon *Jane Austen*	35
from Volpone *Ben Jonson*	37
from Room at the Top *John Braine*	42
Jankin, the clerical seducer *Anon*	46
from The Well of Loneliness *Radclyffe Hall*	48
To his Coy Mistress *Andrew Marvell*	52
Party Piece *Brian Patten*	54

Purposes Mistook

from In the Purely Pagan Sense *John Lehmann*	57
Jupiter and Ganimede *Thomas Heywood*	59
from The Way of the World *William Congreve*	63
from Le Morte d'Arthur (Sir Pelleas and the Lady Ettard) *Thomas Malory*	74

from The Alchemist *Ben Jonson*   78

from Mooncranker's Gift *Barry Unsworth*   84

from Paradise Lost (Book ix: Satan
    tempts Eve) *John Milton*   92

from Cantleman's Spring-Mate
    Wyndham Lewis   103

from Women Beware Women *Thomas*
    Middleton   109

from Arthur Snatchfold *E. M. Forster*   113

from The Country Wife *William*
    Wycherley   118

from Joseph Andrews *Henry Fielding*   124

from The Changeling *Thomas Middleton*
    and William Rowley   129

from Time after Time *Molly Keane*   135

Wise and Foolish Virgins

from The Bell Jar *Sylvia Plath*   139

from Don Juan *George Gordon, Lord Byron*   145

from Sons and Lovers *D. H. Lawrence*   149

The Willing Mistriss *Aphra Behn*   152

from Heroes and Villains *Angela Carter*   153

from Sodom *attributed to John Wilmot,*
    Earl of Rochester   156

from The New Atalantis *Mary de la*
    Riviere Manley   158

Deceptions *Philip Larkin*   166

from Moll Flanders *Daniel Defoe*   167

The Sick Rose *William Blake*   177

from Clarissa *Samuel Richardson*   178

from Measure for Measure *William*
    Shakespeare   188

from The Monk *Matthew G. Lewis*   194

from Virgin Territory *Sara Maitland*   198

from The Lustful Turk *Anon*   206

The Thorn *William Wordsworth*   210

from The Ha-Ha *Jennifer Dawson*   218

from Tess of the d'Urbervilles *Thomas Hardy* 221

The Ruined Maid *Thomas Hardy* 227

Travesties

from Homemade *Ian McEwan* 231

Song (Fair Chloris) *John Wilmot, Earl of Rochester* 238

from Pamela *Samuel Richardson* 240

from Shamela *attributed to Henry Fielding* 244

from Venus and Adonis *William Shakespeare* 247

from Free Fall *William Golding* 252

from Richard III *William Shakespeare* 255

from Paradise Lost (Book v) *John Milton* 263

from Lamia *John Keats* 266

Goblin Market *Christina Rossetti* 272

Song (*from* The Vicar of Wakefield) *Oliver Goldsmith* 288

from The Revenger's Tragedy *Cyril Tourneur* 289

from Point Counter Point *Aldous Huxley* 292

Leda and the Swan *W. B. Yeats* 297

Leda *Lilian Bowes-Lyon* 298

from Dracula *Bram Stoker* 299

Siren Song

from The Book of Genesis 309

from Paradise Lost (Book ix: Eve tempts Adam) *John Milton* 311

from Doctor Faustus *Christopher Marlowe* 317

from Cider with Rosie *Laurie Lee* 320

from The Faerie Queene (Book ii) *Edmund Spenser* 323

from Le Morte d'Arthur (Launcelot is tricked by Dame Brisen) *Thomas Malory* 329

La Belle Dame sans Merci *John Keats* 332

from Antony and Cleopatra *William Shakespeare*   335

from Salomé *Oscar Wilde*   337

from Sir Gawain and the Green Knight *Anon*   342

from Jude the Obscure *Thomas Hardy*   350

The River God *Stevie Smith*   355

What The Pool Said, On Midsummer's Day *Liz Lochhead*   356

Index of Authors and Works   359

Acknowledgements   365

Introduction

Seduction operates somewhere between courtship and rape. At best, with its ritual techniques of persuasion, it promises all the pleasures of courtship while avoiding the consequences. At worst, it is a way of despoiling, only distinguishable from crime because it does not involve brute force. Seduction, unlike a marriage proposal, can never occur between equals. Its inherent imbalance explains why it is always exploitative in one way or another.

For seduction to be possible, one person must want sex more than the other – or else have less to lose by it. But the advantage can shift unpredictably in the struggle for sexual supremacy or possession. The risks of the business are exposed with particular clarity as those engaged in it are obliged to perform beyond the reach of the safety net of courtship. If there is any relationship at all between literature and life, the history of fictional seduction is bound to throw the nature of our sexual politics into sharp relief.

Traditionally there are two main ways of looking at the seduction scene. The first is comic in method. Its entertainment value springs from a display of tactics. Whether or not the seducer gets his or her own way, some kind of happy ending confirms a generally optimistic view of sex. This kind of seduction can be seen as a more adventurous counterpart to what happens in marriage, reaffirming the accepted order of society. The pleasure is in the exercise of power, while the emphasis falls not on what one is, but on what one does. The attitudes operating here are best typified in literature by the Cavalier approach to sex.

The other view of seduction is tragic. People get hurt and, instead of being allowed to choose, they are drawn inevitably to betrayal. Ironically, this goes along with a stress on morality rather than strategy. Resistance to this kind of temptation always leads to loss; while to succumb means the downfall of both seducer

[ix]

and seduced, and perhaps of the whole of society too. Instead of coexisting with marriage, this sort of seduction tends to undermine it. Its power brings not pleasure but knowledge. This is the line of thought that governed the Puritan attitude to sex.

Military campaigns and games – both demanding tactics – are often used as figurative expressions of the comic view of seduction. So is the hunt, with its climax and division of spoils emphasizing the ritualized energy of sexual pursuit. Such metaphors occur in *Sir Gawain and the Green Knight*, many Restoration comedies, *Tom Jones*, and other works whose characters are expected to fend for themselves. In the darker treatment of seduction, which in the English tradition becomes the richer and more complex, the range of metaphors is correspondingly wider. Enchantment (*Le Morte d'Arthur*, 'La Belle Dame sans Merci'); dreaming (*Paradise Lost* Book v); madness (*Le Morte d'Arthur*) and metamorphosis (*The Faerie Queene*, *Paradise Lost* Book iv, 'Lamia', *Dracula*, 'Leda and the Swan') are all used to suggest troubled sexuality. These metaphors may also occur in the comic mode, but only as material for parody.

Sir Gawain and the Green Knight (c. 1375) is typical of the first kind of attitude. There is a hint of complicity between Gawain and the chatelaine. At the customary exchange of winnings with his host, the knight fails to relinquish the girdle she had given him that morning. A serious issue is at stake, as is made clear by the three hunting scenes which parallel the Lady's three attempts to entice her noble guest to turn the game of courtly love into sexual activity. The quarry dies as a result of Bertilak's chase across the frosty morning landscape. Yet the controlling metaphor of the hunt also emphasizes the place of festivity and entertainment. In the chatelaine's final visit to Gawain's bedroom, anthologized here, her sudden entrance, the enthralling boldness of her behaviour, her extreme *décolleté*, back and front, and her impropriety in seating herself on the knight's bed within the curtain all heighten the excitement of the scene.* Later, when we realize that Bertilak is also the Green Knight and that his Lady has been attempting to seduce Gawain with her husband's consent, we see how this kind of seduction can work in conjunction with marriage rather than counter to its interests. The status quo is endorsed by Gawain's

---

*See W. R. J. Barron, *'Trawthe' and treason: the sin of Gawain reconsidered* (1980), p. 26.

refusal to succumb, and his virtue restores the honour of King Arthur's court.

By the time we reach Thomas Malory's *Le Morte d'Arthur* (1470), characteristic of the sombre approach to seduction, the Gawain figure has degenerated into a philanderer who plays a base trick on his fellow knight, Sir Pelleas. His deceitful behaviour with the Lady Ettard contrasts unfavourably with Launcelot's impassioned devotion to Guenever, which is the nearest equivalent here to the *trawthe* of *Sir Gawain and the Green Knight*.

The Gawain-poet's hero of the Round Table's younger days is accorded a choice between dishonour and discourtesy, and we watch him demonstrate his sophistication by contriving to reconcile the two. For Malory's Launcelot, on the other hand, no such opportunity exists. Dame Brisen's magic can empower her to lead Launcelot by the finger to Elaine's bed, only because his identity as a knight is utterly bound up with his adulterous passion for Guenever, to whom he believes he is about to make love. His tragedy is that his allegiance to his 'special good lady' and 'most noble Christian queen' is also an act of betrayal towards his king. On discovering that he has been tricked, he jumps out of the bay window into the thorns that score his naked body, and then runs mad for two years. His anguish foreshadows the inevitable consequences of the secret passion soon to dispeople the Round Table.

In both *Sir Gawain and the Green Knight* and *Le Morte d'Arthur* society's survival depends on the hero's resistance to temptation. Despite his failure, it is Launcelot who takes us forward into the Renaissance, with its recognition that spiritual and temporal values are inextricably mixed in our understanding of sexuality. Seduction scenes on the Elizabethan and Jacobean stage embody a tumult of impulses both sacred and secular, leading to a new definition of ecstasy. Christopher Marlowe's Doctor Faustus is a key figure in the transition from Medieval to Renaissance, torn as he is between a Christian creed and humanist aspirations. In an act of daring he chooses secular power at the expense of the spiritual; or rather, when he asks for a kiss from the demon who has taken Helen of Troy's shape, he hopes, as Launcelot never did, that sexual passion may lead to immortality. He is punished severely for this heterodoxy, but the possibility continues to haunt the seventeenth-century imagination, fuelling the urgent sensuousness that is entering the language.

Angelo in *Measure for Measure* in some ways resembles Marlowe's hero. He, too, is a figure of the Middle Ages in his asceticism, and of the Renaissance in his desires, trying unsuccessfully to write good angel on the devil's horn. Yet Angelo perceives not choice, but paradox, in his urge to seduce Isabella. His deliberations bring about stasis rather than the accelerated time-scheme of Faustus's end, bringing to the drama of seduction a new inwardness, and making Angelo one of the first seducers to scrutinize his own motives:

> What dost thou, or what art thou, Angelo?
> Dost thou desire her foully for those things
> That make her good?

The deadlock between Angelo and Isabella brings the age's conflicting beliefs about the value of virginity into head-on collision. Like Donne in the Paradoxes, Angelo claims that its importance is only relative. Isabella seems a less interesting character, because she is allowed no choice as to how to retain her identity. Her only function is to resist his bullying tactics, even though she is as yet unaware that he has already seduced and betrayed Mariana.

If Angelo, attempting to indulge his 'sweet uncleanness', is willing to try civic authority as a route to sexual power, Shakespeare's Cleopatra reverses the process. Characteristic of the period, the play's rhetoric of seduction is charged with images of conspicuous consumption, as in Enobarbus's description of Cleopatra's strange, invasive perfume uniting sex and wealth, which floats from her barge to render Antony powerless in his empty market-place. The lavish menu Ben Jonson's Volpone proposes for Celia, with its 'heads of parrots, tongues of nightingales, / The brains of peacocks, and of estriches', is of the same order of opulence. In such cases crucial scenes are often elaborately stage-managed by the characters themselves, as when Volpone leaps unexpectedly at the horrified Celia from his pretended deathbed, or Richard III woos the widow of the man he has murdered while she accompanies the bier of her dead father-in-law, or the Lady

Livia orchestrates her telling game of chess in Thomas Middleton's *Women Beware Women*.

On the seventeenth-century stage we see a number of female characters like the independent-minded Livia, whose attempts to gain sexual autonomy constitute a powerful challenge to the traditional values of the open clan system. We are reminded of its male-dominated structure – and of women's attempts to undermine it – in countless seduction scenes. The Duchess in Cyril Tourneur's *The Revenger's Tragedy*, for example, avenges her son's harsh treatment in court at the hands of her second husband by seducing the latter's bastard son. In John Webster's *The White Devil*, Duke Brachiano's man, Flamineo, interprets for the audience the Duke's seduction of Flamineo's sister, Vittoria, through a series of innuendoes ('Excellent! His jewel for her jewel: well put in, duke!'); he also notes the dangers their adultery holds for society ('Excellent devil! She hath taught him in a dream / To make away his duchess and her husband'); while his mother, Cornelia, listening to the same interchange, spells out its dynastic consequences: 'Now find our house / Sinking to ruin'.

Other spirited Renaissance women besides Vittoria and Tourneur's Duchess attempt to circumvent masculine supremacy by putting their sexuality to work – in order to gratify lust, exact revenge or further ambition. But even the most defiant do not escape the mandatory repentance of Act v. Beatrice in Middleton and Rowley's *The Changeling*, Bianca in Middleton's *Women Beware Women* and Vittoria herself are only three among the many rebellious women allowed time, before they die, to beg forgiveness of the patriarchy they have offended.

Female defiance is more fully explored in *Paradise Lost*, which, oddly enough, can also be seen as the first major Puritan apology for the companionate marriage. Satan, a typical Cavalier seducer in his troubled contempt for bourgeois domesticity, finds it easy to exploit this new commitment to love and friendship between husband and wife, and its anomalous relationship to a firmly reiterated insistence on the man's divinely-ordained superiority. Eve, pursuing her solitary gardening, naturally finds attractive the discordant note of power in the serpent's overtures. The first rakehell disguises his insatiate drives in a parody of courtly love that is grotesque and sexual at the same time: 'Oft he bowed / His turret crest, and sleek enamelled neck, / Fawning, and licked the ground whereon she trod.'

The belief that lust was the sin of our first parents has always been part of the exegetical tradition. Indeed, the idea is so persistent that one twentieth-century commentator has remarked that even today every seduction scene is an allegory of the Fall.* Eve's dream of the night before is essential to any discussion of her vulnerability to temptation. Satan, disguised as an angel whose 'dewy locks distilled ambrosia', gives her a summary of the argument he will develop next day: 'Taste this, and be henceforth among the Gods / Thyself a Goddess.' Then he flies her over the 'Earth outstretcht immense, a prospect wide / And various' in an episode analogous to Christ's temptation in the wilderness. The events of the following day show Milton's reworking of the Genesis myth, but the apocryphal vision which precedes it raises more interesting questions about the status of the subconscious in relation to morality ('that I, methought, / Could not but taste').

Clearly the Aristotelian precept that sleep divests the mind of moral responsibility is unhelpful here. By morning Eve has been irrevocably changed as a result of her new knowledge; waking from her dream of seduction, she finds it truth. In general, this convention is used to preserve the heroine's psychological purity throughout the complexities of a sexual interchange. Unconsciousness later plays an important role in, for example, Samuel Richardson's *Pamela* and *Clarissa*, John Keats's 'The Eve of St Agnes', Thomas Hardy's *Tess of the d'Urbervilles* and Bram Stoker's *Dracula*. But in the case of Milton's Eve it suggests that she has an inborn propensity to sin, an impression corroborated by the frequent correspondences the poet establishes between her and Satan. Either way the device differs sharply from the parallel literary convention whereby a man is seduced through magic (as with Launcelot and Dame Brisen, Guyon and Acrasia in Edmund Spenser's *The Faerie Queene*, Keats's 'La Belle Dame sans Merci' and 'Lamia', and Ambrosio and Matilda in Matthew Lewis's *The Monk*). Here fewer distinctions are necessary because there is less danger of moral ambiguity. Nothing short of witchcraft can prevent men from behaving rationally; when they succumb to a

*Robert Meister, *A Literary Guide to Seduction* (1964), p. 20.

woman their change of identity is so radical that their very manhood is at risk.

By making her the heroine of the poem's nocturnal vision, Eve's dream of seduction projects for her a grander destiny than she would have had as Adam's helpmate. Her dream-flight to the Tree of Knowledge reworks the Prometheus myth in a conjugal setting. It is only in the official version of the events that occur the next day that Eve's desire is trivialized as curiosity.* But even here the lessons that she and Adam learn may well seem – to the fallen reader at least – an essential part of growing up. After they have both given way to 'lascivious dalliance', they find out that passion and guilt are often inseparable, and that most sexual pleasures are transitory, only to be enjoyed through a knowledge of their absence.

This is not the first time an English writer has looked at the effect of sexual transgression on the psyche. Angelo, for example, and Beatrice in *The Changeling* are both brought to realize the consequences of yoking an illicit sex drive to the exercise of power. What is different in Milton is his stark focus on the irrevocable effects of new expeience, as opposed to the simpler recognition of the early Renaissance that external forces – court, dynasty, church or law – are too formidably arrayed against the covert desires of the individual.

Paradise Lost pits Satan the Cavalier seducer against the sanctity of Puritan wedlock. But the ambiguities of Milton's treatment of Satan and Eve in particular show that, even in a society as deeply divided as that of the seventeenth century, it is the tension between the two elements that gives English literature its distinctive quality. In some of the most sparkling works of the period the opposing forces are held in equipoise. Andrew Marvell's 'To his Coy Mistress', for instance, reflects a profound understanding of both strains. The Parliamentarian poet allows his Cavalier persona to bring an insistence on immediate gratification into play by reinventing his own opposite: the early Puritan woman who weds sex to the idea of the millenium.

The same imaginative interplay marks the outcome of Resto-

*Gillian Beer, 'Eve was the first scientist . . .', *Women's Review*, Issue 11, September 1986.

ration comedies such as William Congreve's *Love for Love* and *The Way of the World*. Harking back to *Much Ado about Nothing*, and foreshadowing Jane Austen's *Emma*, these plays end with marriages which signify the union of courtly wit with a Puritan commitment to the building of a future. More generally, however, aristocratic values such as daring, poise and eagerness for pleasure predominate in Restoration comedy, where the excitement of seduction is likely to make monogamy look insipid. This is exemplified by Wycherley's *The Country Wife*, where Horner's escapades generate the main excitement.

Generally associated with the upper classes, such sexual behaviour lends itself to burlesque. In *Love for Love*, for instance, Miss Prue's ebullience inadvertently reveals the absurdity of the fop Tattle's formulaic tuition in the art of seduction. Miss Prue has yet to learn how to feign the indifference which allows the more experienced practitioners of latter-day courtly love a route to pleasure while maintaining the appearances of honour. Mrs Foresight's treatment of Scandal after he has seduced her is characteristic:

SCANDAL: This I have heard of before, but never believed. I have been told, she had that admirable quality of forgetting to a man's face in the morning, that she had lain with him all night, and denying that she had done favours with more impudence than she could grant 'em.

Perhaps a growing bourgeois audience was confirmed in its prejudices by witnessing this kind of upper-class duplicity. In the main, however, such compelling portraits of wickedly attractive women are more likely to foster the idea that sex is a game where victory goes to the player who best knows how to bend the rules to advantage.

Women need to play with more circumspection than men because of the double standard. They are obliged to maintain at least the appearances of honour. Horner's feigned impotence in *The Country Wife* is designed primarily to further his own ends, but he is also rewarded by Lady Fidget and her cronies for simultaneously protecting their reputation. We have here a world where women can play with men – or at least cheat with them – on equal terms if they are clever and attractive. Their pursuit of sexual pleasure can be seen as an expression both of autonomy and of a readiness to undermine the possessiveness of husbands like Sir Jasper Fidget, who in the notorious china scene is roundly mocked for his unwitting complaisance. But these wealthy and sophisticated women of the town have no wish to disturb the status quo – which is why camaraderie and discretion are important. The country wife herself inadvertently courts disaster when, after sex with Horner, she jibs at leaving London with her 'musty husband'. In one sense she is the most honest and subversive character in the play; in another, she simply evinces a failure to understand the rules, and deserves her fate.

Young women like Margery, or Miss Prue racing Tattle to the bedroom in *Love for Love*, are satirized rather gently for their display of sexual appetite. With older female characters it is usually different. Lady Fidget and Mrs Squeamish are made to look ridiculous for harassing the depleted Horner in the china scene. Lady Wishfort in *The Way of the World* is likewise subjected to ribald laughter when she tries to seduce Sir Rowland, who later proves to be a butler in disguise, her maid's husband and her enemy's serving-man. The trebly-humiliated Lady Wishfort joins the many women, including Shakespeare's importunate goddess in *Venus and Adonis* and Henry Fielding's Lady Booby in *Joseph Andrews*, mocked for attempting to do what men have done all along – that is, to practise seduction on those who are younger and of a lower social standing.

The characters of Restoration comedy, brittle but never broken by the game of seduction, come close to epitomizing the Cavalier spirit. Their stratagems owe everything to the existence of an apparently immutable social order, where an elaborate code of conduct is scrupulously observed by an exclusive circle. Different codes, however, apply to the rising mercantile classes, upon which, by the beginning of the eighteenth century, an impoverished aristocracy is coming more and more to depend. The Restoration is the first age in which seduction is presented publicly as a possible mode of social intercourse, and also the last.

In the crowded city streets scarcely even visited by the beau monde, seduction is a matter not of pleasure, but of profit. Daniel Defoe's heroine in *Moll Flanders* embodies the new entrepreneurial spirit. Her increasing adroitness at putting her sexuality to work as a business asset may seem at first to betoken a new equality between men and women of the middle classes. But Moll is not necessarily a feminist heroine. Her enterprise springs from economic individualism rather than an understanding of women's oppression. By the end of the novel she is a prosperously married woman who has repented of her sexual irregularities.

For some other novelists of the epoch the situation is different. Women writers have always been slower than men to look on the bright side of seduction, perhaps because as members of the second sex they are more aware of its dangers. In the eighteenth century the seduction tales of many female authors develop an inherently feminist ethic, attacking a society which demands purity of women but not of men.* Charlot, heroine of one of the most important episodes in Mary de la Riviere Manley's *The New Atalantis*, is, like Moll, innocent at the outset. But unlike Defoe's heroine she is indifferent to bribery, and develops into a deeply sexual woman, as passionate as any on the Restoration stage. The consequences of such feeling unallied to a sense of self-preservation are sharply delineated: the Duke soon tires of Charlot, and abandons her in favour of a lucrative bride.

Cautionary tales like this encourage a sympathetic reading of Samuel Richardson's first novel, *Pamela*. Poor but virtuous women need to protect their own interests. Pamela herself is adept at this. All Moll's methods of reckoning up the financial and, later, the spiritual benefits of her adventures are subsumed here into a titillating mixture of Puritanism and prurience as the virtuous serving-maid repels the advances of her employer, Squire B——. Sharing a bed with the housekeeper, Mrs Jervis, Pamela unfortunately fails to look in the bedroom closet according to her usual custom, even though she has heard an inexplicable noise there. In what reads like a travesty of 'The Eve of St Agnes', Pamela describes in a letter how she pulls off her stays, her stockings and her under-petticoat. Not surprisingly, her master chooses this moment to rush out of the closet clad in a rich silk and silver morning gown. Pamela jumps back into bed and the Squire follows her:

*See Jane Spencer, *The Rise of the Woman Novelist* (1986), chapter 4.

I found his hand in my bosom; and when my fright let me know it, I was ready to die; and I sighed and screamed and fainted away. And still he had his arms about my neck; and Mrs Jervis was about my feet, and upon my coat. And all in a cold dewy sweat was I.

Moll Flanders would not have had a second's hesitation here, especially in view of the five hundred pounds Squire B—— is offering. Because Pamela settles for nothing less than marriage, it is not easy to tell who has the upper hand. Of course, Richardson's fairy-tale of rewarded virtue is open to satire and soon provokes it. In Henry Fielding's *Shamela*, virtue becomes 'vartue' through a brief return to the cynical and robust manner of the Restoration stage:

> Mrs Jervis and I are just in bed, and the door unlocked; if my Master should come – Odsbobs! I hear him just coming in at the door. You see I write in the present tense, as Parson Williams says. Well, he is in bed between us, we both shamming a sleep, he steals a hand into my bosom, which I, as if in my sleep, press close to me with mine, and then pretend to awake – I no sooner see him, but I scream out to Mrs Jervis, she feigns likewise but just to come to herself; we both begin, she to becall, and I to bescratch very liberally. After having made a pretty free use of my fingers, without any great regard to the parts I attacked, I counterfeit a swoon. Mrs Jervis then cries out, O, Sir, what have you done, you have murthered poor Pamela: she is gone, she is gone.
> *O what a difficulty it is to keep one's countenance, when a violent laugh desires to burst forth.*

Both *Shamela* and the same author's *Joseph Andrews* show how absurd is the sharp differentiation of sex-roles on which Richardson's fiction depends. While Shamela demonstrates the ease with which the conventions may be manipulated to advantage

> No, Mrs Jervis, nothing under a regular taking into keeping, a settled settlement, for me, and all my heirs, all my whole life-time, shall do the business – or else cross-legged, is the word, faith, with Sham; and then I snapt my fingers [. . .]

Joseph Andrews exposes their arbitrariness by making the belea-guered virgin a man (the eponymous hero is allegedly the brother of Pamela), while Squire B—— becomes the lascivious Lady Booby. In *Joseph Andrews* and, more particularly, *Tom Jones*, Fielding creates a world where, for well-born men at any rate, there are worse crimes than fornication, and a totemic belief in virginity can produce a base and hypocritical spirit.

This kind of mockery appears not to have weakened but to have reinforced Richardson's belief in the power of virginity. In his second novel, *Clarissa*, it is accorded absolute importance – an advance on *Pamela*, where it is too closely involved with consider-ations of status. Here the conflict between Puritan and Cavalier is carried to the death. Imprisoned and drugged by the villainous Lovelace, the heroine is clearly raped and not seduced. Yet *Clarissa* remains one of the most powerful novels of seduction in Europe. This is not because of the initial complicity between Lovelace and Clarissa, their equal facility at letter-writing and her rash entry into a secret correspondence with him; nor is it because of their shared superiority to her bullying mercantile family. There remains a deep-rooted difference between them which simultaneously stimulates Lovelace's desire and makes its fulfil-ment impossible. Clarissa wins the tragic victory for Puritanism that Pamela contrives at a domestic level, when Squire B—— succumbs to her virtue and agrees to marry her.

Lovelace is not by character a rapist but a seducer. For this reason, his violent and degraded assault on Clarissa becomes a measure of his failure, and her utter rejection of his marriage proposal a sign of her triumph. Her subsequent decision to die is fraught with morbid eroticism. Yet it is to be seen in sharp contrast to Lovelace's accidental death in a duel (suitable for an aristocratic seducer). Clarissa differs from many women in litera-ture who are of Lovelace's own class. It is her honour, and not her reputation in the eyes of the world, that is important to her. She becomes the first middle-class woman to lay claim to a tragic destiny. Physically she is violated, but ideologically her victory is complete.

The period after the French Revolution saw the publication of Mary Wollstonecraft's radical novel of seduction *The Wrongs of Woman* in the same year as Wordsworth's and Coleridge's *Lyrical*

Ballads. The traditional forms are now extended to accommodate the experiences of working-class women. Wollstonecraft herself, through her joint heroine, Maria (imprisoned in a madhouse by the husband who has married her for her money) and Maria's wardress, Jemima, shows 'the wrongs of different classes of women, equally oppressive, though from the differences of education, necessarily various'.

In spite of this militant declaration close to the beginning of the century, fallen women in subsequent fiction often figure as rather passive stereotypes, best epitomized by the phrase 'victims of seduction'. This is partly because biology becomes for them, in the age of Darwin, a particularly striking manifestation of destiny. The upper-class women of the two previous centuries appear to have been immune from unwanted pregnancies, which are reserved for members of the lower orders, like Margery in *Love for Love*, who exasperates her aristocratic lover by failing to smother his bastard at birth. The entrepreneurial Moll Flanders is scarcely more sympathetic to female liability than is Valentine, and abandons her own illegitimate children to the wet nurse rather than letting them impede her progress.

Victorian women, in literature at least, seem less resilient. The disastrous consequences of their pregnancies – often occurring after only one unlucky lapse – may indicate a new sensitivity to the conditions which oppressed working women. Elizabeth Gaskell's Ruth, George Eliot's Hetty Sorrel (in *Adam Bede*) and Thomas Hardy's Tess, for instance, are all in one way or another financially dependent on callous or irresponsible seducers who happen to be far their social superiors. In an age when feminine purity was idealized, a minatory note may also have been intended in novels where public shame inevitably follows seduction. And, practically speaking, pregnancy is a convenient way of signalling lost virginity at a time when public notions of decency prevent the frank mention of sex in popular novels.

In spite of such limitations, the fallen woman develops a powerful appeal for the Victorian reader, with her vulnerability serving to heighten her erotic charm. The male seducer, on the other hand, has been difficult to take seriously since the demise of Lovelace, for all the emphasis on the evil results of his actions. Richardson's epistolary mode allows his seducer to speak, scheme and expostulate on his own behalf. The hero of Byron's *Don Juan* is, perhaps, the last seducer likewise involved in his creator's narrative and artistic identity. But the poem is unfinished, and Juan's girlish bashfulness makes him as much a subject for travesty – as when he dresses in a woman's clothes in the harem – as a seducer in the tradition of his namesake Don Giovanni, or of Casanova or other legendary lovers.

Subsequently, the seducer is demoted for a long time to the subplot, as he is in most of Jane Austen's novels, where his machinations serve primarily to offer a contrast to the more orthodox approach of the heroine's suitor. Only in her final, unfinished novel, *Sanditon*, does Austen appear to put the seducer at the centre of the plot in order to anatomize him. After this, the figure remains marginal throughout the nineteenth century. James Steerforth, in *David Copperfield*, begins as a compelling character, but Dickens does not allow us to trace his development into a full-blown seducer. Henry Bellingham in *Ruth* and Arthur Donnithorne in *Adam Bede* are indistinguishable members of the squirearchy. Eugene Wrayburn in *Our Mutual Friend* initially looks like a late manifestation of the Cavalier seducer, a more fully explored version of James Harthouse in *Hard Times*, but Dickens proves more interested in his redemption at the hands of a good woman than in his amatory powers.

Thomas Hardy tries to dissociate Alec d'Urberville from the stock of Victorian melodrama by furnishing him with several contradictory impulses, but the attempt is unsuccessful. Nevertheless, the seduction in *Tess of the d'Urbervilles* is a literary landmark at the end of a century where no such scene has been described outside pornography. The fact that Dickens, Gaskell and Eliot were all condemned by their contemporaries for too great a degree of sexual explicitness shows the magnitude of the problem Hardy faces. His aim is to portray – for the first time since the early eighteenth century – a woman of a deeply sensuous nature.

Hardy feels it necessary to add both the sub-title and a network of references to the heroine's purity at a late stage in the composition of his novel.* The evocation of Tess's 'beautiful

---

*See Penny Boumelha, *Thomas Hardy and women: sexual ideology and narrative form* (1982), p. 129.

feminine tissue, sensitive as gossamer, and practically as blank as snow', arises from Hardy's desire to modify the predictable public outcry. We are never told that Tess's seduction awakes her from her exhausted sleep in the Chase. And yet her situation differs materially from Clarissa's, whose resistance would have been total had she not been drugged. As in *Paradise Lost*, an earlier scene is more psychologically revealing than the event itself. The first encounter, where Alec feeds Tess strawberries, convinces us that her innocent modesty is combined with a sensuality reluctant as yet, but potentially powerful:

> D'Urberville began gathering specimens of the fruit for her, handing them back to her as he stooped; and, presently, selecting a specially fine product of the 'British Queen' variety, he stood up and held it by the stem to her mouth.
>
> 'No – no!' she said quickly, putting her fingers between his hand and her lips. 'I would rather take it in my own hand – '
>
> 'Nonsense!' he insisted; and in a slight distress she parted her lips and took it in.

There is a remarkable resemblance between these lines and Eve's dream in *Paradise Lost*. In Milton's epic the seducer also picks and proffers unnatural fruit (D'Urberville's strawberries are forced in two senses) to the lips of a woman bashful but stirred at the same time:

> So saying, he drew nigh, and to me held,
> Even to my mouth of that same fruit held part
> Which he had pluckt.

And there is a similarity, too, in the woman's troubled acceptance:

> the pleasant savourie smell
> So quicken'd appetite, that I, methought,
> Could not but taste.

Hardy's attitude differs considerably from Milton's because he blames not his heroine, but society, with its arbitrary codes and fetishistic attitude towards female chastity. In his selfish assumption of the *droit de seigneur*, Alec d'Urberville would be a descendant of Lovelace if his claim to distinguished lineage were not as spurious as everything else about him. It is Tess herself who is of noble descent. Hardy has, however, too subtle a social awareness to use this discrepancy as proof that all parvenus are boors. The moral is rather that this is how men will behave with women unable to challenge their authority in social or economic terms: 'Doubtless some of Tess d'Urberville's mailed ancestors rollicking home from a fray had dealt the same measure even more ruthlessly towards peasant girls of their time.' Alec's misfortune is that he is living in an evangelical age when such behaviour is no longer endorsed.

As Tess gazes down on her native village after her fall, Hardy invests his description with a feeling of loss even more profound than at the end of *Paradise Lost*:

> It was always beautiful from here; it was terribly beautiful to Tess to-day, for since her eyes last fell on it she had learnt that the serpent hisses where the sweet birds sing, and her views of life had been totally changed for her by the lesson.

In *Jude the Obscure* an early encounter is, once again, more revealing than the act of seduction itself. Arabella's opening gambit of hurling what in later versions Hardy calls 'the characteristic part of a barrow-pig' at Jude's head is unsophisticated – Kate Millet calls the missile 'a grotesque parody of Cupid's shaft'* – but in this respect Arabella shares the panache of 'The Ruined Maid', rarer in Victorian fiction than in verse where more libertarian attitudes are traditionally allowed expression. In novels women are likelier to be fascinated by displays of male initiative, as Bathsheba is when she is subdued by the phallic sword play of Sergeant Troy in *Far from the Madding Crowd*. In the serial version of *Jude the Obscure*,† anthologized here, Jude impales the pig's penis on a stick. Unnecessarily perhaps, Arabella's friend Anny emphasizes the emblematic importance of the scene when she mocks Arabella for speaking to Jude 'on the bridge, wi' the piece o' pig hanging down between ye – hau-hauḡh!' and adds: 'What a proper thing to court over in these parts!'

Sexual Politics (1977 edn.), p. 130.
†Called 'The Simpletons', *Harpers*, European edition 29 (1894).

The later scene where Arabella inveigles Jude into her bedroom pales by comparison. In both, however, Jude, following the tradition of Joseph Andrews and Bryon's Don Juan, appears all the more ridiculously virginal for being a man. Later his fascination with Arabella's robust vitality gives way to revulsion, and her initiative is shown by implication to be as unnatural as Lady Wishfort's, when Jude discovers that her dimples are contrived and her long thick hair has been supplemented by a hairpiece. He subsequently falls in love with the ethereal Sue Bridehead; but he will never be completely satisfied by either of those women, representing as they do the opposite extremes of fleshliness and febrility.

This opposition between female characters is typical of an age that found it hard to accept that women are sexual beings. In *Dracula* (1897) the split is even more radical. Liberated by the Gothic genre from some of the constraints of socio-realism, Bram Stoker contrives a contrast between virgin and whore that divides not two women but one – Lucy Westenra alive and undead.

Lucy is not seduced at any conscious level – unlike Jonathan Harker, who on his first visit to Transylvania confesses in his diary (but not to his future wife) to feeling a 'languorous ecstasy' at the voluptuous advances of the three female vampires. But underlying the early Lucy's waking self is an eroticism betokened by her privately expressed wish not to confine herself to one husband only, and by her sleepwalking through the streets of Whitby in nightgown and bare feet. By the time Lucy, a vampire now herself, attempts to seduce her former fiancé Arthur in Highgate cemetery, her transformation from the pure ideal of Victorian womanhood to the insatiable monster feared to be lurking underneath is complete. Here she has returned to her coffin:

> She seemed like a nightmare of Lucy as she lay there; the
> pointed teeth, the bloodstained, voluptuous mouth – which
> it made one shudder to see – the whole carnal and
> unspiritual appearance, seeming like a devilish mockery of
> Lucy's sweet purity.

Like Lamia and other metamorphosized temptresses, Lucy illustrates the theory that extreme seductiveness can approach the bounds of horror.* It is Arthur, appropriately enough, who brutally subdues her, hammering into her supine body an undeniably phallic stake. Having died in degrading throes, she is restored to the unsullied self preferred by her rescuers. Her corpse is imprisoned in a little mausoleum to which Arthur keeps the key, where she becomes an apotheosis of the Angel in the House and one of the most damaging distortions of Victorian womanhood.†

Like Tess of the D'Urbervilles, Lucy resembles Milton's Eve. Both Eve and Lucy gain access to immortality – or believe they do – through an oneiric journey, and both are punished relentlessly as a consequence. Eve's courtly seducer squats at her ear by night in the shape of a toad, inspiring her dreams, while the aristocratic Dracula invades the privacy of the middle-class home in the shape of a bat.

Milton remains influential in what may prove to be the definitive twentieth-century treatment of seduction. Notwithstanding T. S. Eliot's attempts to oust Milton from his place in the literary canon, both these poets – the dissenting Whig regicide and the Anglo-Catholic royalist – write within the same Puritan tradition.‡ Like *Paradise Lost*, *The Waste Land* links a series of seduction scenes to suggest the moral disintegration of society.§ But Eliot's treatment of temptation has a greater air of finality about it. Instead of challenging the primal freshness and vigour of the creation, as in Milton's account, his disinherited fornicators can do no more than juggle the fragments of former civilizations.

Travesties of earlier seductions – Cleopatra on her barge, the game of chess in *Women Beware Women*, 'To his Coy Mistress', the song from *The Vicar of Wakefield* – are drained of political and theological meaning, to signify the breakdown of a culture into a series of largely incoherent echoes of individual experience. The national importance of Elizabeth's intrigue with Leicester on the barge dwindles to the anonymity of the supine woman who raises

*George Bataille, 'Eye', in *Visions of Excess: Selected Writings, 1927–1939* (1985), p. 17.
†See Franco Moretti, 'The Dialectic of Fear', in *Signs taken for wonders: essays on the sociology of literary forms* (1983).
‡See Frank Kermode, 'A Babylonish Dialect', in C. B. Cox and Arnold P. Hinchliffe (eds.), *T. S. Eliot: The Waste Land* (1968), p. 227.
§I have not included these scenes in the anthology, as it is not permitted to quote extracts from T. S. Eliot's poems.

her knees on the floor of the narrow canoe on the Thames. If Milton's couple sinned through lust and ambition, in *The Waste Land* the characters' lack of desire is a register of their accidie.

The most outstanding example is that of the typist and the 'young man carbuncular' whose exploring hands meet with no resistance. Their boredom is paralleled in the weariness of the hermaphrodite Tiresias, the all-seeing avatar of the poet. As the young man gropes his way down the unlit stairs at the end (in an earlier draft the sordidness of the occasion is emphasized as he stops to urinate and spit), their encounter fixes itself as one more image of disinheritance in the modern waste land beyond the garden.

After Eliot, it is seldom possible neatly to categorize seduction scenes as either comic or tragic. The topic becomes susceptible to a range of interpretations – the unabashed materialism of John Braine's *Room at the Top*, for instance, or the neo-pastoralism of Laurie Lee's *Cider with Rosie*, or the lesbian eroticism in Sara Maitland's *Virgin Territory*. Sometimes an infringed taboo can still make for an arresting episode, as when a brother seduces a sister (Ian McEwan, 'Homemade'), a married woman has intercourse with an adolescent half-wit (Angela Carter, *Heroes and Villains*), or a blind woman makes an attempt on a man with one eye (Molly Keane, *Time after Time*).

In all these works – apart from the short story – the seduction scene is marginal. William Golding's *Free Fall* is, perhaps, a rare, late example where the subject is treated centrally, and the moral consequences of Sammy Mountjoy's treatment of Beatrice Ifor are fully explored. In a retrospective quest for the moment when he lost his innocence, Sammy as narrator divides his life into events before and after the fall. The novel's title is enough to make it clear that Golding is reinterpreting *Paradise Lost*. Its ambiguity heightens Sammy's resemblance to Eve at the moment of temptation, for it may suggest either a moment of choice, or an unimpeded drop through the air.

As with Adam and Eve, Sammy first discovers his Beatrice after he has inadvertently bestowed life upon her – capturing her on paper in a school art class with a free and authoritative line which has far more vitality than the passive model. The decisive moment of Sammy's loss of innocence occurs, however, in a garden, the spot where he recognizes the lure of the forbidden: 'the angel of the gate of paradise held his sword between me and the spices.' In lines reminiscent of the soliloquies of both Doctor Faustus and Satan in Book IV of *Paradise Lost*, his temptation is defined as specifically sexual:

> In my too susceptible mind sex dressed itself in gorgeous colours, brilliant and evil. I was in that glittering net, then, just as the silk moths were when they swerved and lashed their slim bodies and spurted the pink musk of their mating. Musk, shameful and heady, be thou my good.

From this point Sammy's desire to possess Beatrice grows until he cajoles her into having sex with him. His threatened madness travesties the penitent and solitary passion of lovers like Launcelot, and also Beatrice's own later insanity, which is brought about after Sammy has abandoned her. His impotence registers the futility of his passion. But he does not learn his most important lesson until later, in a German concentration camp, where he comes to realize that to use another person as a means to fulfilment can only lead to betrayal. More complicated, however, is the paradox inherent in Sammy's retelling of his seduction of Beatrice – perhaps because it exposes the central contradiction of morality's struggle to survive in a predominantly determinist climate. Despite his eventual location of a moment of choice – philosophically a dubious notion at best – the momentum of the narrative lends its weight to a growing sense of inevitability: 'Guilty am I; therefore wicked will I be.' This sense of doom is easily assimilated to the Promethean stance often struck by Sammy. Seduction becomes both sin and a recognition that 'consciousness and the guilt which is unhappiness go together'.

Traditionally, descriptions of the act of seduction acknowledge, if only implicitly, the involvement of human sexuality with potentially anti-social drives to power, knowledge, wealth and sensory satisfaction. It may be that Golding's treatment of this theme is one of the last. With the rise of the women's movement, more readily available contraception and greater social mobility, people are, perhaps, less likely to suffer the conflicting attitudes to sex necessary for seduction. As a result, this subject may no longer be crucial to our understanding of sexual politics, and the way they affect society at large. If sex for its own sake is no more than a casual pleasure – as opposed to an act of defiance, betrayal or daring – then it can only prompt the kind of nostalgia we see in Brian Patten's 'Party Piece'. Or else it becomes, as in a recent novel by Malcolm Bradbury, no more than a sort of currency in a world where ideological oppositions have broken down between eastern and western blocs, as between individuals, under the growing pressure of consumerism. Addressing directly a hypothetical sequence of readers characterized briefly by contemporary status symbols, Bradbury asks:

> . . . what are you doing but putting what you like to think of as your self in the pan, bartering your mind and body, your youth and opinions, on the economic frontier, in an attempt to find a meaning, invent a value, find your highest price, trade at the best possible rate of exchange?*

In this anthology I have restricted myself mainly to British literature, in order to create a sense of context and continuity. The extracts themselves are arranged so as to provide unexpected points of contrast and comparison within the tradition. With earlier texts I have provided a modernized version wherever it seemed likely to increase enjoyment in reading. Friends and colleagues who suggested individual items are too numerous to mention here. But Peter Cushing, Glenda Jones, Steve Newman, Paul O'Keeffe, Dorothy and Pamela Sprigings and Gregory Woods gave me particularly helpful lists. I am grateful to the staff of the Bodleian, and particularly of Duke Humfrey's library; to the staff of the Special Collection in the Liverpool University Sidney Jones library; and to Peter Rowley and Margaret Chambers in the Library of the Department of Continuing Education. I would also like to thank Craig Raine for commissioning this anthology, Christopher Reid for his editorial help and encouragement, Nicholas Roe for a meticulous reading of the first draft of the introduction, and Hermione Lee for generous help with the last. My greatest debt is to Dave Evans, who has been closely involved with every stage of this book's preparation.

---

*Malcolm Bradbury, *Rates of Exchange* (1984), p. 9.

The Whole Artillery of Love

William Congreve
1670–1729

from Love for Love

Mrs Foresight and her friend have left the fop Tattle alone with the former's ward, the country girl Miss Prue.

TATTLE: I must make love to you, pretty Miss. Will you let me make love to you?

MISS PRUE: Yes, if you please.

TATTLE: (*Aside*) Frank, egad, at least. What a pox does Mrs Foresight mean by this civility? Is it to make a fool of me? Or does she leave us together out of good morality, and do as she would be done by? Gad, I'll understand it so.

MISS PRUE: Well, and how will you make love to me? Come, I long to have you begin. Must I make love too? You must tell me how.

TATTLE: You must let me speak Miss, you must not speak first. I must ask you questions, and you must answer.

MISS PRUE: What, is it like the catechism? Come then, ask me.

TATTLE: De'e you think you can love me?

MISS PRUE: Yes.

TATTLE: Pooh, pox, you must not say yes already. I shan't care a farthing for you then in a twinkling.

MISS PRUE: What must I say then?

TATTLE: Why you must say no, or you believe not, or you can't tell.

MISS PRUE: Why, must I tell a lie then?

TATTLE: Yes, if you would be well-bred. All well-bred persons lie. Besides, you are a woman, you must never speak what you think. Your words must contradict your thoughts, but your actions may contradict your words. So, when I ask you if you can love me, you must say no, but you must love me too. If I tell you you are handsome, you must deny it,

[3]

and say I flatter you. But you must think yourself more charming than I speak you, and like me, for the beauty which I say you have, as much as if I had it myself. If I ask you to kiss me, you must be angry, but you must not refuse me. If I ask you for more, you must be more angry, but more complying. And as soon as ever I make you say you'll cry out, you must be sure to hold your tongue.

MISS PRUE: O Lord, I swear this is pure. I like it better than our old-fashioned country way of speaking one's mind. And must not you lie too?

TATTLE: Hum – yes. But you must believe I speak truth.

MISS PRUE: O Gemini! Well, I always had a great mind to tell lies, but they frighted me, and said it was a sin.

TATTLE: Well, my pretty creature, will you make me happy by giving me a kiss?

MISS PRUE: No, indeed, I'm angry at you. (*Runs and kisses him.*)

TATTLE: Hold, hold, that's pretty well, but you should not have given it me, but have suffered me to take it.

MISS PRUE: Well, we'll do it again.

TATTLE: With all my heart. Now then, my little angel. (*Kisses her.*)

MISS PRUE: Pish.

TATTLE: That's right. Again, my charmer. (*Kisses again.*)

MISS PRUE: O fie, nay, now I can't abide you.

TATTLE: Admirable! That was as well as if you had been born and bred in Covent-Garden all the days of your life. And won't you shew me, pretty Miss, where your bed-chamber is?

MISS PRUE: No, indeed won't I. But I'll run there, and hide myself from you behind the curtains.

TATTLE: I'll follow you.

MISS PRUE: Ah, but I'll hold the door with both hands and be angry – and you shall push me down before you come in.

TATTLE: No, I'll come in first, and push you down afterwards.

MISS PRUE: Will you? Then I'll be more angry, and more complying.

TATTLE: Then I'll make you cry out.

MISS PRUE: Oh, but you shan't, for I'll hold my tongue.

TATTLE: O my dear apt scholar.

MISS PRUE: Well, now I'll run and make more haste than you. (*Exit* MISS PRUE.)

TATTLE: You shall not fly so fast as I'll pursue. (*Exit after her.*)

John Donne
1571/2–1631

Going to Bed

Come, Madam, come, all rest my powers defie,
Until I labour, I in labour lie.
The foe oft-times having the foe in sight,
Is tir'd with standing though he never fight.
Off with that girdle, like heavens Zone glittering,
But a far fairer world incompassing.
Unpin that spangled breastplate which you wear,
That th'eyes of busie fooles may be stopt there.
Unlace your self, for that harmonious chyme,
Tells me from you, that now it is bed time.
Off with that happy busk, which I envie,
That still can be, and still can stand so nigh.
Your gown going off, such beautious state reveals,
As when from flowry meads th'hills shadow steales.
Off with that wyerie Coronet and shew
The haiery Diademe which on you doth grow:
Now off with those shooes, and then safely tread
In this loves hallow'd temple, this soft bed.
In such white robes, heaven's Angels us'd to be
Receavd by men; Thou Angel bringst with thee
A heaven like Mahomets Paradise; and though
Ill spirits walk in white, we easly know,
By this these Angels from an evil sprite,
Those set our hairs, but these our flesh upright.
    Licence my roaving hands, and let them go,
Before, behind, between, above, below.
O my America! my new-found-land,
My kingdome, safeliest when with one man man'd,
My Myne of precious stones, My Emperie,
How blest am I in this discovering thee!

To enter in these bonds, is to be free;
Then where my hand is set, my seal shall be.
    Full nakedness! All joyes are due to thee,
As souls unbodied, bodies uncloth'd must be,
To taste whole joyes. Gems which you women use
Are like Atlanta's balls, cast in mens views,
That when a fools eye lighteth on a Gem,
His earthly soul may covet theirs, not them.
Like pictures, or like books gay coverings made
For lay-men, are all women thus array'd;
Themselves are mystick books, which only wee
(Whom their imputed grace will dignifie)
Must see reveal'd. Then since that I may know;
As liberally, as to a Midwife, shew
Thy self: cast all, yea, this white lynnen hence,
There is no pennance due to innocence.
    To teach thee, I am naked first; why than
What needst thou have more covering then a man.

Graham Greene
1904–

Chagrin in Three Parts

It was February in Antibes. Gusts of rain blew along the ramparts, and the emaciated statues on the terrace of the Château Grimaldi dripped with wet, and there was a sound absent during the flat blue days of summer, the continual rustle below the ramparts of the small surf. All along the Côte the summer restaurants were closed, but lights shone in Flix au Port and one Peugeot of the latest model stood in the parking-rank. The bare masts of the abandoned yachts stuck up like tooth-picks and the last plane in the winter-service dropped, in a flicker of green, red and yellow lights, like Christmas-tree baubles, towards the airport of Nice. This was the Antibes I always enjoyed; and I was disappointed to find I was not alone in the restaurant as I was most nights of the week.

Crossing the road I saw a very powerful lady dressed in black who stared out at me from one of the window-tables, as though she were willing me not to enter, and when I came in and took my place before the other window, she regarded me with too evident distaste. My raincoat was shabby and my shoes were muddy and in any case I was a man. Momentarily, while she took me in, from balding top to shabby toe, she interrupted her conversation with the *patronne* who addressed her as Madame Dejoie.

Madame Dejoie continued her monologue in a tone of firm disapproval: it was unusual for Madame Volet to be late, but she hoped nothing had happened to her on the ramparts. In winter there were always Algerians about, she added with mysterious apprehension, as though she were talking of wolves, but nonetheless Madame Volet had refused Madame Dejoie's offer to be fetched from her home. 'I did not press her under the circumstances. Poor Madame Volet.' Her hand clutched a huge pepper-mill like a bludgeon, and I pictured Madame Volet as a weak

[8]

timid old lady, dressed too in black, afraid even of protection by so formidable a friend.

How wrong I was. Madame Volet blew suddenly in with a gust of rain through the side door beside my table, and she was young and extravagantly pretty, in her tight black pants, and with a long neck emerging from a wine-red polo-necked sweater. I was glad when she sat down side by side with Madame Dejoie, so that I need not lose the sight of her while I ate.

'I am late,' she said, 'I know that I am late. So many things have to be done when you are alone, and I am not yet accustomed to being alone,' she added with a pretty little sob which reminded me of a cut-glass Victorian tear-bottle. She took off thick winter gloves with a wringing gesture which made me think of handkerchiefs wet with grief, and her hands looked suddenly small and useless and vulnerable.

'*Pauvre cocotte*,' said Madame Dejoie, 'be quiet here with me and forget awhile. I have ordered a *bouillabaisse* with *langouste*.'

'But I have no appetite, Emmy.'

'It will come back. You'll see. Now here is your *porto* and I have ordered a bottle of *blanc de blancs*.'

'You will make me *tout à fait saoule*.'

'We are going to eat and drink and for a little while we are both going to forget everything. I know exactly how you are feeling, for I too lost a beloved husband.'

'By death,' little Madame Volet said. 'That makes a great difference. Death is quite bearable.'

'It is more irrevocable.'

'Nothing can be more irrevocable than my situation. Emmy, he loves the little bitch.'

'All I know of her is that she has deplorable taste – or a deplorable hairdresser.'

'But that was exactly what I told him.'

'You were wrong. I should have told him, not you, for he might have believed me, and in any case my criticism would not have hurt his pride.'

'I love him,' Madame Volet said, 'I cannot be prudent,' and then she suddenly became aware of my presence. She whispered something to her companion, and I heard the reassurance, '*Un anglais*.' I watched her as covertly as I could – like most of my fellow writers I have the spirit of a *voyeur* – and I wondered how stupid married men could be. I was temporarily free, and I very much wanted to console her, but I didn't exist in her eyes, now she knew that I was English, nor in the eyes of Madame Dejoie. I was less than human – I was only a reject from the Common Market.

I ordered a small *rouget* and a half bottle of Pouilly and tried to be interested in the Trollope I had brought with me. But my attention strayed.

'I adored my husband,' Madame Dejoie was saying, and her hand again grasped the pepper-mill, but this time it looked less like a bludgeon.

'I still do, Emmy. That is the worst of it. I know that if he came back . . .'

'Mine can never come back,' Madame Dejoie retorted, touching the corner of one eye with her handkerchief and then examining the smear of black left behind.

In a gloomy silence they both drained their *portos*. Then Madame Dejoie said with determination, 'There is no turning back. You should accept that as I do. There remains for us only the problem of adaptation.'

'After such a betrayal I could never look at another man,' Madame Volet replied. At that moment she looked right through me. I felt invisible. I put my hand between the light and the wall to prove that I had a shadow, and the shadow looked like a beast with horns.

'I would never suggest another man,' Madame Dejoie said. 'Never.'

'What then?'

'When my poor husband died from an infection of the bowels I thought myself quite inconsolable, but I said to myself, Courage, courage. You must learn to laugh again.'

'To laugh,' Madame Volet exclaimed. 'To laugh at what?' But before Madame Dejoie could reply, Monsieur Félix had arrived to perform his neat surgical operation upon the fish for the *bouillabaisse*. Madame Dejoie watched with real interest; Madame Volet, I thought, watched for politeness' sake while she finished a glass of *blanc de blancs*.

When the operation was over Madame Dejoie filled the glasses and said, 'I was lucky enough to have *une amie* who taught me not to mourn for the past.' She raised her glass and cocking a finger as I had seen men do, she added, '*Pas de mollesse.*'

'*Pas de mollesse,*' Madame Volet repeated with a wan enchanting smile.

I felt decidedly ashamed of myself – a cold literary observer of human anguish. I was afraid of catching poor Madame Volet's eyes (what kind of a man was capable of betraying her for a woman who took the wrong sort of rinse?) and I tried to occupy myself with sad Mr Crawley's courtship as he stumped up the muddy lane in his big clergyman's boots. In any case the two of them had dropped their voices; a gentle smell of garlic came to me from the *bouillabaisse*, the bottle of *blanc de blancs* was nearly finished, and, in spite of Madame Volet's protestation, Madame Dejoie had called for another. 'There are no half bottles,' she said. 'We can always leave something for the gods.' Again their voices sank to an intimate murmur as Mr Crawley's suit was accepted (though how he was to support an inevitably large family would not appear until the succeeding volume). I was startled out of my forced concentration by a laugh: a musical laugh: it was Madame Volet's.

'*Cochon,*' she exclaimed. Madame Dejoie regarded her over her glass (the new bottle had already been broached) under beetling brows. 'I am telling you the truth,' she said. 'He would crow like a cock.'

'But what a joke to play!'

'It began as a joke, but he was really proud of himself. *Après seulement deux coups . . .*'

'*Jamais trois?*' Madame Volet asked and she giggled and splashed a little of her wine down her polo-necked collar.

'*Jamais.*'

'*Je suis saoule.*'

'*Moi aussi, cocotte.*'

Madame Volet said, 'To crow like a cock – at least it was a *fantaisie*. My husband has no *fantaisies*. He is strictly classical.'

'*Pas de vices.*'

'And yet you miss him?'

'He worked hard,' Madame Volet said and giggled. 'To think that at the end he must have been working hard for both of us.'

'You found it a little boring?'

'It was a habit – how one misses a habit. I wake now at five in the morning.'

'At five?'

'It was the hour of his greatest activity.'

'My husband was a very small man,' Madame Dejoie said. 'Not in height of course. He was two metres high.'

'Oh, Paul is big enough – but always the same.'

'Why do you continue to love that man?' Madame Dejoie sighed and put her large hand on Madame Volet's knee. She wore a signet-ring which perhaps had belonged to her late husband. Madame Volet sighed too and I thought melancholy was returning to the table, but then she hiccuped and both of them laughed.

'*Tu es vraiment saoule, cocotte.*'

'Do I truly miss Paul, or is it only that I miss his habits?' She suddenly met my eye and blushed right down into the wine-coloured wine-stained polo-necked collar.

Madame Dejoie repeated reassuringly, '*Un anglais – ou un américain.*' She hardly bothered to lower her voice at all. 'Do you know how limited my experience was when my husband died? I loved him when he crowed like a cock. I was glad he was so pleased. I only wanted him to be pleased. I adored him, and yet in those days – *j'ai peutêtre joui trois fois par semaine.* I did not expect more. It seemed to me a natural limit.'

'In my case it was three times a day,' Madame Volet said and giggled again. '*Mais toujours d'un façon classique.*' She put her hands over her face and gave a little sob. Madame Dejoie put an arm round her shoulders. There was a long silence while the remains of the *bouillabaisse* were cleared away.

2

'Men are curious animals,' Madame Dejoie said at last. The coffee had come and they divided one *marc* between them, in turn dipping lumps of sugar which they inserted into one another's mouths. 'Animals too lack imagination. A dog has no *fantaisie.*'

'How bored I have been sometimes,' Madame Volet said. He would talk politics continually and turn on the news at eight in the morning. At eight! What do I care for politics? But if I asked his advice about anything important he showed no interest at all. With you I can talk about anything, about the whole world.'

'I adored my husband,' Madame Dejoie said, 'yet it was only after his death I discovered my capacity for love. With Pauline. You never knew Pauline. She died five years ago. I loved her more than I ever loved Jacques, and yet I felt no despair when she died. I knew that it was not the end, for I knew by then my capacity.'

'I have never loved a woman,' Madame Volet said.

'*Chérie*, then you do not know what love can mean. With a woman you do not have to be content with *une façon classique* three times a day.'

'I love Paul, but he is so different from me in every way . . .'

'Unlike Pauline, he is a man.'

'Oh Emmy, you describe him so perfectly. How well you understand. A man!'

'When you really think of it, how comic that little object is. Hardly enough to crow about, one would think.'

Madame Volet giggled and said, '*Cochon*.'

'Perhaps smoked like an eel one might enjoy it.'

'Stop it. Stop it.' They rocked up and down with little gusts of laughter. They were drunk, of course, but in the most charming way.

3

How distant now seemed Trollope's muddy lane, the heavy boots of Mr Crawley, his proud shy courtship. In time we travel a space as vast as any astronaut's. When I looked up Madame Volet's head rested on Madame Dejoie's shoulder. 'I feel so sleepy,' she said.

'Tonight you shall sleep, *chérie*.'

'I am so little good to you. I know nothing.'

'In love one learns quickly.'

'But am I in love?' Madame Volet asked, sitting up very straight and staring into Madame Dejoie's sombre eyes.

'If the answer were no, you wouldn't ask the question.'

'But I thought I could never love again.'

'Not another man,' Madame Dejoie said. '*Chérie*, you are almost asleep. Come.'

'The bill?' Madame Volet said as though perhaps she were trying to delay the moment of decision.

'I will pay tomorrow. What a pretty coat this is – but not warm enough, *chérie*, in February. You need to be cared for.'

'You have given me back my courage,' Madame Volet said. 'When I came in here I was *si démoralisée* . . .'

'Soon – I promise – you will be able to laugh at the past . . .'

'I have already laughed,' Madame Volet said. 'Did he really crow like a cock?'

'Yes.'

'I shall never be able to forget what you said about smoked eel. Never. If I saw one now . . .' She began to giggle again and Madame Dejoie steadied her a little on the way to the door.

I watched them cross the road to the car-park. Suddenly Madame Volet gave a little hop and skip and flung her arms around Madame Dejoie's neck, and the wind, blowing through the archway of the port, carried the faint sound of her laughter to me where I sat alone *chez* Félix. I was glad she was happy again. I was glad that she was in the kind reliable hands of Madame Dejoie. What a fool Paul had been, I reflected, feeling chagrin myself now for so many wasted opportunities.

John Webster
1580?–1625?

from The White Devil

*Flamineo is acting as the pandar of his employer, Duke Brachiano, to his
sister, Vittoria Corombona. This is the occasion of the Duke's first visit.
Zanche is Vittoria's maid, and Cornelia is her mother.*

(*Enter* FLAMINEO *and* VITTORIA.)

FLAMINEO: Come, sister; darkness hides your blush. Women
    are like curst dogs: civility keeps them tied all daytime, but
    they are let loose at midnight; then they do most good, or
    most mischief. – My lord, my lord!
    (*Enter* BRACHIANO. ZANCHE *brings out a carpet, spreads it, and
    lays on it two fair cushions.*)

BRACH: Give credit, I could wish time would stand still,
    And never end this interview, this hour:
    But all delight doth itself soon'st devour.
    (*Enter* CORNELIA *behind, listening.*)
    Let me into your bosom, happy lady,
    Pour out, instead of eloquence, my vows:
    Loose me not, madam; for, if you forgo me,
    I am lost eternally.

VIT. COR: Sir, in the way of pity,
    I wish you heart-whole.

BRACH: You are a sweet physician.

VIT. COR: Sure, sir, a loathed cruelty in ladies
    Is as to doctors many funerals;
    It takes away their credit.

BRACH: Excellent creature!
    We call the cruel fair: what name for you
    That are so merciful?

ZAN: See, now they close.

FLAM: Most happy union.

[15]

COR: My fears are fall'n upon me: O, my heart!
My son the pandar! now I find our house
Sinking to ruin. Earthquakes leave behind,
Where they have tyranniz'd, iron, lead, or stone;
But, woe to ruin, violent lust leaves none!

BRACH: What value is this jewel?

VIT. COR: 'Tis the ornament
Of a weak fortune.

BRACH: In sooth, I'll have it; nay, I will but change
My jewel for your jewel.

FLAM: Excellent!
His jewel for her jewel: – well put in, duke.

BRACH: Nay, let me see you wear it.

VIT. COR: Here, sir?

BRACH: Nay, lower, you shall wear my jewel lower.

FLAM: That's better; she must wear his jewel lower.

VIT. COR: To pass away the time, I'll tell your grace
A dream I had last night.

BRACH: Most wishedly.

VIT. COR: A foolish idle dream.
Methought I walk'd about the mid of night
Into a church-yard, where a goodly yew-tree
Spread her large root in ground. Under that yew,
As I sate sadly leaning on a grave
Chequer'd with cross sticks, there came stealing in
Your duchess and my husband: one of them
A pick-axe bore, the other a rusty spade;
And in rough terms they gan to challenge me
About this yew.

BRACH: That tree?

VIT. COR: This harmless yew:
They told me my intent was to root up
That well-grown yew, and plant i'the stead of it
A wither'd black-thorn; and for that they vow'd
To bury me alive. My husband straight
With pick-axe gan to dig, and your fell duchess
With shovel, like a Fury, voided out
The earth, and scatter'd bones. Lord, how, methought,
I trembled! and yet, for all this terror,

I could not pray.

FLAM: No; the devil was in your dream.

VIT. COR: When to my rescue there arose, methought,
A whirlwind, which let fall a massy arm
From that strong plant;
And both were struck dead by that sacred yew,
In that base shallow grave that was their due.

FLAM: Excellent devil! she hath taught him in a dream
To make away his duchess and her husband.

BRACH: Sweetly shall I interpret this your dream.
You are lodg'd within his arms who shall protect you
From all the fevers of a jealous husband;
From the poor envy of our phlegmatic duchess.
I'll seat you above law, and above scandal;
Give to your thoughts the invention of delight,
And the fruition; nor shall government
Divide me from you longer than a care
To keep you great: you shall to me at once
Be dukedom, health, wife, children, friends, and all.

COR: (*Coming forward*) Woe to light hearts, they still fore-run our
fall!

FLAM: What Fury rais'd thee up? – Away, away!
(*Exit* ZANCHE.)

COR: What make you here, my lord, this dead of night?
Never dropp'd mildew on a flower here
Till now.

FLAM: I pray, will you go to bed, then,
Lest you be blasted?

COR: O, that this fair garden
Had with all poison'd herbs of Thessaly
At first been planted; made a nursery
For witchcraft, rather than a burial plot
For both your honours!

VIT. COR: Dearest mother, hear me.

COR: O, thou dost make my brow bend to the earth,
Sooner than nature! See, the curse of children!
In life they keep us frequently in tears;
And in the cold grave leave us in pale fears.

BRACH: Come, come, I will not hear you.

[17]

VIT. COR: Dear, my lord –

COR: Where is thy duchess now, adulterous duke?
   Thou little dreamd'st this night she is come to Rome.

FLAM: How! come to Rome!

VIT. COR: The duchess!

BRACH: She had been better –

COR: The lives of princes should like dials move,
   Whose regular example is so strong,
   They make the times by them go right or wrong.

FLAM: So; have you done?

COR: Unfortunate Camillo!

VIT. COR: I do protest, if any chaste denial,
   If any thing but blood could have allay'd
   His long suit to me –

COR: I will join with thee,
   To the most woeful end e'er mother kneel'd:
   If thou dishonour thus thy husband's bed,
   Be thy life short as are the funeral tears
   In great men's –

BRACH: Fie, fie, the woman's mad.

COR: Be thy act, Judas-like, – betray in kissing:
   Mayst thou be envied during his short breath;
   And pitied like a wretch after his death!

VIT. COR: O me accurs'd (*Exit.*)

FLAM: Are you out of your wits, my Lord!
   I'll fetch her back again.

BRACH: No, I'll to bed:
   Send Doctor Julio to me presently –
   Uncharitable woman: thy rash tongue
   Hath raised a fearful and prodigious storm:
   Be thou the cause of all ensuing harm.
   (*Exit.*)

Henry Fielding
1707–54

---

from Tom Jones

Tom Jones, the hero of this picaresque novel, has been banished from the presence of Sophia, whom he loves. On his travels he meets Mrs Waters, destitute through a series of misadventures. He brings her to the inn at Upton, where they have a meal.

Now Mrs Waters and our hero had no sooner sat down together, than the former began to play this artillery upon the latter. But here, as we are about to attempt a description hitherto unassayed either in prose or verse, we think proper to invoke the assistance of certain aerial beings, who will, we doubt not, come kindly to our aid on this occasion.

'Say then, ye Graces! you that inhabit the heavenly mansions of Seraphina's countenance; for you are truly divine, are always in her presence, and well know all the arts of charming; say, what were the weapons now used to captivate the heart of Mr Jones.'

'First, from two lovely blue eyes, whose bright orbs flashed lightning at their discharge, flew forth two pointed ogles. But, happily for our hero, hit only a vast piece of beef which he was then conveying into his plate, and harmless spent their force. The fair warrior perceived their miscarriage, and immediately from her fair bosom drew forth a deadly sigh. A sigh, which none could have heard unmoved, and which was sufficient at once to have swept off a dozen beaux; so soft, so sweet, so tender, that the insinuating air must have found its subtle way to the heart of our hero, had it not luckily been driven from his ears by the coarse bubbling of some bottled ale, which at that time he was pouring forth. Many other weapons did she assay; but the god of eating (if there be any such deity, for I do not confidently assert it) preserved his votary; or perhaps it may not be *dignus vindice nodus*, and the present security of Jones may be accounted for by natural

[19]

means; for as love frequently preserves from the attacks of hunger, so may hunger possibly, in some cases, defend us against love.

'The fair one, enraged at her frequent disappointments, determined on a short cessation of arms. Which interval she employed in making ready every engine of amorous warfare for the renewing of the attack, when dinner should be over.

'No sooner then was the cloth removed, than she again began her operations. First, having planted her right eye sidewise against Mr Jones, she shot from its corner a most penetrating glance; which, though great part of its force was spent before it reached our hero, did not vent itself absolutely without effect. This the fair one perceiving, hastily withdrew her eyes, and levelled them downwards, as if she was concerned for what she had done; though by this means she designed only to draw him from his guard, and indeed to open his eyes, through which she intended to surprise his heart. And now, gently lifting up those two bright orbs which had already begun to make an impression on poor Jones, she discharged a volley of small charms at once from her whole countenance in a smile. Not a smile of mirth, nor of joy; but a smile of affection, which most ladies have always ready at their command, and which serves them to show at once their good-humour, their pretty dimples, and their white teeth.

'This smile our hero received full in his eyes, and was immediately staggered with its force. He then began to see the designs of the enemy, and indeed to feel their success. A parley now was set on foot between the parties; during which the artful fair so slily and imperceptibly carried on her attack, that she had almost subdued the heart of our hero, before she again repaired to acts of hostility. To confess the truth, I am afraid Mr Jones maintained a kind of Dutch defence, and treacherously delivered up the garrison, without duly weighing his allegiance to the fair Sophia. In short, no sooner had the amorous parley ended, and the lady had unmasked the royal battery, by carelessly letting her handkerchief drop from her neck, than the heart of Mr Jones was entirely taken, and the fair conqueror enjoyed the usual fruits of her victory.'

Delight in Disorder

A sweet disorder in the dress
Kindles in clothes a wantonness:
A lawn about the shoulders thrown
Into a fine distraction:
An erring lace, which here and there
Enthrals the crimson stomacher:
A cuff neglectful, and thereby
Ribbands to flow confusedly:
A winning wave (deserving note)
In the tempestuous petticoat:
A careless shoestring, in whose tie
I see a wild civility:
Do more bewitch me, than when art
Is too precise in every part.

Malcolm Bradbury
1932–

from Rates of Exchange

Petworth, a university linguist, visits Slaka – the capital of an imaginary Eastern European country – to lecture for two weeks. There he meets the writer, Katya Princip. When he visits her at her flat she persuades him to take a shower.

'Well, very well,' says Petworth, getting up from the sofa. 'And take please your time, my dear,' says Princip, smiling at him, 'We are lucky, this is our afternoon, you do not need to hurry. I can put away these plates and tidy for you my room, I did not expect such a visitor. Do you find it? You go through the kitchen and there is a little white door.' Petworth goes, through the kitchen, through the white door, into a small, tiled bathroom with bare pipes and a great green mirror. In the mirror his body glints as he undresses, hanging his safari suit behind the door. A dull gloom goes with him, as he thinks of his confession, the admission of his wanting sexuality. He stands in the tub, turns the taps, feels the surge of water come over him, cold first, and then turning to hot; he thinks of his dark wife, who dyes her hair, and paints dark paintings in the lumber room, and stays silent, a dull dark anima at the end of a long tunnel. Like wasted words the water splashes over him; the heat grows, the mirror where his body shone fades and blurs. There is no shower curtain; the thick pipes roar; the flood washes over his face. He turns his head away, to realize that, in the steamed room, a person is standing there. 'Who is it?' he asks. 'You don't mind I come in?' says Katya Princip, 'You see after a cake, I like always to weigh, and my machine is here.' 'Please,' says Petworth. 'I hope the shower makes you fresh after your lecture?' says Princip, a vague shape in the steam. 'Yes, it does,' says Petworth, naked and white. 'Here is my machine,' says Princip, 'Now, do I get fatter? My weigh, fifty five kilos, that is not so bad.

My high, one meter sixty five, that does not change. Other traits, grey eyes, blonde hair, all as usual. Special marks, not any. Rate of pulsation, normal, except when I look at you. You do not mind I look at you?' 'No,' says Petworth. 'The soap, do you like it?' asks Princip, close to his side in the steam, 'It is special, a present from France.' 'It's very nice,' says Petworth. 'And this water, it makes itself hot enough for you?' 'Yes, just right,' says Petworth. 'Often it does not work so well,' says Princip, 'I just try it with my hand. You are my guest here, it is not right that you burn your shoulders. Oh, it is good today, perhaps a little hot, you are sure it is not too much?' 'No, it's just right,' says Petworth, politely, standing there bedraggled in the steaming shower. 'Oh, look at you, my dear,' says Princip, 'Such a thin man, doesn't it hurt to be so thin?' 'Not at all,' says Petworth, 'I've always been like this.'

'Oh, you think I criticize the way you look, please, I do not,' says Princip, 'Really you look so nice there in the water, your wet body, very nice. But I hope you admit your lecture was open to an ideological criticism?' 'Too pragmatic?' asks Petworth. 'Exactly,' says Princip, 'Do you like me to soap you, and we can talk also about your deviations?' 'Well, yes,' says Petworth, 'It seems a good idea.' 'Perhaps it is easy if I come there in the tub with you,' says Princip, 'I do not want to get wet with this dress, do you like it, I paid for it much money?' 'I love it,' says Petworth. 'Yes, I am nice in it,' says Princip, fading into the steam. 'But I am nice without it too. We must not be bound by fetishism of the commodities. I hang it up and come back to you.' Without it, Princip emerges again from the steam, her naked back a blur in the mirror. 'Make please a room for me,' says Princip, 'It is not such a big tub. Yes, you are easily disproved. Stand still, please, I put this soap on you, oh, what a soft skin. Yes, you see, my dear, in our histories, we both have an old grey man.' 'Do we?' asks Petworth. 'Is good? You like?' asks Princip, 'Oh, yes, one is Marx, and the other Freud. Naturally my thinking has much of Marx. My husband the apparatchik, he talked to me much of Marx.' 'Does he have to be here?' asks Petworth. 'My husband is nowhere, Marx everywhere,' says Princip, 'Of course he is here. My dear, it is you should not be here. You know if I make you a guest in my apartment, if I give you some terrible coffee and a nice shower, I should report this contact to the authorities? That is our law, of course I do not do it.

Don't you wash me now, I think you are very clean.' 'Yes,' says Petworth, 'Certainly.' 'You do not know Marx, but I think you know Freud,' says Princip, 'Isn't this water very nice?'

'Yes, I do,' says Petworth, his hands moving over the soft contours of no-longer batik-clad magical realist novelist Katya Princip. 'Marx explains the historical origins of consciousness,' she says, 'Freud quite ignores this, neglecting the ideological foundations of the mind. Yet it must be admitted he made some essential discoveries. He knew that it is nice to put a certain thing you have into a certain thing that is mine. For this he made a contribution to the progress of thought, don't you say?' 'Yes,' says Petworth. 'So you are deviationist, but not entirely to be condemned,' says Princip, 'Both thought-systems have their deficiencies. Do you think it is possible to make a dialectical synthesis? If we do it well, it might not produce a false consciousness. Do you like to try it? Oh, Petwit, look at you there, already I think you do. No, no, wait, my dear, my dear, I do not think we succeed like this, do you? For some problems in philosophy, Plato shows it is best to think lying down. Don't we go back there to my bed, isn't it better, oh, what do you do to me now, my dear, oh do you, oh do you really, oh isn't it nice, perhaps I am wrong, perhaps we stay, isn't it too wet, don't we fall down, no, we don't, I think we stay, yes, we stay, yes, yes.' 'Yes, yes,' says Petworth, an unattached signifier amid steam. 'Da, da,' says Princip, 'Da, da, da, da.' The water showers over them; for a moment there are no words. 'Oh, yes,' says Princip, a little later, 'This was a real contribution to thought. But now I bring you your nice towel and we dry. I think we go back to my little room and consider again our positions. Oh, Petwit, you are lovely.'

'I am sorry I do not have a nice little bedroom for you to lie in,' says Princip, back in the sitting-room, 'Here for everyone only so many metres of space. I am lucky, I am approved writer, I have certain privileges. But only so much space, others are not so lucky even. My sofa is my bed, I make magic and it changes. Look, I just press here and now you have a bed to lie on. Lie, please, it is very comfortable. You must make strong again. Remember, you are only just started here. There are many more things for you to do in my country. Oh, our music has stopped. Were we so long at the shower? Well, I put some more on before I come to you, what do you like better, the woods or the strings? Here is some army songs, I don't think you like to hear that. Here is Vivaldi, here Janaček? Do you like charming or sad? Of course, you told me your taste, it is Vivaldi for you. Now I come to you, my dear. Are you warm? No, don't move, I just like to kneel here and look down at you. So thin, really there is not much of you. Your nice wet hairs, a thin white chest, so neat the thigh, is that what you call it, and what a good present for me in the middle. You know, you are just a little bit beautiful, Petwit. And me, do you like me? I am very good at the top, I think, but perhaps too fat for you at the stomach. Here we think a fatness there is just a little erotic. That is our cultural characteristic, but not so much in the West. All the ladies flat like a table, don't forget I have been there. Well, in any case, my dear, my weigh goes down. So perhaps I please you more when we meet again, do you think? Do you believe it, we meet again? Or do you go home away soon to your country and forget all about me? Yes, I think you do, it is natural.'

'No,' says Petworth, lying there on the sofa which has so magically become a bed, his head against books, looking up at Princip, big over him as she leans on one elbow to stare down into his face. 'Oh, listen, you are so sure,' says Princip, 'Well I am not. There is a world out there, my dear Petwit, do you forget it? Of course we have made a very nice exchange, each one gives the other something, all so simple. Oh, such nice touchings and chattings, but they do not last long, not like history. Sex is good, but is not information. Here, you see me, I look at you, and what do I know? I know you have a sad wife, I think you are sad too, perhaps you have many problems. I know you are not character in the world historical sense, I try to make you better, but I don't think I do. You are confused, you are good person, you have a desire, or you would not come with me, you are a little bit in my heart. And you look at me, and what do you know, I could be anyone, your good witch or your bad. You know I have had four husbands, and I have written a book you could not read. Now you know I have a body that you can read, it has been your book and you have read it in a certain way, for the pleasure. Well, I hope it was a good pleasure, but did you learn much, do you think you will pass the examination? Well, perhaps it does not matter. Often the best relations are between the peoples who do not know each other so well. Perhaps it is silly that people get to know each other very well, often it is nothing but disappointment. Who is ever as interesting as ourselves? Who can love us enough to drive away all the lonely and the terror? And to be known, that is often dangerous, especially in my country. No, I think I am a thing that happens to you once, in a foreign place, not a part of time, not a part of your true life.'

'I don't think so,' says Petworth, 'You're more than that.' 'Well, of course, it is possible to reach in a sudden into a soul, and find a friend,' says Princip, 'This is what I felt when I saw you at the awful lunch of Tankic. Such an apparatchik, I know that kind. Did you know at once I wanted you then, I felt an ache? Perhaps you made me a little foolish, you know I did not behave well. But something happened, I wanted you in my life, I wanted to give you a story, make you a character. And I think you wanted that too, you are not a character, not yet, but there is something in your eyes, always looking. Yes, we liked each other, I believe that. Of course we did, or we would not do these things. But what is liking when it is so easy? Oh, we made the bad world go away for a minute, that really is what love is for, but when it comes back, we have of course to live in it. Make all the loves you like and you still do not escape. Most lives are a prison, here in my country of course, you know, but I know also in yours. Do not forget, I have been there. If yours is not, you are very lucky. And all the lovings in the world, they do not make these things go away. The sad wife in your bed at home. The black car that waits outside, did you see it? The water that dries here on your skin that is like me going away. Oh, yes, my dear, we have made our nice secret, all so natural. But of course it is not so natural. As my grey father Marx tells, it is also cultural and ideological, economical and sexual. It is part of all the systems, and each time you choose or you do, you enter one of them. I make you a certain kind of man, you make me a certain kind of woman. What a nice bed this would be if it was not in the world, but it is. Petwit, do you listen, do you go to sleep?'

'No,' says Petworth, 'I listen very carefully.' 'But you don't like what I say,' says Princip, 'No, this is why love is sad, this is why people after love lie on beds like we do, and do not feel happy. My dear, excuse me, please. In my country, after an event, we make always an analysis. That is our cultural characteristic. But you see, my dear, I want to give you a better sense of existence. Petwit, you know, to exist, that is not so very fantastic. Any fool can do this. All that is needed is for two people to make the nice little secret, just like you and me, and pouf, another in the world. I don't think this happens this time, Petwit, don't look so bad, of course I make a certain protection. But so we come into existence. And the problem is not to exist at all, it is to make importance of it. We are not just stones that sit in a field. I don't think so. Are you a stone, Petwit? I am not. Don't we have to find a desire, make a will? Don't we go always somewhere toward something? Of course to do it is hard as well as nice, it is even dangerous. No teacher is pure. No witch is safe. Oh, Petwit, my dear, I upset you. Now, I see it, you are the one who is sad. Well, perhaps I meaned it. Not to hurt you but to learn you. Stay quite still, please, one minute, I just do something to you. Do you like it? I kiss your feet. It is something we do here. Perhaps not in your country? Well, it was worth your travels. Oh, Petwit, you go soon, I don't like it. I wish I could keep you here for always. Perhaps you do not wish it also. Well, remember, a witch is not so easy to lose. I will not be far away when you go into the forest. And even if you do not come back, you will not really forget me.'

'I won't,' says Petworth, 'I really won't.' 'Listen, I think I tell you just one more story,' says Princip, 'Not a very interesting story, it is just about me, a true story, how I became writer. I was married then, with one of my husbands, not the best one. It was the one I told you, the minister, the apparatchik. He sat all the day in an office, with fat secretary, he drove inside the official cars with the curtains, he was high in the party, at all the meetings, he came home each night nice in a dark suit. I was student then, I read many books, I was clever. I studied with him his work, I advised his awful decisions, all those corrupt things. But always he told, please, be a good wife, an apparatchik must have a good wife. Well, he was not such a good man, but I was pretty good wife. I made the dinner parties, I sat at the table, not this one here, of course then there was an apartment, very good, I said amusing things, I spoke in Russian and English, I talked the music and the art. Not the politics of course, oh no, not permitted. Well, on a certain night, he brought round our table some very important men, to talk about a national affair. I knew all about these things then, I listened, I understood, I wanted to say something. Well, I made mistake, I began to talk. These men, they were not so bad, they listened quite politely. But they turned round and round their glasses, they looked at each other in a certain way, I knew of course they want me to stop. Well, at first the things I said were sensible, but then they became foolish, because, you see, they were not wanted. But I knew if I stopped they would all turn right away, and I did not want it, so I could not stop. My face was red, but I talked and talked, and then I got up from there and ran to the door and outside, and always still talking. I went out into the park, and I waited till the cars came for those men. Then I turned back to my husband, he stood in the room in his nice suit, and so angry. Do you know what he told me?'

'No,' says Petworth. 'He told, when you give a party again, you say nothing, never again do you speak in this way,' says Princip, 'Well, he came home the next day in his nice suit, and I expect he called for me, but I was not there. I was somewhere else, with someone else, and already I was writer. I could not live in a world where you think words you cannot speak. Of course, if people make of reality a prison, then others will wish to escape from it. I wrote down my words, the nonsense and the not nonsense, the words I could speak and the words I was trying to learn to speak, the words that were not yet words. I learned then a certain sense of existence. This is what I thought. But in case you think it is easy, no, it is not, because those words are like love, they do not go out of history. I feel toward the free, but I am not free. And no one is free, which is why the words are as sad as the love. My life is not better, but it is mine. I am sorry, my dear, really it is a very dull story. The others were much better. It is boring to be true.' 'What happened to your husband?' asks Petworth. 'This one, the apparatchik?' asks Princip, 'Oh, there was a political change in my country. What was right was now wrong. Who was in now was out. Well, we had been given some nice privileges. We builded a nice dacha, a little house, out in the forest, not so far from here. One day he went there in his nice suit, and he shot himself. He was allowed to be a hunter and to keep a gun. It was better for him than a trial and a prison. This also is remembered about me, by those who do not like me. For him, I am afraid I was not such good witch. For you, I hope I am much better. Now you see why I can tell so much about history. I have learned in the best places.'

'Should we have done this?' asks Petworth, looking at her, as they lie there in the small room, where a faint wind blows the net curtains, and rustles the papers on the desk, and the light begins to fade down in the sky beyond. 'Now you think you commit a crime against the state,' says Princip, 'Now you wish it had not happened. Well, it is not a real offence, even under Marx. Not if you do it with a good ideological attitude. Of course, if you find your position is not correct . . .' 'Well,' says Petworth, looking at their bodies infolded into each other, 'It looks quite good to me.' 'I think so,' says Princip, laughing, 'Perhaps you like to improve it some more? You see now I know how to teach you.' 'Yes,' says Petworth. 'Then I will help you,' says Princip, 'I told you you had many things still to do in my country. Hold me so, see me please as a comrade-of-arms of the struggle. Think with your mind you build a great and startling project. Feel with your heart you reach the great laws of human universality. Know with your strong you contribute to the historic advance of the proletariat.' Live grey eyes are staring into his face; a body beside him is a fundamental mass with a living motion; there are hands on his own body, drawing its shape and a design, drawing it out of shape and design. 'Yes, something is happening to you, do you feel it,' says Katya, eyes, hair, flesh leaning over him. 'Oh, Katya,' says Petworth, looking at the face, alert, moving, the eyes open, reaching out to touch the mass and feel its architecture, the bone order beneath the fleshly pads, 'Katya.' 'Oh, Petwit, do you remember my name?' says Princip, 'You have not said it before. Do you call me a person? Well, perhaps I am Katya, someone like that, but please, it is not the person, it is cause that matters. Take me into yourself, do you do it better if I come on top of you, don't you say?'

There is a body elevated above him, shaped against the light. 'Petwit, now I am magicking you,' says Princip, 'I will take you somewhere, on a nice journey, I am your guide.' 'Oh,' says Petworth, 'Oh my god.' 'Petwit, please, no god,' says Princip, swinging the top of her body across his face, 'Don't you know our task is secular? Try please to relate your subjective to your objective, your spirit to history. In this way you will grow free of errors. Yes, I am your guide, we make it together, our special journey. Do you remember Stupid, do you think you know now how he climbed the tower, perhaps he did what you do, perhaps he found the witch was the princess also. Well, I am your sex princess, I am witching you, I am taking you where you cannot go, think of a word you do not know, I am that word, try to understand it, do you come nearer?' Above him is skin in its long planes, hollowed here, puffed there, the outward thrust of breasts, the inward tuck of the navel, the feel of an intricate yielding crease. 'Yes, you come nearer,' says Princip, 'is there a meaning, is there a place, you go into that place, I put you in that place, you come there and I come there with you, and we are together. You don't have a sad wife, you have me only, no other, all the bodies are my body, do you feel it happen, I do, you do, I know you do, yes, yes.' There is light and dark, inside and outside, arrest, explosion, light following dark, a room of books where curtains blow. 'Wasn't it my best story?' says Princip, 'Didn't I magic you nicely?' 'It was better,' says Petworth. 'Of course,' says Princip, 'Only one thing wrong.' 'What's that?' asks Petworth. 'Look at you,' says Princip, 'Nowhere to pin on you your medal. Petwit, do you think we found a place that is ours?' Petworth leaps up; with a dull, dragging, mechanical note, the telephone on the desk under the blowing curtains begins to ring.

'Oh, no,' says Princip, looking at him, 'Who is this? Quick, go please and put on clothes. Wait, what is time?' 'Time?' asks Petworth. 'On your watch,' says Princip. 'It's a quarter to six,' says Petworth, hurrying, heart beating, into the bathroom. The steam is fading slowly off the green mirror, a naked Petworth refracts emptily at him, the pipes in the tub rattle and groan, Katya Princip's batik dress swings loose on the hook behind the door. Dressing quickly, tugging up clothes, he can hear, beyond the thin wall, the stop and start of a voice, in rapid irregular conversation in the language he still does not know. Telephones and time are of this world; something in the world, half-remembered, presses on him, a worry. In the other room, the telephone clicks down; then Princip, big, naked, her face sad, stands in the door. 'Oh, Petwit, be quick, you must go now,' she says, 'Someone comes here soon, I cannot stop it. Find please my dress.' 'Here,' says Petworth, handing it to her, watching her body scurry, become disorderly, as she pulls it on to her. 'Oh, why don't we have time?' she says, 'And now you will go away, and perhaps I will not see you again.' 'We have to,' says Petworth, 'I'm back in Slaka in ten days.' 'Ten days, it is long,' says Princip, 'And things will happen on your journey, perhaps you will not want then to see me. And you have not been good visitor today, they will watch you, it will not be easy. Oh, I know how it is done, they will make you suddenly busy, they will change your programme. Or they will perhaps invite me to make a little journey from the town. All of a sudden they need my new book, go, please, to the dacha for writers in the country, it is all arranged. For people not to meet, that is easy to fix, we are experts. Wait, your hair, borrow please this comb, you must not look like that when you go. Oh, look, you are in my mirror, I wish I keep you in there. I have a love for you, Petwit, I don't know why, and no time to say it.' 'I have it too,' says Petworth.

Christopher Marlowe
1564–93

from Hero and Leander

Leander has swum the River Hellespont to see Hero, the young woman he loves.

By this Leander being near the land,
Cast down his weary feet, and felt the sand.
Breathless albeit he were, he rested not
Till to the solitary tower he got;
And knock'd, and call'd; at which celestial noise
The longing heart of Hero much more joys
Than nymphs and shepherds when the timbrel rings,
Or crooked dolphin when the sailor sings;
She stayed not for her robes, but straight arose,
And drunk with gladness, to the door she goes;
Where seeing a naked man, she screech'd for fear,
Such sights as this to tender maids are rare,
And ran into the dark herself to hide;
Rich jewels in the dark are soonest spied.
Unto her was he led, or rather drawn,
By those white limbs which sparkled through the lawn.
The nearer that he came, the more she fled,
And seeking refuge, slipt into her bed.
Whereon Leander sitting, thus began,
Through numbing cold all feeble, faint and wan:
'If not for love, yet, love, for pity sake,
Me in thy bed and maiden bosom take;
At least vouchsafe these arms some little room,
Who hoping to embrace thee, cheerly swum.
This head was beat with many a churlish billow,
And therefore let it rest upon thy pillow.'
Herewith affrighted Hero shrunk away,

And in her lukewarm place Leander lay,
Whose lively heat, like fire from heaven fet,
Would animate gross clay, and higher set
The drooping thoughts of base declining souls,
Than dreary Mars carousing nectar bowls.
His hands he cast upon her like a snare,
She overcome with shame and sallow fear,
Like chaste Diana when Actæon spied her,
Being suddenly betrayed, div'd down to hide her.
And as her silver body downward went,
With both her hands she made the bed a tent,
And in her own mind thought herself secure,
O'ercast with dim and darksome coverture.
And now she lets him whisper in her ear,
Flatter, entreat, promise, protest, and swear,
Yet ever as he greedily assay'd
To touch those dainties, she the harpy play'd,
And every limb did as a soldier stout
Defend the fort, and keep the foeman out.
For though the rising ivory mount he scal'd,
Which is with azure circling lines empal'd,
Much like a globe (a globe may I term this,
By which Love sails to regions full of bliss),
Yet there with Sisyphus he toil'd in vain,
Till gentle parley did the truce obtain.
Wherein Leander on her quivering breast,
Breathless spoke something, and sigh'd out the rest;
Which so prevail'd, as he with small ado
Enclos'd her in his arms, and kiss'd her too;
And every kiss to her was as a charm,
And to Leander as a fresh alarm;
So that the truce was broke, and she alas,
Poor silly maiden, at his mercy was.
Love is not full of pity, as men say,
But deaf and cruel where he means to prey.
Even as a bird, which in our hands we wring,
Forth plungeth, and oft flutters with her wing,
She trembling strove; this strife of hers (like that
Which made the world) another world begat

Of unknown joy. Treason was in her thought,
And cunningly to yield herself she sought.
Seeming not won, yet won she was at length,
In such wars women use but half their strength.
Leander now, like Theban Hercules,
Enter'd the orchard of th' Hesperides;
Whose fruit none rightly can describe but he
That pulls or shakes it from the golden tree.

Jane Austen
1775–1817

from Sanditon

Charlotte Heywood is visiting Sanditon, a seaside resort. There she meets Sir Edward Denham, an impoverished local baronet, whose home is in the grounds of his rich aunt, Lady Denham. The latter has recently taken the young and beautiful Clara Brereton as a companion. A meeting between Sir Edward and Charlotte outside the local library provides the author with the occasion for the following analysis.

The truth was that Sir Edward, whom circumstances had confined very much to one spot, had read more sentimental novels than agreed with him. His fancy had been early caught by all the impassioned, and most exceptionable parts of Richardson's; and such authors as have since appeared to tread in Richardson's steps, so far as man's determined pursuit of woman in defiance of every opposition of feeling and convenience is concerned, had since occupied the greater part of his literary hours, and formed his character.

With a perversity of judgement, which must be attributed to his not having by nature a very strong head, the graces, the spirit, the sagacity, and the perseverance, of the villain of the story outweighed all his absurdities and all his atrocities with Sir Edward. With him, such conduct was genius, fire and feeling. It interested and inflamed him; and he was always more anxious for its success and mourned over its discomfitures with more tenderness than could ever have been contemplated by the authors.

Though he owed many of his ideas to this sort of reading, it were unjust to say that he read nothing else, or that his language were not formed on a more general knowledge of modern literature. He read all the Essays, Letters, Tours and Criticisms of the day – and with the same ill-luck which made him derive only false principles from lessons of morality, and incentives to vice from the history of its overthrow, he gathered only hard words and involved sentences from the style of our most approved writers.

Sir Edward's great object was to be seductive. With such personal advantages as he knew himself to possess, and such talents as he did also give himself credit for, he regarded it as his duty. He felt that he was formed to be a dangerous man – quite in the line of the Lovelaces. The very name of Sir Edward, he thought, carried some degree of fascination with it. To be generally gallant and assiduous about the fair, to make fine speeches to every pretty girl, was but the inferior part of the character he had to play. Miss Heywood, or any other young woman with any pretensions to beauty, he was entitled (according to his own views of society) to approach with high compliment and rhapsody on the slightest acquaintance; but it was Clara alone on whom he had serious designs; it was Clara whom he meant to seduce. Her seduction was quite determined on. Her situation in every way called for it. She was his rival in Lady Denham's favour, she was young, lovely and dependent. He had very early seen the necessity of the case, and had now been long trying with cautious assiduity to make an impression on her heart, and to undermine her principles. Clara saw through him, and had not the least intention of being seduced – but she bore with him patiently enough to confirm the sort of attachment which her personal charms had raised.

A greater degree of discouragement indeed would not have affected Sir Edward. He was armed against the highest pitch of disdain or aversion. If she could not be won by affection, he must carry her off. He knew his business. Already had he had many musings on the subject. If he *were* constrained so to act, he must naturally wish to strike out something new, to exceed those who had gone before him – and he felt a strong curiosity to ascertain whether the neighbourhood of Tombuctoo might not afford some solitary house adapted for Clara's reception; but the expense alas! of measures in that masterly style was ill-suited to his purse, and prudence obliged him to prefer the quietest sort of ruin and disgrace for the object of his affections, to the more renowned.

Ben Jonson
1572–1637

from Volpone

*Corvino has just left his young wife Celia alone in Volpone's presence. He has
been duped into believing that Volpone is on the point of death, and against
Celia's wishes he is attempting to prostitute her to him in the hope of a
substantial reward from Volpone's will. Bonario, who delays his entrance for
an inexplicably long time, is an honourable young man hiding in Volpone's
room in an attempt to find out if his father has disinherited him.*

CELIA: O God, and his good angels! whither, whither,
    Is shame fled human breasts? that with such ease
    Men dare put off your honours, and their own?
    Is that, which ever was a cause of life,
    Now placed beneath the basest circumstance,
    And modesty an exile made, for money?
VOLPONE: Ay, in Corvino, and such earth-fed minds,
    (*He leaps off from the couch.*)
    That never tasted the true heaven of love.
    Assure thee, Celia, he that would sell thee,
    Only for hope of gain, and that uncertain,
    He would have sold his part of Paradise
    For ready money, had he met a cope-man.
    Why art thou 'mazed to see me thus revived?
    Rather applaud thy beauty's miracle;
    'Tis thy great work, that hath, not now alone,
    But sundry times raised me in several shapes,
    And, but this morning, like a mountebank,
    To see thee at thy window. Ay, before
    I would have left my practice for thy love,
    In varying figures I would have contended
    With the blue Proteus, or the hornèd flood.
    Now, art thou welcome.

CELIA: Sir!

VOLPONE: Nay, fly me not,
    Nor let thy false imagination
    That I was bed-rid, make thee think I am so:
    Thou shalt not find it. I am, now, as fresh,
    As hot, as high, and in as jovial plight
    As when, in that so celebrated scene,
    At recitation of our comedy,
    For entertainment of the great Valois,
    I acted young Antinous, and attracted
    The eyes and ears of all the ladies present,
    T' admire each graceful gesture, note, and footing.

                    Song
    Come, my Celia, let us prove,
    While we can, the sports of love;
    Time will not be ours forever,
    He, at length, our good will sever;
    Spend not then his gifts in vain.
    Suns that set may rise again;
    But if once we lose this light,
    'Tis with us perpetual night.
    Why should we defer our joys?
    Fame and rumour are but toys.
    Cannot we delude the eyes
    Of a few poor household spies?
    Or his easier ears beguile,
    Thus removèd by our wile?
    'Tis no sin love's fruits to steal,
    But the sweet thefts to reveal:
    To be taken, to be seen,
    These have crimes accounted been.

CELIA: Some serene blast me, or dire lightning strike
    This my offending face.

VOLPONE: Why droops my Celia?
    Thou hast in place of a base husband found
    A worthy lover; use thy fortune well,
    With secrecy and pleasure. See, behold,
    What thou art queen of; not in expectation,

As I feed others, but possessed and crowned.
See, here, a rope of pearl, and each more orient
Than that the brave Egyptian queen caroused;
Dissolve and drink 'em. See, a carbuncle
May put out both the eyes of our St Mark;
A diamond would have bought Lollia Paulina
When she came in like star-light, hid with jewels
That were the spoils of provinces; take these,
And wear, and lose 'em; yet remains an ear-ring
To purchase them again, and this whole state.
A gem but worth a private patrimony
Is nothing: we will eat such at a meal.
The heads of parrots, tongues of nightingales,
The brains of peacocks, and of estriches
Shall be our food, and, could we get the phœnix,
Though nature lost her kind, she were our dish.
CELIA: Good sir, these things might move a mind affected
With such delights; but I, whose innocence
Is all I can think wealthy, or worth th' enjoying,
And which, once lost, I have nought to lose beyond it,
Cannot be taken with these sensual baits.
If you have conscience –
VOLPONE: 'Tis the beggar's virtue.
If thou hast wisdom, hear me, Celia.
Thy baths shall be the juice of July-flowers,
Spirit of roses, and of violets,
The milk of unicorns, and panthers' breath
Gathered in bags and mixed with Cretan wines.
Our drink shall be preparèd gold and amber,
Which we will take until my roof whirl round
With the vertigo; and my dwarf shall dance,
My eunuch sing, my fool make up the antic.
Whilst we, in changèd shapes, act Ovid's tales,
Thou like Europa now, and I like Jove,
Then I like Mars, and thou like Erycine;
So of the rest, till we have quite run through,
And wearied all the fables of the gods.
Then will I have thee in more modern forms,
Attirèd like some sprightly dame of France,

Brave Tuscan lady, or proud Spanish beauty;
Sometimes unto the Persian Sophy's wife,
Or the Grand Signior's mistress; and, for change,
To one of our most artful courtesans,
Or some quick Negro, or cold Russian;
And I will meet thee in as many shapes;
Where we may so transfuse our wand'ring souls
Out at our lips and score up sums of pleasures,
           That the curious shall not know
                How to tell them as they flow;
           And the envious, when they find
                What their number is, be pined.
CELIA: If you have ears that will be pierced, or eyes
    That can be opened, a heart may be touched,
    Or any part that yet sounds man about you;
    If you have touch of holy saints, or heaven,
    Do me the grace to let me 'scape. If not,
    Be bountiful and kill me. You do know
    I am a creature hither ill betrayed
    By one whose shame I would forget it were.
    If you will deign me neither of these graces,
    Yet feed your wrath, sir, rather than your lust,
    (It is a vice comes nearer manliness)
    And punish that unhappy crime of nature,
    Which you miscall my beauty: flay my face,
    Or poison it with ointments for seducing
    Your blood to this rebellion. Rub these hands
    With what may cause an eating leprosy,
    E'en to my bones and marrow; anything
    That may disfavour me, save in my honour,
    And I will kneel to you, pray for you, pay down
    A thousand hourly vows, sir, for your health;
    Report, and think you virtuous –
VOLPONE: Think me cold,
    Frozen, and impotent, and so report me?
    That I had Nestor's hernia thou wouldst think.
    I do degenerate and abuse my nation
    To play with opportunity thus long;
    I should have done the act, and then have parleyed.

Yield, or I'll force thee.

(*He seizes her.*)

CELIA: O! just God!

VOLPONE: In vain –

BONARIO: Forbear, foul ravisher! libidinous swine!

(*He leaps out from where* MOSCA *had placed him.*)

Free the forced lady, or thou diest, impostor.
But that I am loath to snatch thy punishment
Out of the hand of justice, thou shouldst yet
Be made the timely sacrifice of vengeance,
Before this altar, and this dross, thy idol.
Lady, let's quit the place, it is the den
Of villainy; fear nought, you have a guard;
And he ere long shall meet his just reward.

(*Exeunt* BONARIO *and* CELIA.)

John Braine
1922–86

from Room at the Top

*Susan, an attractive young woman from a powerful and wealthy family, has
fallen in love with Joe, who wants to belong to that world. Joe has already
embarked on a passionate and tender love affair with Alice, an unhappily
married older woman.*

'Gosh, isn't it hot?' Susan said.

We were lying in a clearing in the bracken above the Folly; the
afternoon sun beat down on us like a pleasurable *peine forte et dure*.

'*You* shouldn't feel hot,' I said, looking at her off-the-shoulder
blouse and cotton skirt. 'You've nothing on.'

'*Wicked!*' she said, and pulled up the blouse till it covered her
shoulders. 'Happy now? Joety happy now his Susan back?'

I pulled her blouse off her shoulders again. I kissed each
shoulder gently. 'Happy now. Only happy now I'm with you.'

Women over thirty look younger at dusk or by candlelight; a girl
of nineteen looks younger, childish almost, in the hard glare of the
midday sun: at that moment Susan looked no more than fourteen.
Her lipstick had been kissed away, her powder had disappeared;
her lips were still red, her skin flawless.

'It was a *lovely* letter,' she said. 'Oh Joe, I was so miserable until
I got it. It was the best surprise I've ever had in my whole life.'

Charles had helped me to write it, after a long argument, in the
course of which he'd called me, among other things, a sex-besotted
moron and an unsuccessful gigolo. 'There now,' he'd said when I
signed it, 'that should bring the silly bitch running back with the
lovelight in her eyes. You can always depend upon your Uncle
Charles.'

Indeed I could; and there was Susan to prove it. I'd been back
from Dorset a week and she'd only just returned from Cannes;
she'd phoned me the minute she'd read the letter. The sour smoky

[42]

smell of the bracken caught at my throat; I raised myself on my elbow and looked down at Warley in the valley below. I could see it all: the Town Hall with the baskets of flowers above the entrance, the boats on the river at Snow Park, the yellow buses crawling out of the station, the big black finger of Tebbut's Mills in Sebastopol Street, the pulse of traffic in Market Street with its shops whose names I could recite in a litany – Wintrip the jeweller with the beautiful gold and silver watches that made my own seem cheap, Finlay the tailor with the Daks and the Vantella shirts and the Jaeger dressing-gowns, Priestley the grocer with its smell of cheese and roasting coffee, Robbins the chemist with the bottles of Lenthéric after-shave lotion and the beaver shaving-brushes – I loved it all, right down to the red-brick front of the Christadel-phian reading-room and the posters outside the Coliseum and Royal cinemas, I couldn't leave it. And if I married Alice I'd be forced to leave it. You can only love a town if it loves you, and Warley would never love a co-respondent. I had to love Warley properly too, I had to take all she could give me; it was too late to enjoy merely her warm friendship, a life with a Grade Six girl perhaps, a life spent in, if I were lucky, one of the concrete boxes of houses on the new Council estate. People could be happy in those little houses with their tiny gardens and one bathroom and no garage. They could be happy on my present income, even on a lot less. But it wasn't for me; if the worst came to the worst, I would accept it sooner than not live in Warley at all, but I had to force the town into granting me the ultimate intimacy, the power and privilege and luxury which emanated from T'Top.

'Joe,' said Susan. 'You're very naughty. You're not listening.'

'I am, honey,' I said. 'It wasn't a lovely letter, though. I was too agitated when I wrote it. I was frightened that you'd recognize the writing and throw it away. I haven't had a happy moment since you told me it was all over between us.'

'You promised me never to see Alice again. Have you told her?'

'You know she's in hospital. She's very ill too.'

Susan's face was very hard; she didn't look like a schoolgirl now, but more like one of those female magistrates who are always sending someone to jail without the option so that no one will be able to accuse them of womanly soft-heartedness.

'You must tell her now.' She looked like her mother: the soft curves of her face seemed to change to straight lines and her mouth became tight and disciplined – not exactly cruel, but set in an expression of judgement.

Alice had come home the day before me and had been taken to hospital in the middle of the night. I never did find out what the illness was; it wasn't cancer but it was some kind of internal swelling that was quite serious – serious enough for an operation – but not serious enough for the doctors to give her the dope necessary to keep away the pain. She was waiting for the operation now, and wasn't allowed any visitors except for family. I hadn't written her because she'd sent me a note saying that it was wisest not to; but my conscience troubled me about it because I knew that she didn't really expect me to take her at her word.

'Do you hear me, Joe?' Susan's voice had a shrill note. 'Tell her now. She's not going to die. If you don't write to her straightaway I really have finished with you this time. I mean it.'

'Shut up. I'll do what I promised – I'll finish the affair once and for all. When she comes out of hospital. And face to face. Not by letter. That's cowardly.'

Susan stood up. 'You're absolutely hateful and despicable. You won't do anything I ask you to, and now you're going back to this – this old woman just because she's supposed to be ill. I wish I'd never met you. You've spoilt France for me and now that I'm happy again you're doing *this*. I hate you, I hate you, I hate you – ' She burst into tears. 'I'm going. I don't want to see you again. You never loved me – '

I took hold of her roughly, then slapped her hard on the face. She gave a little cry of surprise, then flew at me with her nails. I held her off easily.

'You're not going,' I said. 'And I'm not going to do what you asked me either. I love you, you silly bitch, and I'm the one who says what's to be done. Now and in the future.'

'Let me go,' she said. 'I'll scream for help. You can't make me stay against my will.' She started to struggle. Her black hair was dishevelled and her brown eyes were gleaming with anger, changed into a tigerish topaz. I shook her as hard as I could. I'd done it in play before, when she'd asked me to hurt her, please hurt her; but this time I was in brutal earnest, and when I'd finished she was breathless and half-fainting. Then I kissed her, biting her

[44]

lip till I tasted blood. Her arms tightened round my neck and she let herself fall to the ground. This time she did not play the frightened virgin; this time I had no scruples, no horizon but the hot lunacy of my own instincts.

'You hurt me,' she said when I came to my sense afterwards, my whole body empty and exhausted. 'You hurt me and you took all my clothes – look, I'm bleeding here – and here – and here. Oh Joe, I love you with all of me now, every little bit of me is yours. You won't need *her* any more, will you?'

She laughed. It was a low gurgling laugh. It was full of physical contentment. 'Tell her when she comes out of hospital if you like, darling. You won't need her any more. I know that.' She smiled at me; the smile radiated an almost savage well-being.

'I won't need her any more,' I repeated dully. There was a taste of blood in my mouth and my hand was bleeding where she'd scratched it. The sun was hurting my eyes now, and the bracken round the clearing seemed actually to be growing taller and closing in on me.

Anon
early 15th century

Jankin, the clerical seducer

Kyrie, so kyrie,
Jankin singeth merye,
With Aleison.

As I went on Yol Day
In oure prosession,
Knew I joly Jankin
By his mery ton,
Kyrieleyson.

Jankin began the offis
On the Yol Day,
And yit me thinketh it does me good
So merye gan he say,
'Kyrieleyson'.

Jankin red the Pistle
Full faire and full well,
And yit me thinketh it dos me good
As evere have I sel,
Kyrieleyson.

Jankin at the Sanctus
Craketh a merye note,
And yit me thinketh it dos me good –
I payed for his cote,
Kyrieleyson.

Jankin craketh notes
An hundered on a knot,
And yit he hacketh hem smallere
Than wortes to the pot,
Kyrieleyson.

Jankin at the Agnus
Bereth the pax-brede:
He twinkled but said nowt,
And on my fot he trede,
Kyrieleyson.

Benedicamus Domino,
Christ fro shame me shilde:
Deo gracias, therto –
Alas! I go with childe,
Kyrieleyson.

Radclyffe Hall
1886–1943

from The Well of Loneliness

Twenty-one-year-old Stephen Gordon lives with her mother, Anna, and her retired governess, Miss Puddleton (Puddle) at Morton, her country home. She has recently met the newcomer, Angela Crossby, over a dogfight in the local town.

On a beautiful evening three weeks later, Stephen took Angela over Morton. They had had tea with Anna and Puddle, and Anna had been coldly polite to this friend of her daughter's, but Puddle's manner had been rather resentful – she deeply mistrusted Angela Crossby. But now Stephen was free to show Angela Morton, and this she did gravely, as though something sacred were involved in this first introduction to her home, as though Morton itself must feel that the coming of this small, fair-haired woman was in some way momentous. Very gravely, then, they went over the house – even into Sir Philip's old study.

From the house they made their way to the stables, and still grave, Stephen told her friend about Raftery. Angela listened, assuming an interest she was very far from feeling – she was timid of horses, but she liked to hear the girl's rather gruff voice, such an earnest young voice, it intrigued her. She was thoroughly frightened when Raftery sniffed her and then blew through his nostrils as though disapproving, and she started back with a sharp exclamation, so that Stephen slapped him on his glossy grey shoulder: 'Stop it, Raftery, come up!' And Raftery, disgusted, went and blew on his oats to express his hurt feelings.

They left him and wandered away through the gardens, and quite soon poor Raftery was almost forgotten, for the gardens smelt softly of night-scented stock, and of other pale flowers that smell sweetest at evening, and Stephen was thinking that Angela

[48]

Crossby resembled such flowers – very fragrant and pale she was, so Stephen said to her gently:

'You seem to belong to Morton.'

Angela smiled a slow, questioning smile: 'You think so, Stephen?'

'And Stephen answered: 'I do, because Morton and I are one,' and she scarcely understood the portent of her words; but Angela, understanding, spoke quickly:

'Oh, I belong nowhere – you forget I'm the stranger.'

'I know that you're you,' said Stephen.

They walked on in silence while the light changed and deepened, growing always more golden and yet more elusive. And the birds, who loved that strange light, sang singly and then all together: 'We're happy, Stephen!'

And turning to Angela, Stephen answered the birds: 'Your being here makes me so happy.'

'If that's true, then why are you so shy of my name?'

'Angela – ' mumbled Stephen.

Then Angela said: 'It's just over three weeks since we met – how quickly our friendship's happened. I suppose it was meant, I believe in Kismet. You were awfully scared that first day at The Grange; why were you so scared?'

Stephen answered slowly: 'I'm frightened now – I'm frightened of you.'

'Yet you're stronger than I am – '

'Yes, that's why I'm so frightened, you make me feel strong – do you want to do that?'

'Well – perhaps – you're so very unusual, Stephen.'

'Am I?'

'Of course, don't you know that you are? Why, you're altogether different from other people.'

Stephen trembled a little: 'Do you mind?' she faltered.

'I know that you're you,' teased Angela, smiling again, but she reached out and took Stephen's hand.

Something in the queer, vital strength of that hand stirred her deeply, so that she tightened her fingers: 'What in the Lord's name are you?' she murmured.

'I don't know. Go on holding like that to my hand – hold it tighter – I like the feel of your fingers.'

[49]

'Stephen, don't be absurd!'

'Go on holding my hand, I like the feel of your fingers.'

'Stephen, you're hurting, you're crushing my rings!'

And now they were under the trees by the lakes, their feet falling softly on the luminous carpet. Hand in hand they entered that place of deep stillness, and only their breathing disturbed the stillness for a moment, then it folded back over their breathing.

'Look,' said Stephen, and she pointed to the swan called Peter, who had come drifting past on his own white reflection. 'Look,' she said, 'this is Morton, all beauty and peace – it drifts like that swan does, on calm, deep water. And all this beauty and peace is for you, because now you're a part of Morton.'

Angela said: 'I've never known peace, it's not in me – I don't think I'd find it here, Stephen.' And as she spoke she released her hand, moving a little away from the girl.

But Stephen continued to talk on gently; her voice sounded almost like that of a dreamer: 'Lovely, oh, lovely it is, our Morton. On evenings in winter these lakes are quite frozen, and the ice looks like slabs of gold in the sunset, when you and I come and stand here in the winter. And as we walk back we can smell the log fires long before we can see them, and we love that good smell because it means home, and our home is Morton – and we're happy, happy – we're utterly contented and at peace, we're filled with the peace of this place – '

'Stephen – don't!'

'We're both filled with the old peace of Morton, because we love each other so deeply – and because we're perfect, a perfect thing, you and I – not two separate people but one. And our love has lit a great, comforting beacon, so that we need never be afraid of the dark any more – we can warm ourselves at our love, we can lie down together, and my arms will be round you – '

She broke off abruptly, and they stared at each other.

'Do you know what you're saying?' Angela whispered.

And Stephen answered: 'I know that I love you, and that nothing else matters in the world.'

Then, perhaps because of that glamorous evening, with its spirit of queer, unearthly adventure, with its urge to strange, unendurable sweetness, Angela moved a step nearer to Stephen, then another, until their hands were touching. And all that she was, and all that she had been and would be again, perhaps even tomorrow, was fused at that moment into one mighty impulse, one imperative need, and that need was Stephen. Stephen's need was now hers, by sheer force of its blind and uncomprehending will to appeasement.

Then Stephen took Angela into her arms, and she kissed her full on the lips, as a lover.

Andrew Marvell
1621–78

To his Coy Mistress

Had we but world enough, and time,
This coyness, lady, were no crime.
We would sit down, and think which way
To walk, and pass our long love's day.
Thou by the Indian Ganges' side
Shouldst rubies find: I by the tide
Of Humber would complain. I would
Love you ten years before the flood,
And you should, if you please, refuse
Till the conversion of the Jews;
My vegetable love should grow
Vaster than empires and more slow;
An hundred years should go to praise
Thine eyes, and on thy forehead gaze;
Two hundred to adore each breast,
But thirty thousand to the rest;
An age at least to every part,
And the last age should show your heart.
For, lady, you deserve this state,
Nor would I love at lower rate.
 But at my back I always hear
Time's wingèd chariot hurrying near,
And yonder all before us lie
Deserts of vast eternity.
Thy beauty shall no more be found,
Nor, in thy marble vault, shall sound
My echoing song; then worms shall try
That long-preserved virginity,
And your quaint honour turn to dust,
And into ashes all my lust:

The grave's a fine and private place,
But none, I think, do there embrace.
    Now therefore, while the youthful hue
Sits on thy skin like morning dew,
And while thy willing soul transpires
At every pore with instant fires,
Now let us sport us while we may,
And now, like amorous birds of prey,
Rather at once our time devour,
Than languish in his slow-chapt power.
Let us roll all our strength and all
Our sweetness up into one ball,
And tear our pleasures with rough strife,
Thorough the iron gates of life;
Thus, though we cannot make our sun
Stand still, yet we will make him run.

Party Piece

He said:

'Let's stay here
Now this place has emptied
And make gentle pornography with one another,
While the partygoers go out
And the dawn creeps in,
Like a stranger.

Let us not hesitate
Over what we know
Or over how cold this place has become,
But let's unclip our minds
And let tumble free
The mad, mangled crocodile of love.'

So they did,
There among the woodbines and guinness stains,
And later he caught a bus and she a train
And all there was between them then
was rain.

❧

Purposes Mistook

———————————————

John Lehmann
1907–

from In the Purely Pagan Sense

The absent Duncan is the friend and lover of the young narrator, whom he has recently introduced to Babington, an old and famous novelist. The narrator goes to dinner at Babington's home, in the belief that both he and Duncan have been invited.

When I reached Babington's house on the night appointed, I found to my surprise that Duncan was not there. 'He's just rung up to say he has a bad cold, and can't come,' Babington announced in his rather squeaky voice, 'but he begged me not to send you away. It's a shame, but I think we'll enjoy ourselves without him, don't you?' He squeezed my arm. Duncan's cold surprised me, as I had been with him the night before, and had not noticed anything. Afterwards he swore that he had even had a temperature, but I was never completely convinced; especially as after a time I began to discover Duncan's skill in telling white lies without a blush.

After we had had some gin, Babington took me off to a French restaurant in Soho, and ordered what struck me as a very expensive meal. He seemed a little tongue-tied and uncertain of himself at first, but as the wine began to circulate in our veins and he became aware of my doglike attention to everything he said, he talked more and more without restraint, imitating some of the dons I had encountered at Cambridge with hilariously comic effect, making malicious comments about my seniors in the V & A whom he seemed to know, ridiculing, in a completely devastating way, two or three of the more highly thought-of authors of the day, and above all discoursing with a brilliance that completely dazzled me of the French writers of the seventeenth and eighteenth centuries, whose works had been among my undergraduate studies. Never had I listened to such conversation, in which wit and learning and imagination were so effortlessly blended. Nor was his attitude that of masterly lecturer to humble listener: he continually drew me in, with questions and jokes about my own generation, and showed a gentle deference to my haltingly expressed opinions.

After we had finished our coffee and brandy, he suggested we should go back to his house for a final whisky and soda. By that time his attitude towards me had become distinctly intimate. He had discovered my sexual inclinations without actually putting any point-blank questions to me, and as soon as we were sitting side by side on the sofa he began to question me playfully about my lovers, whom he suggested must be legion. I told him, between rather embarrassed giggles, that I had hardly had any lovers so far. He then leaned over me and started to fondle me and kiss me on the cheek, and proposed that we should go to bed together. I was not so tipsy or fuddled as to be unable to avoid a direct answer, but he became more and more insistent, and when his hand began to stray over my trousers a totally unexpected thing happened. I had become completely fascinated by Babington as mind and person during the evening, but physically he not only did not attract me, but in fact repelled me. The beard, the lanky unathletic figure, the limp manner – all these were utterly remote from my erotic dreams. The combination of the two emotions under his caresses, however, revealed itself as violently potent. While his hand renewed its attention to my flies, I came in my trousers.

I could hardly understand it myself. 'Too late!' I exclaimed. 'It's too late!' 'Why?' he asked, puzzled. 'It's all over!' I gasped. It took him some time to grasp what had happened, and even then I'm not sure he believed it. But he knew he was beaten, for that evening at least.

Thomas Heywood
1574?–1641

Jupiter and Ganimede

The Argument of the Dialogue entitled Jupiter and Ganimede

Jove's masculine love this fable reprehends,
And wanton dotage on the Trojan boy.
Shaped like an eagle, he from th'earth ascends,
And bears through th'air his new Delight and Joy.
   In Ganimed's expressed a simple swain
   Who would leave Heaven, to live on Earth again.

The Dialogue

JUPITER: Now kiss me, lovely Ganimede, for see,
   We are at length arrived where we would be:
   I have no crooked beak, no talons keen,
   No wings or feathers are about me seen;
   I am not such as I but late appeared.
GANIMEDE: But were you not that eagle who late feared,
   And snatched me from my flock? where is become
   That shape? you speak now, who but late were dumb.
JUPITER: I am no man, fair youth, as I appear,
   Nor eagle, to astonish thee with fear:
   But King of all the gods, who for some reason
   Have by my power transhaped me for a season.
GANIMEDE: What's that you say? you are not Pan, I know:
   Where's then your pipe? or where your horns, should grow
   Upon your temples? where your hairy thighs?
JUPITER: Thinks Ganimede that godhead only lies
   In rural Pan?
GANIMEDE: Why not? I know him one:

We shepherds sacrifice to him alone.
A spotted goat into some cave we drive,
And then he seizeth on the beast alive.
Thou art but some child-stealer, that's thy best.
JUPITER: Hast thou not heard of any man contest
By Jove's great name? nor his rich altar viewed
In Gargarus, with plenteous showers bedewed?
There seen his fire and thunder?
GANIMEDE: Do you then
Affirm yourself the same who on us men
Of late poured hail-stones? he that dwells above us,
And there makes noise; yet some will say doth love us?
To whom my father did observance yield,
And sacrificed the best ram in the field.
Why then (if you of all the gods be chief)
Have you, by stealing me, thus played the thief;
When in my absence the poor sheep may stray,
Or the wild ravenous wolves snatch them away?
JUPITER: Yet hast thou care of lambs, of folds, of sheep;
That now art made immortal, and must keep
Society with us.
GANIMEDE: I no way can
Conceive you. Will you play the honest man,
And bear me back to Ida?
JUPITER: So in vain
I shaped me like an eagle, if again
I should return thee back.
GANIMEDE: My father, he
By this hath made inquiry after me;
And if the least of all the flock be eaten
I in his rage am most sure to be beaten.
JUPITER: Where shall he find thee?
GANIMEDE: That's the thing I fear,
He never can climb up to meet me here,
But if thou beest a good god, let me pass
Into the mount of Ida where I was:
And then I'll offer, in my thankful piety,
Another well-fed goat unto thy deity,
(As price of my redemption) three years old,

[60]

And now the chief and prime in all the fold.

JUPITER: How simple is this innocent lad? a mere
Innocuous child. But Ganimede now hear:
Bury the thoughts of all such terren dross,
Think Ida and thy father's flocks no loss:
Thou now art heavenly, and much grace mayst do
Unto thy father and thy country too.
No more of cheese and milk from henceforth think,
Ambrosia thou shalt eat, and nectar drink,
Which thy fair hands in flowing cups shalt fill
To me and others, but attend us still;
And (that which most should move thee) make thy abode
Where thou art now, thou shalt be made a god,
No more be mortal, and thy glorious star
Shine with refulgence, and be seen from far.
Here thou art ever happy.

GANIMEDE: But I pray,
When I would sport me, who is here to play?
For when in Ida I did call for any,
Both of my age and growth it yielded many.

JUPITER: Play-fellows for thee I will likewise find,
Cupid, with divers others to thy mind,
And such as are of both thy years and size,
To sport with thee all what thou canst devise.
Only be bold and pleasant, and then know
Thou shalt have need of nothing that's below.

GANIMEDE: But here no service I can do indeed,
Unless in heaven you had some flocks to feed.

JUPITER: Yes, thou to me shalt fill celestial wine,
And wait upon me when in state I dine:
Then learn to serve in banquets.

GANIMEDE: That I can
Already, without help of any man:
For I use ever when we dine or sup,
To pour out milk, and crown the pastoral cup.

JUPITER: Fie, how thou still remember'st milk and breasts,
As if thou wert to serve at mortal feasts.
Know, this is heaven, be merry then and laugh;
When thou art thirsty thou shalt nectar quaff.

GANIMEDE: Is it so sweet as milk?

JUPITER: Prized far before,
Which tasted once, milk thou wilt ask no more.

GANIMEDE: Where shall I sleep a nights? what, must I lie
With my companion Cupid?

JUPITER: So then I
In vain had raped thee: but I from thy sheep
Of purpose stole thee, by my side to sleep.

GANIMEDE: Can you not lie alone? but will your rest
Seem sweeter, if I nuzzle on your breast?

JUPITER: Yes, being a child so fair.

GANIMEDE: How can you think
Of beauty, whilst you close your eyes and wink?

JUPITER: It is a sweet enticement, to increase
Contented rest, when our desire's at peace.

GANIMEDE: I, but my father every morn would chide,
And say, those nights he lodged me by his side
I much disturbed his rest; tumbling and tossing
Athwart the bed, my little legs still crossing
His: either kicking this way, that way sprawling,
Or if he but removed me, straightways yawling:
Then grumbling in my dreams, (for so he said)
And oft times sent me to my mother's bed:
And then she would complain upon me worse.
Then if for that you stole me, the best course
Is even to send me back again; for I
Am ever so unruly where I lie,
Wallowing and tumbling, and such coil I keep,
That I shall but disturb you in your sleep.

JUPITER: In that the greater pleasure I shall take,
Because I love still to be kept awake.
I shall embrace and kiss thee then the ofter,
And by that means my bed seem much the softer.

GANIMEDE: But whilst you wake I'll sleep.

JUPITER: Mercury, see
This lad straight taste of immortality;
And making him of service capable,
Let him be brought to wait on us at table.

William Congreve
1670–1729

from The Way of the World

Mirabell is in love with Millamant, Lady Wishfort's niece. He incurred the elderly lady's enmity when she discovered that his supposed passion for her was merely to divert her attention from his courtship of Millamant, whom Lady Wishfort will disinherit if she marries without her approbation. Now Mirabell is scheming with Lady Wishfort's maid, Foible, as Lady Wishfort herself suspects until Foible cleverly allays her doubts. The plan is to have Lady Wishfort succumb to Sir Rowland, who is really Waitwell, Mirabell's serving-man and Foible's husband, in disguise. Lady Wishfort sees marriage to Sir Rowland as a way of disinheriting Millamant.

A room in LADY WISHFORT'S *house.* LADY WISHFORT *is at her toilet and* FOIBLE, *her maid, is waiting on her.*

LADY: O Foible, where hast thou been? what hast thou been doing?

FOIB: Madam, I have seen the party.

LADY: But what hast thou done?

FOIB: Nay, 'tis your ladiship has done, and are to do; I have only promised. But a man so enamoured – so transported. Well, if worshipping of pictures be a sin – poor Sir Rowland, I say.

LADY: The miniature has been counted like – But hast thou not betrayed me, Foible? Hast thou not detected me to that faithless Mirabell? – What hadst thou to do with him in the Park? Answer me, has he got nothing out of thee?

FOIB: So, the devil has been beforehand with me, what shall I say? – Alas, madam, could I help it, if I met that confident thing? Was I in fault? If you had heard how he used me, and all upon your ladiship's account, I'm sure you would not suspect my fidelity. Nay, if that had been the worst I could have born: but he had a fling at your ladiship too; and then I could not hold: but i'faith I gave him his own.

LADY: Me? What did the filthy fellow say?

FOIB: O madam; 'tis a shame to say what he said – with his taunts and his fleers, tossing up his nose. Humh (says he), what you are a hatching some plot (says he), you are so early abroad, or catering (says he), ferreting for some disbanded officer, I warrant – half pay is but thin subsistance (says he) – Well, what pension does your lady propose? Let me see (says he), what she must come down pretty deep now, she's superannuated (says he) and –

LADY: Ods my life, I'll have him, I'll have him murdered. I'll have him poisoned. Where does he eat? I'll marry a drawer to have him poisoned in his wine. I'll send for Robin from Lockets – immediately.

FOIB: Poison him? Poisoning's too good for him. Starve him, madam, starve him; marry Sir Rowland, and get him disinherited. O you would bless yourself, to hear what he said.

LADY: A villain, superannuated!

FOIB: Humh (says he), I hear you are laying designs against me too (says he), and Mrs Millamant is to marry my uncle (he does not suspect a word of your ladiship); but (says he) I'll fit you for that, I warrant you (says he), I'll hamper you for that (says he), you and your old frippery too (says he), I'll handle you –

LADY: Audacious villain! handle me, would he durst – Frippery? old frippery! Was there ever such a foul-mouthed fellow? I'll be married tomorrow, I'll be contracted tonight.

FOIB: The sooner the better, madam.

LADY: Will Sir Rowland be here, say'st thou? when, Foible?

FOIB: Incontinently, madam. No new sheriff's wife expects the return of her husband after knighthood, with that impatience in which Sir Rowland burns for the dear hour of kissing your ladiship's hand after dinner.

LADY: Frippery! superannuated frippery! I'll frippery the villain; I'll reduce him to frippery and rags: a tatterdemallion – I hope to see him hung with tatters, like a Long-Lane pent-house, or a gibbet-thief. A slander-mouthed railer: I warrant the spendthrift prodigal's in debt as much as the million lottery, or the whole court upon a birthday. I'll spoil his credit with his tailor. Yes, he shall have my niece with her fortune, he shall.

FOIB: He! I hope to see him lodge in Ludgate first, and angle into Black-Fryars for brass farthings, with an old mitten.

LADY: Ay, dear Foible; thank thee for that, dear Foible. He has put me out of all patience. I shall never recompose my features to receive Sir Rowland with any oeconomy of face. This wretch has fretted me that I am absolutely decayed. Look, Foible.

FOIB: Your ladiship has frowned a little too rashly, indeed, madam. There are some cracks discernible in the white vernish.

LADY: Let me see the glass – Cracks, say'st thou? Why, I am arrantly fleaed – I look like an old peeled wall. Thou must repair me, Foible, before Sir Rowland comes; or I shall never keep up to my picture.

FOIB: I warrant you, madam; a little art once made your picture like you; and now a little of the same art must make you like your picture. Your picture must sit for you, madam.

LADY: But art thou sure Sir Rowland will not fail to come? Or will a not fail when he does come? Will he be importunate, Foible, and push? For if he should not be importunate – I shall never break decorums – I shall die with confusion, if I am forced to advance – Oh no, I can never advance – I shall swoon if he should expect advances. No, I hope Sir Rowland is better bred, than to put a lady to the necessity of breaking her forms. I won't be too coy neither – I won't give him despair – but a little disdain is not amiss; a

[65]

little scorn is alluring.

FOIB: A little scorn becomes your ladiship.

LADY: Yes, but tenderness becomes me best – a sort of a dyingness – You see that picture has a sort of a – Ha, Foible? A swimmingness in the eyes – Yes, I'll look so – my niece affects it; but she wants features. Is Sir Rowland handsome? Let my toilet be removed – I'll dress above. I'll receive Sir Rowland here. Is he handsome? Don't answer me. I won't know: I'll be surprized. I'll be taken by surprize.

FOIB: By storm, madam. Sir Rowland's a brisk man.

LADY: Is he! O then he'll importune, if he's a brisk man. I shall save decorums if Sir Rowland importunes. I have a mortal terror at the apprehension of offending against decorums. O I'm glad he's a brisk man. Let my things be removed, good Foible.

(*Later the same day*)

LADY: Is Sir Rowland coming, say'st thou, Foible? and are things in order?

FOIB: Yes, madam. I have put wax-lights in the sconces; and placed the footmen in a row in the hall, in their best liveries, with the coachman and postilion to fill up the equipage.

LADY: Have you pullvilled the coachman and postilion, that they may not stink of the stable, when Sir Rowland comes by?

FOIB: Yes, madam.

LADY: And are the dancers and the music ready, that he may be entertained in all points with correspondence to his passion?

FOIB: All is ready, madam.

LADY: And – well – and how do I look, Foible?

FOIB: Most killing well, madam.

LADY: Well, and how shall I receive him? In what figure shall I give his heart the first impression? There is a great deal in the first impression. Shall I sit? – No, I won't sit – I'll walk – ay, I'll walk from the door upon his entrance; and then turn full upon him – No, that will be too sudden. I'll lye – ay, I'll lye down – I'll receive him in my little dressing-room, there's a couch – yes, yes, I'll give the first impression on a couch – I won't lye neither, but loll and lean upon one elbow; with one foot a little dangling off, jogging in a thoughtful way – yes – and then as soon as he appears, start, ay, start and be surprized, and rise to meet him in a pretty disorder – yes – O, nothing is more alluring than a levee from a couch in some confusion – it shews the foot to advantage, and furnishes with blushes, and re-composing airs beyond comparison. Hark! There's a coach.

FOIB: 'Tis he, madam.

(*Exit* FOIBLE.)

(*Enter* WAITWELL, disguised as SIR ROWLAND.)

LADY: Dear Sir Rowland, I am confounded with confusion at the retrospection of my own rudeness – I have more pardons to ask than the pope distributes in the year of jubile. But I hope where there is likely to be so near an alliance, we may unbend the severity of decorum, and dispense with a little ceremony.

WAIT: My impatience, madam, is the effect of my transport; – and 'till I have the possession of your adorable person, I am tantalised on the rack; and do but hang, madam, on the tenter of expectation.

LADY: You have excess of gallantry, Sir Rowland; and press things to a conclusion, with a most prevailing vehemence – But a day or two for decency of marriage –

WAIT: For decency of funeral, madam. The delay will break my heart – or if that should fail, I shall be poisoned. My nephew will get an inkling of my designs, and poison me, – and I would willingly starve him before I die – I would gladly go out of the world with that satisfaction – That would be some comfort to me, if I could but live so long as to be revenged on that unnatural viper.

LADY: Is he so unnatural, say you? Truly I would contribute much both to the saving of your life, and the accomplishment of your revenge – not that I respect myself; though he has been a perfidious wretch to me.

[67]

WAIT: Perfidious to you!

LADY: O Sir Rowland, the hours that he has died away at my
feet, the tears that he has shed, the oaths that he has
sworn, the palpitations that he has felt, the trances and the
tremblings, the ardors and the ecstacies, the kneelings, and
the risings, the heart-heavings and the hand-grippings, the
pangs and the pathetick regards of his protesting eyes! Oh,
no memory can register.

WAIT: What, my rival! Is the rebel my rival? a' dies.

LADY: No, don't kill him at once, Sir Rowland, starve him
gradually inch by inch.

WAIT: I'll do't. In three weeks he shall be bare-foot; in a month
out at knees with begging an alms – he shall starve upward
and upward, 'till he has nothing living but his head,
and then go out in a stink like a candle's end upon a
save-all.

LADY: Well, Sir Rowland, you have the way – you are no
novice in the labyrinth of love – you have the clue – But
as I am a person, Sir Rowland, you must not attribute
my yielding to any sinister appetite, or indigestion of
widow-hood; nor impute my complacency to any lethargy
of continence – I hope you do not think me prone to
any iteration of nuptials –

WAIT: Far be it from me –

LADY: If you do, I protest I must recede – or think that I have
made a prostitution of decorums, but in the vehemence of
compassion, and to save the life of a person of so much
importance –

WAIT: I esteem it so –

LADY: Or else you wrong my condescension –

WAIT: I do not, I do not –

LADY: Indeed you do.

WAIT: I do not, fair shrine of virtue.

LADY: If you think the least scruple of carnality was an
ingredient –

WAIT: Dear madam, no. You are all camphire and
frankincense, all chastity and odour.

LADY: Or that –
    (*Enter* FOIBLE.)

FOIB: Madam, the dancers are ready, and there's one with a
    letter, who must deliver it into your own hands.
LADY: Sir Rowland, will you give me leave? Think favourably,
    judge candidly, and conclude you have found a person who
    would suffer racks in honour's cause, dear Sir Rowland,
    and will wait on you incessantly.
    (*Exit* LADY WISHFORT.)
WAIT: Fie, fie! – What a slavery have I undergone; spouse,
    hast thou any cordial, I want spirits.
FOIB: What a washy rogue art thou, to pant thus for a quarter
    of an hour's lying and swearing to a fine lady?
WAIT: O, she is the antidote to desire. Spouse, thou wilt fare
    the worse for't – I shall have no appetite to iteration of
    nuptials this eight and forty hours – By this hand I'd
    rather be a chairman in the dog-days, than act Sir
    Rowland 'till this time to-morrow.
    (*Enter* LADY *with a letter.*)
LADY: Call in the dancers; – Sir Rowland, we'll sit, if you
    please, and see the entertainment.
    (*Dance.*)
    Now with your permission, Sir Rowland, I will peruse my
    letter – I would open it in your presence, because I would
    not make you uneasie. If it should make you uneasie I
    would burn it – speak if it does – but you may see, the
    superscription is like a woman's hand.
FOIB: By heaven! Mrs Marwood's,* I know it, – my heart akes
    – get it from her –
    (*To him.*)
WAIT: A woman's hand? No, madam, that's no woman's hand,
    I see that already. That's somebody whose throat must be
    cut.
LADY: Nay, Sir Rowland, since you give me a proof of your
    passion by your jealousie, I promise you I'll make a return,
    by a frank communication – You shall see it – we'll open it
    together – look you here. (*Reads*) 'Madam, though

---

*Enemy to Mirabell (Ed.).

unknown to you,' – Look you there, 'tis from nobody that I
know – 'I have that honour for your character, that I think
myself obliged to let you know you are abused. He who
pretends to be Sir Rowland is a cheat and a rascal – ' Oh
heavens! what's this?

FOIB: Unfortunate, all's ruined.

WAIT: How, how, let me see, let me see (*reading*). 'A rascal and
disguised, and suborned for that imposture,' – O villany!
O villany – 'by the contrivance of – '

LADY: I shall faint, I shall die, oh!

FOIB: (*To him*) Say 'tis your nephew's hand. – Quickly, his plot,
swear, swear it.

WAIT: Here's a villain! Madam, don't you perceive it, don't you
see it?

LADY: Too well, too well. I have seen too much.

WAIT: I told you at first I knew the hand – A woman's hand?
The rascal writes a sort of a large hand; your Roman hand
– I saw there was a throat to be cut presently. If he were
my son, as he is my nephew, I'd pistol him –

FOIB: O treachery! But are you sure, Sir Rowland, it is his
writing?

WAIT: Sure? Am I here? do I live? do I love this pearl of India?
I have twenty letters in my pocket from him, in the same
character.

LADY: How!

FOIB: O what luck it is, Sir Rowland, that you were present at
this juncture! This was the business that brought Mr
Mirabell disguised to Madam Millamant this afternoon. I
thought something was contriving, when he stole by me
and would have hid his face.

LADY: How, how! – I heard the villain was in the house
indeed; and now I remember, my niece went away
abruptly, when Sir Wilfull was to have made his
addresses.

FOIB: Then, then, madam, Mr Mirabell waited for her in her
chamber; but I would not tell your ladiship to discompose
you when you were to receive Sir Rowland.

WAIT: Enough, his date is short.

FOIB: No, good Sir Rowland, don't incur the law.

WAIT: Law! I care not for law. I can but die, and 'tis in a good
cause – my lady shall be satisfied of my truth and
innocence, though it cost me my life.

LADY: No, dear Sir Rowland, don't fight, if you should be killed
I must never show my face; or hanged – O consider my
reputation, Sir Rowland – No, you shan't fight. – I'll go in
and examine my niece; I'll make her confess. I conjure you,
Sir Rowland, by all your love, not to fight.

WAIT: I am charmed, madam, I obey. But some proof you must
let me give you; – I'll go for a black box, which contains
the writings of my whole estate, and deliver that into your
hands.

LADY: Ay, dear Sir Rowland, that will be some comfort, bring
the black box.

WAIT: And may I presume to bring a contract to be signed this
night? May I hope so far?

LADY: Bring what you will; but come alive, pray come alive. O
this is a happy discovery.

WAIT: Dead or alive I'll come – and married we will be in
spight of treachery; ay, and get an heir that shall defeat the
last remaining glimpse of hope in my abandoned nephew.
Come, my buxom widow:

> E'er long you shall substantial proof receive
> That I'm an arrant knight –

FOIB: Or arrant knave.

(*The scene continues.*)

LADY: Out of my house, out of my house, thou viper, thou
serpent, that I have fostered; thou bosom traitress, that I
raised from nothing – begone, begone, go, go, – that I took
from washing of old gause and weaving of dead hair, with a
bleak blue nose, over a chafing-dish of starved embers, and
dining behind a traver's rag, in a shop no bigger than a
bird-cage, – go, go, starve again, do, do.

FOIB: Dear madam, I'll beg pardon on my knees.

LADY: Away, out, out, go set up for yourself again – do, drive a
trade, do, with your threepenny-worth of small ware,
flaunting upon a packthread, under a brandy-feller's bulk,

or against a dead wall by a ballad-monger. Go, hang out an old frisoneer-gorget with a yard of yellow colberteen again; do; an old gnawed mask, two rows of pins and a child's fiddle; a glass necklace with the beads broken, and a quilted nightcap with one ear. Go, go, drive a trade. – These were your commodities, you treacherous trull, this was the merchandize you dealt in, when I took you into my house, placed you next myself, and made you governante of my whole family. You have forgot this, have you, now you have feathered your nest?

FOIB: No, no, dear madam. Do but hear me, have but a moment's patience – I'll confess all. Mr Mirabell seduced me; I am not the first that he has wheadled with his dissembling tongue; your ladiship's own wisdom has been deluded by him, then how should I, a poor ignorant, defend myself? O madam, if you knew but what he promised me, and how he assured me your ladiship should come to no damage – or else the wealth of the Indies should not have bribed me to conspire against so good, so sweet, so kind a lady as you have been to me.

LADY: No damage? What, to betray me, to marry me to a cast-serving-man; to make me a receptacle, an hospital for a decayed pimp? No damage? O thou frontless impudence, more than a big-bellied actress.

FOIB: Pray do but hear me, madam, he could not marry your ladiship, madam – no indeed, his marriage was to have been void in law; for he was married to me first, to secure your ladiship. He could not have bedded your ladiship; for if he had consummated with your ladiship, he must have run the risque of the law, and been put upon his clergy – Yes indeed, I enquired of the law in that case before I would meddle or make.

LADY: What, then I have been your property, have I? I have been convenient to you, it seems – while you were catering for Mirabell; I have ben broaker for you? What, have you made a passive bawd of me? – This exceeds all precedent; I am brought to fine uses, to become a botcher of second-hand marriages between Abigails and Andrews! I'll couple you. Yes, I'll baste you together, you and your Philander.

I'll Duke's Place you, as I'm a person. Your turtle is in custody already: you shall coo in the same cage, if there be constable or warrant in the parish.

FOIB: O that ever I was born, O that I was ever married, – a bride, ay, I shall be a Bridewell-bride. Oh!

Thomas Malory
d. 1471

from Le Morte d'Arthur

Sir Pelleas and the Lady Ettard

And so Sir Pelleas chose the Lady Ettard for his sovereign lady, and never to love other but her, but she was so proud that she had scorn of him, and said that she would never love him though he would die for her. Wherefore all ladies and gentlewomen had scorn of her that she was so proud, for there were fairer than she, and there was none that was there but an Sir Pelleas would have proffered them love, they would have loved him for his noble prowess. And so this knight promised the Lady Ettard to follow her into this country, and never to leave her till she loved him. And thus he is here the most part nigh her, and lodged by a priory, and every week she sendeth knights to fight with him. And when he hath put them to the worse, then will he suffer them wilfully to take him prisoner, because he would have a sight of this lady. And always she doth him great despite, for sometime she maketh her knights to tie him to his horse's tail, and some to bind him under the horse's belly; thus in the most shamefullest ways that she can think he is brought to her. And all she doth it for to cause him to leave this country, and to leave his loving; but all this cannot make him to leave, for an he would have fought on foot he might have had the better of the ten knights as well on foot as on horseback. Alas, said Sir Gawaine, it is great pity of him; and after this night I will seek him tomorrow, in this forest, to do him all the help I can. So on the morn Sir Gawaine took his leave of his host Sir Carados, and rode into the forest; and at the last he met with Sir Pelleas, making great moan out of measure, so each of them saluted other, and asked him why he made such sorrow. And as it is above rehearsed, Sir Pelleas told Sir Gawaine: But always I suffer her knights to fare so with me as ye saw yesterday, in trust at the last to

[74]

win her love, for she knoweth well all her knights should not lightly win me, an me list to fight with them to the uttermost. Wherefore an I loved her not so sore, I had liefer die an hundred times, an I might die so oft, rather than I would suffer that despite; but I trust she will have pity upon me at the last, for love causeth many a good knight to suffer to have his entent, but alas I am unfortunate. And therewith he made so great dole and sorrow that unnethe he might hold him on horseback.

Now, said Sir Gawaine, leave your mourning and I shall promise you by the faith of my body to do all that lieth in my power to get you the love of your lady, and thereto I will plight you my troth. Ah, said Sir Pelleas, of what court are ye? tell me, I pray you, my good friend. And then Sir Gawaine said, I am of the court of King Arthur, and his sister's son, and King Lot of Orkney was my father, and my name is Sir Gawaine. And then he said, My name is Sir Pelleas, born in the Isles, and of many isles I am lord, and never have I loved lady nor damosel till now in an unhappy time; and, sir knight, since ye are so nigh cousin unto King Arthur, and a king's son, therefore betray me not but help me, for I may never come by her but by some good knight, for she is in a strong castle here, fast by within this four mile, and over all this country she is lady of. And so I may never come to her presence, but as I suffer her knights to take me, and but if I did so that I might have a sight of her, I had been dead long or this time; and yet fair word had I never of her, but when I am brought to-fore her she rebuketh me in the foulest manner. And then they take my horse and harness and put me out of the gates, and she will not suffer me to eat nor drink; and always I offer me to be her prisoner, but that she will not suffer me, for I would desire no more, what pains so ever I had, so that I might have a sight of her daily. Well, said Sir Gawaine, all this shall I amend an ye will do as I shall devise: I will have your horse and your armour, and so will I ride unto her castle and tell her that I have slain you, and so shall I come within her to cause her to cherish me, and then shall I do my true part that ye shall not fail to have the love of her.

And therewith Sir Gawaine plight his troth unto Sir Pelleas to be true and faithful unto him; so each one plight their troth to other, and so they changed horses and harness, and Sir Gawaine departed, and came to the castle whereas stood the pavilions of this lady without the gate. And as soon as Ettard had espied Sir Gawaine she fled in toward the castle. Sir Gawaine spake on high, and bade her abide, for he was not Sir Pelleas; I am another knight that have slain Sir Pelleas. Do off your helm, said the Lady Ettard, that I may see your visage. And so when she saw that it was not Sir Pelleas, she bade him alight and led him unto her castle, and asked him faithfully whether he had slain Sir Pelleas. And he said her yea, and told her his name was Sir Gawaine of the court of King Arthur, and his sister's son. Truly, said she, that is great pity, for he was a passing good knight of his body, but of all men alive I hated him most, for I could never be quit of him; and for ye have slain him I shall be your woman, and to do anything that might please you. So she made Sir Gawaine good cheer. Then Sir Gawaine said that he loved a lady and by no means she would love him. She is to blame, said Ettard, an she will not love you, for ye that be so well born a man, and such a man of prowess, there is no lady in the world too good for you. Will ye, said Sir Gawaine, promise me to do all that ye may, by the faith of your body, to get me the love of my lady? Yea, sir, said she, and that I promise you by the faith of my body. Now, said Sir Gawaine, it is yourself that I love so well, therefore I pray you hold your promise. I may not choose, said the Lady Ettard, but if I should be forsworn; and so she granted him to fulfil all his desire.

So it was then in the month of May that she and Sir Gawaine went out of the castle and supped in a pavilion, and there was made a bed, and there Sir Gawaine and the Lady Ettard went to bed together, and in another pavilion she laid her damosels, and in the third pavilion she laid part of her knights, for then she had no dread of Sir Pelleas. And there Sir Gawaine lay with her in that pavilion two days and two nights. And on the third day, in the morning early, Sir Pelleas armed him, for he had never slept since Sir Gawaine departed from him; for Sir Gawaine had promised him by the faith of his body, to come to him unto his pavilion by that priory within the space of a day and a night.

Then Sir Pelleas mounted upon horseback, and came to the pavilions that stood without the castle, and found in the first pavilion three knights in three beds, and three squires lying at their feet. Then went he to the second pavilion and found four gentlewomen lying in four beds. And then he yede to the third pavilion and found Sir Gawaine lying in bed with his Lady Ettard, and either clipping other in arms, and when he saw that his heart well-nigh brast for sorrow, and said: Alas! that ever a knight should be found so false; and then he took his horse and might not abide no longer for pure sorrow. And when he had ridden nigh half a mile he turned again and thought to slay them both; and when he saw them both so lie sleeping fast, unnethe he might hold him on horseback for sorrow, and said thus to himself, Though this knight be never so false, I will never slay him sleeping, for I will never destroy the high order of knighthood; and therewith he departed again. And or he had ridden half a mile he returned again, and thought then to slay them both, making the greatest sorrow that ever man made. And when he came to the pavilions, he tied his horse unto a tree, and pulled out his sword naked in his hand, and went to them thereas they lay, and yet he thought it were shame to slay them sleeping, and laid the naked sword overthwart both their throats, and so took his horse and rode his way.

And when Sir Pelleas came to his pavilions he told his knights and his squires how he had sped, and said thus to them, For your true and good service ye have done me I shall give you all my goods, for I will go unto my bed and never arise until I am dead. And when that I am dead I charge you that ye take the heart out of my body and bear it her betwixt two silver dishes, and tell her how I saw her lie with the false knight Sir Gawaine. Right so Sir Pelleas unarmed himself, and went unto his bed making marvellous dole and sorrow.

Ben Jonson
1572–1637

from The Alchemist

Face has duped Sir Epicure Mammon into believing that his fellow trickster Doll Common is a lord's sister turned mad by the study of divinity. Sir Epicure, who thinks that Subtle, the 'alchemist' of the title and Face's colleague, is turning his metal into gold, finally meets the 'lady'.

MAMMON: (*Alone*)   Now, Epicure,
    Heighten thyself, talk to her all in gold;
    Rain her as many showers as Jove did drops
    Unto his Danaë, show the god a miser,
    Compared with Mammon. What! the Stone will do't.
    She shall feel gold, taste gold, hear gold, sleep gold;
    Nay, we will *concumbere* gold. I will be puissant
    And mighty in my talk to her.
    (*Re-enter* FACE *with* DOL, *richly dressed.*)
                                Here she comes.
FACE: (*Aside*) To him, Dol, suckle him. – This is the noble
    knight I told your ladyship –
MAMMON: Madam, with your pardon,
    I kiss your vesture.
DOL COMMON: Sir, I were uncivil
    If I would suffer that; my lip to you, sir.
MAMMON: I hope my Lord your brother be in health, lady.
DOL COMMON: My Lord my brother is, though I no lady, sir.
FACE: (*Aside*) Well said, my Guinea-bird.
MAMMON: Right noble madam –
FACE: (*Aside*) O, we shall have most fierce idolatry.
MAMMON: 'Tis your prerogative.
DOL COMMON: Rather your courtesy.
MAMMON: Were there nought else t'enlarge your virtues to me,
    These answers speak your breeding and your blood.

DOL COMMON: Blood we boast none, sir; a poor baron's
    daughter.
MAMMON: Poor! and gat you? Profane not. Had your father
    Slept all the happy remnant of his life
    After the act, lien but there still, and panted,
    He'd done enough to make himself, his issue,
    And his posterity noble.
DOL COMMON: Sir, although
    We may be said to want the gilt and trappings,
    The dress of honour, yet we strive to keep
    The seeds and the materials.
MAMMON: I do see
    The old ingredient, virtue, was not lost,
    Nor the drug, money, used to make your compound.
    There is a strange nobility i' your eye,
    This lip, that chin! Methinks you do resemble
    One o' the Austriac princes.
FACE: (Aside)   Very like!
    Her father was an Irish costermonger.
MAMMON: The house of Valois just had such a nose,
    And such a forehead yet the Medici
    Of Florence boast.
DOL COMMON: Troth, and I have been lik'ned
    To all these princes.
FACE: (Aside)   I'll be sworn, I heard it.
MAMMON: I know not how! it is not any one,
    But e'en the very choice of all their features.
FACE: (Aside) I'll in, and laugh. (Exit.)
MAMMON: A certain touch, or air,
    That sparkles a divinity beyond
    An earthly beauty!
DOL COMMON: O, you play the courtier.
MAMMON: Good lady, gi' me leave –
DOL COMMON: In faith, I may not,
    To mock me, sir.
MAMMON: To burn i' this sweet flame;
    The phœnix never knew a nobler death.
DOL COMMON: Nay, now you court the courtier, and destroy
    What you would build. This art, sir, i' your words,

Calls your whole faith in question.

MAMMON: By my soul —

DOL COMMON: Nay, oaths are made o' the same air, sir.

MAMMON: Nature
Never bestowed upon mortality
A more unblamed, a more harmonious feature;
She played the step-dame in all faces else.
Sweet madam, le' me be particular —

DOL COMMON: Particular, sir! I pray you, know your distance.

MAMMON: In no ill sense, sweet lady, but to ask
How your fair graces pass the hours? I see
Y' are lodged here, i' the house of a rare man,
An excellent artist; but what's that to you?

DOL COMMON: Yes, sir. I study here the mathematics,
And distillation.

MAMMON: O, I cry your pardon.
He's a divine instructor! can extract
The souls of all things by his art; call all
The virtues and the miracles of the sun
Into a temperate furnace; teach dull nature
What her own forces are. A man, the Emp'ror
Has courted above Kelly; sent his medals
And chains t'invite him.

DOL COMMON: Ay, and for his physic, sir —

MAMMON: Above the art of Æsculapius,
That drew the envy of the Thunderer!
I know all this, and more.

DOL COMMON: Troth, I am taken, sir,
Whole with these studies that contemplate nature.

MAMMON: It is a noble humour. But this form
Was not intended to so dark a use.
Had you been crookèd, foul, of some coarse mould,
A cloister had done well; but such a feature,
That might stand up the glory of a kingdom,
To live recluse is a mere solecism,
Though in a nunnery. It must not be.
I muse, my Lord your brother will permit it!
You should spend half my land first, were I he.
Does not this diamond better on my finger

[80]

Than i' the quarry?

DOL COMMON: Yes.

MAMMON: Why, you are like it
You were created, lady, for the light.
Here, you shall wear it; take it, the first pledge
Of what I speak, to bind you to believe me.

DOL COMMON: In chains of adamant?

MAMMON: Yes, the strongest bands.
And take a secret, too: here, by your side,
Doth stand this hour the happiest man in Europe.

DOL COMMON: You are contented, sir?

MAMMON: Nay, in true being,
The envy of princes and the fear of states.

DOL COMMON: Say you so, Sir Epicure?

MAMMON: Yes, and thou shalt
prove it.
Daughter of honour. I have cast mine eye
Upon thy form, and I will rear this beauty
Above all styles.

DOL COMMON: You mean no treason, sir?

MAMMON: No, I will take away that jealousy.
I am the lord of the Philosopher's Stone,
And thou the lady.

DOL COMMON: How, sir! ha' you that?

MAMMON: I am the master of the mastery.
This day the good old wretch here o' the house
Has made it for us. Now he's at projection.
Think therefore thy first wish now, let me hear it;
And it shall rain into thy lap, no shower,
But floods of gold, whole cataracts, a deluge,
To get a nation on thee.

DOL COMMON: You are pleased, sir,
To work on the ambition of our sex.

MAMMON: I'm pleased the glory of her sex should know
This nook here of the Friars is no climate
For her to live obscurely in, to learn
Physic and surgery, for the constable's wife
Of some odd hundred in Essex; but come forth,
And taste the air of palaces; eat, drink

[81]

The toils of emp'rics, and their boasted practice;
Tincture of pearl, and coral, gold, and amber;
Be seen at feasts and triumphs; have it asked,
What miracle she is; set all the eyes
Of court a-fire, like a burning-glass,
And work 'em into cinders, when the jewels
Of twenty states adorn thee, and the light
Strikes out the stars; that, when thy name is mentioned,
Queens may look pale; and, we but showing our love,
Nero's Poppæa may be lost in story!
Thus will we have it.
DOL COMMON: I could well consent, sir.
But in a monarchy, how will this be?
The Prince will soon take notice, and both seize
You and your Stone, it being a wealth unfit
For any private subject.
MAMMON: If he knew it.
DOL COMMON: Yourself do boast it, sir.
MAMMON: To thee, my life.
DOL COMMON: O, but beware, sir! You may come to end
The remnant of your days in a loathed prison,
By speaking of it.
MAMMON: 'Tis no idle fear!
We'll therefore go with all, my girl, and live
In a free state, where we will eat our mullets,
Soused in high-country wines, sup pheasants' eggs,
And have our cockles boiled in silver shells;
Our shrimps to swim again, as when they lived,
In a rare butter made of dolphins' milk,
Whose cream does look like opals; and with these
Delicate meats set ourselves high for pleasure,
And take us down again, and then renew
Our youth and strength with drinking the elixir,
And so enjoy a perpetuity
Of life and lust! And thou shalt ha' thy wardrobe
Richer than Nature's, still to change thyself,
And vary oft'ner for thy pride than she,
Or Art, her wise and almost-equal servant.
(*Enter* FACE.)

FACE: Sir, you are too loud. I hear you, every word,
    Into the laboratory. Some fitter place –
    The garden, or great chamber above. (*Aside*) How like you
        her?
MAMMON: Excellent, Lungs! There's for thee.
    (*Gives him money.*)
FACE: But do you hear?
    Good sir, beware, no mention of the rabbins.
MAMMON: We think not on 'em.
FACE: O, it is well sir.
    (*Exeunt* MAMMON *and* DOL.)

Barry Unsworth
1930–

from Mooncranker's Gift

Mrs Pritchett and Miranda have been on a morning expedition up the mountainside from the hot springs near Ephesus where they are staying. The young man James Farnaby is also visiting the same place.

'No, no, no,' exclaimed Mrs Pritchett in her well-bred, strangled contralto, holding up one hand in humorous protest; a capable hand, broad-palmed, fingers slightly spatulate; the knuckles somewhat scraped-looking after her fracas earlier that morning, though she had in the interim rubbed them with her special handcream. She always took care of her hands. Hands show our age like almost nothing else, she was fond of saying, hands and throat. In her other one now was a bottle of glinting liquid, amber in the light, ripe fig colour in the shelter of her creamed, creased palm.

'No, no,' she said, 'I insist.' Full of business on the threshold of Miranda's cabin, this kindly bustle disguising a certain languorous disturbance within, experienced since the brilliant idea had come to her, of not simply lending the bottle to Miranda as she had promised, but volunteering her own fingers to rub it well in with. 'You don't know, you don't know, how positively lethal this sun can be.' Inside the room now, like her own in every outward respect, yet what a change was effected by an alien hairbrush, for example. Odours of talcum powder and lemon balm. Miranda – backing somewhat awkwardly in the narrow confines of the cabin, obliged for the moment to play hostess. Mrs Pritchett took her in with a series of smiling glances: hair carelessly pinned up, exposing the soft, rather long neck; full underlip curving in a faint embarrassed smile; the belted waist of her cream and brown cotton dress.

'Take the word of an old campaigner,' Mrs Pritchett said

playfully, holding up in deprecation of any further protest the bottle of sun-tan oil ruddy and glinting in the light that shafted down on to it from the high square window. '*Ambre Solaire*,' she said, in an archly exaggerated accent. She controlled her breathing, concealed her interior disarray from her young friend, turning and closing the cabin door slowly and carefully. When she looked round again Miranda was standing against the bed, still awkwardly smiling.

'You shouldn't have bothered,' she said.

'No bother at all, my dear,' Mrs Pritchett said, with a sort of domineering jocularity, and she nodded her head at Miranda. 'This will do the trick.'

'Well, thank you very much. Are you in a hurry for it?'

'What *can* you mean?'

'Well, I thought, if you were, I could bring it back as soon as I've finished with it.'

'Oh, no, no, *no*,' Mrs Pritchett said firmly. 'You need someone to rub it well in. You can't reach your own back, now can you?' She paused for a moment. 'It is medicinal too,' she said, 'you see. It tones you up. But it must be rubbed in well, that is essential. It must get into the pores.'

Roguishly, finger and thumb poised delicately over the bottle, she paused, smiling at Miranda. Then with the same playful delicacy she nipped the white cone-shaped top and tried to turn it, but it wouldn't turn and it still wouldn't when she tried harder. Meanwhile, Miranda, realizing that Mrs Pritchett intended to do this service for her, wondered if her bra was very grubby and watched with some concern the other's increasingly violent efforts to remove the bottle top. Smile gone, a pallor of exertion at the temples, Mrs Pritchett was holding the bottle in a convulsive grip against her tummy, and twisting.

'The blasted top won't come off,' she muttered.

'Shall I have a try?' offered Miranda, but Mrs Pritchett yanked the blouse out of her skirt to help her get a grip and with a great effort managed to unscrew the top at last.

'*Finalmente*,' she said, panting. 'The threads had got crossed somehow.' She summoned a smile. 'These things are sent to try us,' she said. But to Miranda, this open-mouthed, audibly breathing woman, blouse hanging unheeded, savagely out of skirt band, was alarming, bringing back to her mind the whirlwind attacker on the hilltop, those breathless vituperations, that upturned bleeding face. She realized that she was afraid of Mrs Pritchett . . .

'Just unbutton your dress and slip it over your shoulders,' Mrs Pritchett said, advancing on Miranda, holding the bottle as if it were a syringe. 'I think that would be the best way. Oh, I see, there's a zip there, is there, well in that case dear I should just take it off altogether, yes, that's right. My goodness, just look at you, you would certainly have had blisters. You are like a lobster on your shoulders and back. Didn't you feel it at the time?'

'Not really.' Miranda was sitting on the bed in her bra and pants with her back to Mrs Pritchett. She shivered involuntarily at the first touch of the cool oil along her shoulders and Mrs Pritchett's velvety yet imperious fingertips stroking firmly from the tops of the shoulder-blades outwards.

'No, it's the water,' Mrs Pritchett said. 'You don't notice at the time how hot the sun is. Even as late in the year as this.' She raised the bottle, tilted it, and poured a drop or two of the thick fluid into the downy declivity between Miranda's shoulder-blades, imme- diately below the girl's nape. Both hands flat, fingers slightly splayed, she moved her palms with a firm pressure outwards over the squarish, unexpectedly compact and athletic shoulders – the girl was much more robust than she seemed when clothed; perhaps it was her posture that was deceptive, or the burdened- seeming neck – rested a moment there, then down, with oily adhesiveness, down the outsides of the forearms to the elbows.

'It has to be rubbed well in,' Mrs Pritchett said, rather thickly.

Miranda felt a warm tingling sensation across her back where Mrs Pritchett's fingers were plying. It was a healing-burning sort of feeling, by no means unpleasant. However, sitting there so awkwardly, her back chastely towards the other lady, her legs over the side of the bed, hands in her lap, she had only her own vertical posture to resist the pressure of Mrs Pritchett's palms, nothing at all to hold on to. Consequently, after the first few passes, she was hard put to it to maintain herself upright. This was partly because, as it seemed to her, Mrs Pritchett was increasing the pressure from moment to moment. Miranda sensed an urgency in those hands and set it down to Mrs Pritchett's healing fervour, though with less than complete conviction. In any case, whatever it was, it was now pushing her forward each time, driving her to perform an apparent obeisance towards the window, the source of light. Up she felt the slippery soft hands go, slowly outwards to the shoulder, nudging her forward to her periodic reverence, slipping down the arms, bringing her upright again.

'It would be better, dear, if you lay down, I think. On your tummy.'

'But haven't you finished yet?' Miranda said, in a sort of rebellion, half turning towards her solicitous masseuse. She was flushed and her voice sounded sleepy or dazed, as if she were divided by veils from full consciousness.

'Finished? Oh dear, no.' There was the slightest of snaps in Mrs Pritchett's voice, denoting hurt perhaps at this attempt to curtail her ministrations. 'It has to penetrate to the subcutaneous fat,' she explained, after a moment. She patted the bed. 'Just you lie here and relax,' she said. 'Leave the rest to me.'

Miranda, divided between reluctance and compliance, looked for some seconds at Mrs Pritchett's face. It was deeply flushed, brilliant-eyed, slightly smiling. 'Come on now,' Mrs Pritchett said, holding up hands shiny with oil. 'We mustn't keep nurse waiting, must we?'

She had adopted by some instinct of insight exactly the right tone for lulling Miranda, breaking down the girl's residual resistance; playful, basically threatening, transporting her to school sickrooms, not so very far behind, when illness was regarded as weakness in the moral fibre somehow, perhaps even something to be ashamed of, and the way to reinstatement was unswerving, uncomplaining cooperation in all the details of treatment . . . Obediently, and without another word, Miranda stretched herself downward on the bed. She felt after a moment Mrs Pritchett's hands stroking the thin tissue that sheathed her shoulder-blades. A strange smell had begun to expand in the cabin, like the exudation of some mammalian gland, attractive or rebuttive: the odour of the sun-tan oil. Miranda heard the other's voice above her talking in richly elegiac tones about Mark, her former fiancé and how she had walked away from Mark along the darkening river bank, past scented fields where cattle grazed . . .

[87]

Without pausing in her massage or her speech, Mrs Pritchett looked down at the girl's body. She could now with impunity dwell on the rounded, polished shoulders, the blunt sprouting of shoulder-blades, sheathed buttons of the spine. The skin was not really red as she had told Miranda except just along the shoulders, but reddish gold, like dark wheat – the girl had a depth, almost a duskiness in the skin which would always prevent that lobster redness. She was not yet completely relaxed, Mrs Pritchett noted: the arms were tensed, still held close to her sides and there was a slight, periodic clenching of the buttocks beneath the thin white cotton knickers. She continued her massaging movement, catching each time the thin fold of flesh which rippled into her hand, escaped again at the shoulder. And while she worked, with an obscure, slowly mounting excitement, on Miranda's flesh, feeling the girl's body more relaxed every moment, she continued the saga of Mark.

To Miranda the voice of Mrs Pritchett and the gentle yet remorseless pressure of her hands were becoming meshed, like a soft harness or a net. She was entering the territory that lies between sleep and waking, though sleep seemed dangerous at first, like a sudden descent into a dark place, or like some sort of submergence, and she resisted it, though sinking further and further into sleep and a sort of warmly sensuous desolation. She did not drown, the voice and the hands kept her from drowning, she was moving still, not gliding now, but flowing along a dark river, the voice leading her, the hands conducting, the river was bearing her. There were black cows on the banks, completely black, and she heard the breaths of the cows, the splashing of their feet in the black water, soft tearing of grass as they grazed along the banks . . . .

'Your bra is rather in the way, dear,' Mrs Pritchett said, and with oily fingers undid the two little hooks from their eyes. Then she dexterously slipped the shoulder straps down to the girl's elbows. She now had the whole of Miranda's naked back to work on, divided into two zones of darker and paler gold by the thin white line where the bra strap had been, the whole expanse gleaming and lustrous with oil. She could follow with her hands the long curve inward of the torso to the waist, and even below this to the compensatory initial convexities of the nates, before the thin

[88]

band of the knickers stayed her. Miranda, in relaxing her arms, had moved them out some few inches from her sides, enabling Mrs Pritchett to see the launching outer curves of each breast. She ventured her hands along the exposed flanks, beginning at the armpit, rubbing lightly with the tips of her fingers along the outer curve of the breasts. This, since there was no flinching, no abatement of the girl's deep, slumbrous inertia, she incorporated into the massaging movement, which was now a great cunning sweep, beginning at the hollowed base of the spine, proceeding outwards to the shoulders, returning via the flanks to the tops of the knickers in which each time her fingers caught and tugged a little.

Thus circumspectly she extended her range. And when she realized, from the girl's heaviness under her hands, and from the complete relaxation, indeed abandonment, of her body – that virginal clench of the bottom quite gone – that she was tranced, resistless, Mrs Pritchett pressed her own hot thighs together and, while not pausing even for a moment in the massaging and caressing of Miranda, encouraged her own increasingly lively feelings by setting up a frictive movement there.

'We must get into the subcutaneous fat, we absolutely must,' gabbled Mrs Pritchett, forgetting Mark as she experienced the approach of sensations never connected with him, but knowing by a sort of instinct that she must at all costs go on talking to Miranda so as not to break the spell. 'That is the secret of it.' She raced on, dry-mouthed, rubbing her robust thighs together. 'Oh!' she cried, with a preliminary pang of pleasure. 'Oh, dear, yes, we absolutely must get below the surface, that is where the healing soothing balm is fully and to best advantage – ah!' A further slight ejaculation, a sort of buzzing sound escaped her. She edged the elastic band of the knickers down slightly, revealing the initial cleft of the buttocks. More than this was not possible for the moment because of the weight of the girl's body. Nevertheless she persevered, with each sweeping massage plucking a little at the band.

Miranda lay face down in fathomless indolence, her body tingling, yet heavy and inert, drugged by the monologue and by the repeated massaging movement, words and hands holding her as in a net, drawing her netted through dark water very slowly, more slowly than the flow of water; banks and fields were moving slowly too, nothing was still but the fisherman, Mark, standing there in midstream, black, immovable. Not swimming, not floating, but *towed*, she moved towards him, outdistanced continuously by the water but drawing nearer, and passing saw it was James Farnaby; the river changed, silvered over, there was a wreckage of birds' nests on the bank and she felt a sleepy tenderness for the boy's serious face, left behind now; the silver water flowed past and around her, endlessly inventive and circumventive, waylaid at the edges, trapped in eddies and swirls and pointless scummy sidings but never ultimately blocked in its career to the sea, minutely to sweeten that salt immensity. The hands massaging her duplicated that ceaseless current, caught however, briefly cluttered, like water in a blocked channel over and over again, in the elastic of her knickers, tugging down slightly, freeing themselves, caught again, a reiterated intolerable blockage. Breathing deeply, a slight impatience troubling her as at some temporary obstacle in a dream, Miranda arched her rump clear of the bed, remaining thus, under the dream-like duress, long enough for Mrs Pritchett to reach round and pull the knickers down at the front, down to the girl's knees.

Sighing, Miranda settled down again, feeling the long flow of the hands from her nape to the backs of her legs without let or hindrance. She heard a brief buzzing sound above her. At that moment there was a brisk knock on the cabin door and a man's voice shouted, 'Anyone at home?' Miranda recognized it at once for Farnaby's, and it brought her full awake. She sat up quickly, reaching for her wrap, which lay across the foot of the bed.

'Don't answer,' said Mrs Pritchett, but Miranda answered almost immediately, in a voice full of gaiety and alertness. 'Yes, is it you, James? I shan't be a minute.' She went towards the door.

Mrs Pritchett sat helpless, a prey to violent emotion, and saw the door being opened. Then she rose. She heard Miranda utter some bright form of greeting, heard the pleasure in the girl's voice, saw with hatred a tall gangling male form, its arms occupied with foodstuffs. 'I thought we might have a picnic,' she heard this creature say and saw the look of delight on the equine face as he looked down at Miranda in her pretty flowered wrap. She saw Miranda hesitating, out of politeness to her presumably, she obviously wanted to go – this was the fellow, almost certainly, who had been occupying her thoughts all morning. Mrs Pritchett moved towards the door. 'I'll leave the oil with you,' she said.

John Milton
1608–74

from Paradise Lost, Book ix

Satan tempts Eve

For now, and since first break of dawne the Fiend,
Meer Serpent in appearance, forth was come,
And on his Quest, where likeliest he might finde
The onely two of Mankinde; but in them
The whole included Race, his purposd prey.
In Bowre and Field he sought, where any tuft
Of Grove or Garden-Plot more pleasant lay,
Thir tendance or Plantation for delight,
By Fountain or by shadie Rivulet
He sought them both, but wish'd his hap might find
Eve separate, he wish'd, but not with hope
Of what so seldom chanc'd, when to his wish,
Beyond his hope, *Eve* separate he spies,
Veild in a Cloud of Fragrance, where she stood,
Half spi'd, so thick the Roses bushing round
About her glowd, oft stooping to support
Each Flour of slender stalk, whose head though gay
Carnation, Purple, Azure, or spect with Gold,
Hung drooping unsustaind, them she upstaies
Gently with Mirtle band, mindless the while,
Her self, though fairest unsupported Flour,
From her best prop so farr, and storm so nigh.
Neerer he drew, and many a walk travers'd
Of stateliest Covert, Cedar, Pine, or Palme,
Then voluble and bold, now hid, now seen
Among thick-wov'n Arborets and Flours
Imborderd on each Bank, the hand of *Eve*:
Spot more delicious then those Gardens feign'd

Or of reviv'd *Adonis*, or renownd
Alcinous, host of old *Laertes* Son,
Or that, not Mystic, where the Sapient King
Held dalliance with his faire *Egyptian* Spouse.
Much hee the Place admir'd, the Person more.
As one who long in populous City pent,
Where Houses thick and Sewers annoy the Aire,
Forth issuing on a Summers Morn to breathe
Among the pleasant Villages and Farmes
Adjoynd, from each thing met conceaves delight,
The smell of Grain, or tedded Grass, or Kine,
Or Dairie, each rural sight, each rural sound;
If chance with Nymphlike step fair Virgin pass,
What pleasing seemd, for her now pleases more,
She most, and in her look summs all Delight.
Such Pleasure took the Serpent to behold
This Flourie Plat, the sweet recess of *Eve*
Thus earlie, thus alone; her Heav'nly forme
Angelic, but more soft, and Feminine,
Her graceful Innocence, her every Aire
Of gesture or lest action overawd
His Malice, and with rapine sweet bereav'd
His fierceness of the fierce intent it brought:
That space the Evil one abstracted stood
From his own evil, and for the time remaind
Stupidly good, of enmitie disarm'd,
Of guile, of hate, of envie, of revenge;
But the hot Hell that alwayes in him burnes,
Though in mid Heav'n, soon ended his delight,
And tortures him now more, the more he sees
Of pleasure not for him ordain'd: then soon
Fierce hate he recollects, and all his thoughts
Of mischief, gratulating, thus excites.
    Thoughts, whither have ye led me, with what sweet
Compulsion thus transported to forget
What hither brought us, hate, not love, nor hope
Of Paradise for Hell, hope here to taste
Of pleasure, but all pleasure to destroy,
Save what is in destroying, other joy

To me is lost. Then let me not let pass
Occasion which now smiles, behold alone
The Woman, opportune to all attempts,
Her Husband, for I view far round, not nigh,
Whose higher intellectual more I shun,
And strength, of courage hautie, and of limb
Heroic built, though of terrestrial mould,
Foe not informidable, exempt from wound,
I not; so much hath Hell debas'd, and paine
Infeebl'd me, to what I was in Heav'n.
Shee fair, divinely fair, fit Love for Gods,
Not terrible, though terrour be in Love
And beautie, not approacht by stronger hate,
Hate stronger, under shrew of Love well feign'd,
The way which to her ruin now I tend.
    So spake the Enemie of Mankind, enclos'd
In Serpent, Inmate bad, and toward *Eve*
Address'd his way, not with indented wave,
Prone on the ground, as since, but on his reare,
Circular base of rising foulds, that tour'd
Fould above fould a surging Maze, his Head
Crested aloft, and Carbuncle his Eyes;
With burnisht Neck of verdant Gold, erect
Amidst his circling Spires, that on the grass
Floted redundant: pleasing was his shape,
And lovely, never since of Serpent kind
Lovelier, not those that in *Illyria* chang'd
Hermione and *Cadmus*, or the God
In *Epidaurus*; nor to which transformd
Ammonian Jove, or *Capitoline* was seen,
Hee with *Olympias*, this with her who bore
Scipio the highth of *Rome*. With tract oblique
At first, as one who sought access, but feard
To interrupt, side-long he works his way.
As when a Ship by skilful Stearsman wrought
Nigh Rivers mouth or Foreland, where the Wind
Veres oft, as oft so steers, and shifts her Saile;
So varied hee, and of his tortuous Traine
Curld many a wanton wreath in sight of *Eve*,

To lure her Eye; shee busied heard the sound
Of rusling Leaves, but minded not, as us'd
To such disport before her through the Field,
From every Beast, more duteous at her call,
Then at *Circean* call the Herd disguis'd.
Hee boulder now, uncall'd before her stood;
But as in gaze admiring: Oft he bowd
His turret Crest, and sleek enamel'd Neck,
Fawning, and lick'd the ground whereon she trod.
His gentle dumb expression turnd at length
The Eye of *Eve* to mark his play; he glad
Of her attention gaind, with Serpent Tongue
Organic, or impulse of vocal Air,
His fraudulent temptation thus began.
   Wonder not, sovran Mistress, if perhaps
Thou canst, who art sole Wonder, much less arm
Thy looks, the Heav'n of mildness, with disdain,
Displeas'd that I approach thee thus, and gaze
Insatiate, I thus single, nor have feard
Thy awful brow, more awful thus retir'd.
Fairest resemblance of thy Maker faire,
Thee all things living gaze on, all things thine
By gift, and thy Celestial Beautie adore
With ravishment beheld, there best beheld
Where universally admir'd; but here
In this enclosure wild, these Beasts among,
Beholders rude, and shallow to discerne
Half what in thee is fair, one man except,
Who sees thee? (and what is one?) who shouldst be seen
A Goddess among Gods, ador'd and serv'd
By Angels numberless, thy daily Train.
   So gloz'd the Tempter, and his Proem tun'd;
Into the Heart of *Eve* his words made way,
Though at the voice much marveling; at length
Not unamaz'd she thus in answer spake.
What may this mean? Language of Man pronounc't
By Tongue of Brute, and human sense exprest?
The first at lest of these I thought deni'd
To Beasts, whom God on thir Creation-Day

Created mute to all articulat sound;
The latter I demurre, for in thir looks
Much reason, and in thir actions oft appeers.
Thee, Serpent, suttlest beast of all the field
I knew, but not with human voice endu'd;
Redouble then this miracle, and say,
How cam'st thou speakable of mute, and how
To me so friendly grown above the rest
Of brutal kind, that daily are in sight?
Say, for such wonder claims attention due.
    To whom the guileful Tempter thus reply'd.
Empress of this fair World, resplendent *Eve*,
Easie to mee it is to tell thee all
What thou commandst, and right thou shouldst be obeyd:
I was at first as other Beasts that graze
The trodden Herb, of abject thoughts and low,
As was my food, nor aught but food discern'd
Or Sex, and apprehended nothing high:
Till on a day roaving the field, I chanc'd
A goodly Tree farr distant to behold
Loaden with fruit of fairest colours mixt,
Ruddie and Gold: I nearer drew to gaze;
When from the boughes a savorie odour blow'n,
Grateful to appetite, more pleas'd my sense
Then smell of sweetest Fenel or the Teats
Of Ewe or Goat dropping with Milk at Eevn,
Unsuckt of Lamb or Kid, that tend thir play.
To satisfie the sharp desire I had
Of tasting those fair Apples, I resolv'd
Not to deferr; hunger and thirst at once,
Powerful perswaders, quick'nd at the scent
Of that alluring fruit, urg'd me so keene.
About the mossie Trunk I wound me soon,
For high from ground the branches would require
Thy utmost reach or *Adams*: Round the Tree
All other Beasts that saw, with like desire
Longing and envying stood, but could not reach.
Amid the Tree now got, where plenty hung
Tempting so nigh, to pluck and eat my fill

I spar'd not, for such pleasure till that hour
At Feed or Fountain never had I found.
Sated at length, ere long I might perceave
Strange alteration in me, to degree
Of Reason in my inward Powers, and Speech
Wanted not long, though to this shape retain'd.
Thenceforth to Speculations high or deep
I turnd my thoughts, and with capacious mind
Considerd all things visible in Heav'n,
Or Earth, or Middle, all things fair and good;
But all that fair and good in thy Divine
Semblance, and in thy Beauties heav'nly Ray
United I beheld; no Fair to thine
Equivalent or second, which compel'd
Mee thus, though importune perhaps, to come
And gaze, and worship thee of right declar'd
Sovran of Creatures, universal Dame.
So talk'd the spirited sly Snake; and *Eve*
Yet more amaz'd unwarie thus reply'd.

Serpent, thy overpraising leaves in doubt
The vertue of that Fruit, in thee first prov'd:
But say, where grows the Tree, from hence how far?
For many are the Trees of God that grow
In Paradise, and various, yet unknown
To us, in such aboundance lies our choice,
As leaves a greater store of Fruit untoucht,
Still hanging incorruptible, till men
Grow up to thir provision, and more hands
Help to disburden Nature of her Bearth.

To whom the wilie Adder, blithe and glad.
Empress, the way is readie, and not long,
Beyond a row of Myrtles, on a Flat,
Fast by a Fountain, one small Thicket past
Of blowing Myrrh and Balme; if thou accept
My conduct, I can bring thee thither soon.

Lead then, said *Eve.* Hee leading swiftly rowld
In tangles, and made intricate seem strait,
To mischief swift. Hope elevates, and joy
Bright'ns his Crest, as when a wandring Fire,

Compact of unctuous vapor, which the Night
Condenses, and the cold invirons round,
Kindl'd through agitation to a Flame,
Which oft, they say, some evil Spirit attends
Hovering and blazing with delusive Light,
Misleads th' amaz'd Night-wanderer from his way
To Boggs and Mires, and oft through Pond or Poole,
There swallow'd up and lost, from succour farr.
So glister'd the dire Snake, and into fraud
Led *Eve* our credulous Mother, to the Tree
Of prohibition, root of all our woe;
Which when she saw, thus to her guide she spake.

   Serpent, we might have spar'd our coming hither,
Fruitless to mee, though Fruit be here to excess,
The credit of whose vertue rest with thee,
Wondrous indeed, if cause of such effects.
But of this Tree we may not taste nor touch;
God so commanded, and left that Command
Sole Daughter of his voice; the rest, we live
Law to our selves, our Reason is our Law.

   To whom the Tempter guilefully repli'd.
Indeed? hath God then said that of the Fruit
Of all these Garden Trees ye shall not eate,
Yet Lords declar'd of all in Earth or Aire?

   To whom thus *Eve* yet sinless. Of the Fruit
Of each Tree in the Garden we may eate,
But of the Fruit of this fair Tree amidst
The Garden, God hath said, Ye shall not eate
Thereof, nor shall ye touch it, least ye die.

   She scarse had said, though brief, when now more bold
The Tempter, but with shew of Zeale and Love
To Man, and indignation at his wrong,
New part puts on, and as to passion mov'd,
Fluctuats disturbd, yet comely and in act
Rais'd, as of som great matter to begin.
As when of old som Orator renound
In *Athens* or free *Rome*, where Eloquence
Flourishd, since mute, to som great cause addrest,
Stood in himself collected, while each part,

Motion, each act won audience ere the tongue,
Somtimes in highth began, as no delay
Of Preface brooking through his Zeal of Right.
So standing, moving, or to highth upgrown
The Tempter all impassiond thus began.

   O Sacred, Wise, and Wisdom-giving Plant,
Mother of Science, Now I feel thy Power
Within me cleere, not onely to discerne
Things in thir Causes, but to trace the wayes
Of highest Agents, deemd however wise.
Queen of this Universe, doe not believe
Those rigid threats of Death; ye shall not Die:
How should ye? by the Fruit? it gives you Life
To Knowledge? By the Threatner, look on mee,
Mee who have touch'd and tasted, yet both live,
And life more perfet have attaind then Fate
Meant mee, by ventring higher then my Lot.
Shall that be shut to Man, which to the Beast
Is open? or will God incense his ire
For such a petty Trespass, and not praise
Rather your dauntless vertue, whom the pain
Of Death denounc't, whatever thing Death be,
Deterrd not from atchieving what might leade
To happier life, knowledge of Good and Evil;
Of good, how just? of evil, if what is evil
Be real, why not known, since easier shunnd?
God therefore cannot hurt ye, and be just;
Not just, not God; not feard then, nor obeyd:
Your feare it self of Death removes the feare.
Why then was this forbid? Why but to awe,
Why but to keep ye low and ignorant,
His worshippers; he knows that in the day
Ye Eate thereof, your Eyes that seem so cleere,
Yet are but dim, shall perfetly be then
Op'nd and cleerd, and ye shall be as Gods,
Knowing both Good and Evil as they know.
That ye should be as Gods, since I as Man,
Internal Man, is but proportion meet,
I of brute human, yee of human Gods.

So ye shall die perhaps, by putting off
Human, to put on Gods, death to be wisht,
Though threat'nd, which no worse then this can bring.
And what are Gods that Man may not become
As they, participating God-like food?
The Gods are first, and that advantage use
On our belief, that all from them proceeds;
I question it, for this fair Earth I see,
Warm'd by the Sun, producing every kind,
Them nothing: If they all things, who enclos'd
Knowledge of Good and Evil in this Tree,
That whoso eats thereof, forthwith attains
Wisdom without their leave? and wherein lies
Th' offence, that Man should thus attain to know?
What can your knowledge hurt him, or this Tree
Impart against his will if all be his?
Or is it envie, and can envie dwell
In heav'nly breasts? these, these and many more
Causes import your need of this fair Fruit.
Goddess humane, reach then, and freely taste.

     He ended, and his words replete with guile
Into her heart too easie entrance won:
Fixt on the Fruit she gaz'd, which to behold
Might tempt alone, and in her ears the sound
Yet rung of his perswasive words, impregn'd
With Reason, to her seeming, and with Truth;
Mean while the hour of Noon drew on, and wak'd
An eager appetite, rais'd by the smell
So savorie of that Fruit, which with desire,
Inclinable now grown to touch or taste,
Sollicited her longing eye; yet first
Pausing a while, thus to her self she mus'd.

     Great are thy Vertues, doubtless, best of Fruits,
Though kept from Man, and worthy to be admir'd,
Whose taste, too long forborn, at first assay
Gave elocution to the mute, and taught
The Tongue not made for Speech to speak thy praise:
Thy praise hee also who forbids thy use,

Conceales not from us, naming thee the Tree
Of Knowledge, knowledge both of good and evil;
Forbids us then to taste, but his forbidding
Commends thee more, while it inferrs the good
By thee communicated, and our want:
For good unknown, sure is not had, or had
And yet unknown, is as not had at all.
In plain then, what forbids he but to know,
Forbids us good, forbids us to be wise?
Such prohibitions binde not. But if Death
Bind us with after-bands, what profits then
Our inward freedom? In the day we eate
Of this fair Fruit, our doom is, we shall die.
How dies the Serpent? hee hath eat'n and lives,
And knows, and speaks, and reasons, and discerns,
Irrational till then. For us alone
Was death invented? or to us deni'd
This intellectual food, for beasts reserv'd?
For Beasts it seems: yet that one Beast which first
Hath tasted, envies not, but brings with joy
The good befall'n him, Author unsuspect,
Friendly to man, farr from deceit or guile.
What fear I then, rather what know to feare
Under this ignorance of good and Evil,
Of God or Death, of Law or Penaltie?
Here grows the Cure of all, this Fruit Divine,
Fair to the Eye, inviting to the Taste,
Of vertue to make wise: what hinders then
To reach, and feed at once both Bodie and Mind?
    So saying, her rash hand in evil hour
Forth reaching to the Fruit, she pluck'd, she eat:
Earth felt the wound, and Nature from her seat
Sighing through all her Works gave signs of woe,
That all was lost. Back to the Thicket slunk
The guiltie Serpent, and well might, for *Eve*
Intent now wholly on her taste, naught else
Regarded, such delight till then, as seemd,
In Fruit she never tasted, whether true

Or fansied so, through expectation high
Of knowledge, nor was God-head from her thought.
Greedily she ingorg'd without restraint,
And knew not eating Death.

Wyndham Lewis
1884–1957

from Cantleman's Spring-Mate

Cantleman walked in the strenuous fields, steam rising from them as though from an exertion, dissecting the daisies specked in the small wood, the primroses on the banks, the marshy lakes, and all God's creatures. The heat of a heavy premature Summer was cooking a little narrow belt of earth-air, causing everything innocently to burst its skins, bask abjectly and profoundly. Everything was enchanted with itself, and with everything else. The horse considered the mares immensely appetizing masses of quivering shiny flesh; was there not something of 'je ne sais quoi' about a mare, that no other beast's better half possessed? The birds with their little gnarled feet, and beaks made for fishing worms out of the mould, or the river, would have considered Shelley's references to the skylark – or any other poet's paeans to their species – as lamentably inadequate to describe the beauty of birds! The female bird, for her particular part, reflected that, in spite of the ineptitude of her sweetheart's latest song, which he insisted on deafening her with, never seemed to tire of, and was so persuaded that she liked as much as he did himself, and although outwardly she remained critical and vicious: that all the same and nevertheless, chock, chock, peep, peep, he was a fluffy object from which certain satisfaction could be derived! And both the male and the female reflected together as they stood a foot or so apart looking at each other with one eye, and at the landscape with the other, that of all nourishment the red earth-worm was the juiciest and sweetest! The sow, as she watched her hog, with his splenetic energy, and guttural articulation, a sound between content and complaint, not noticing the untidy habits of both of them, gave a sharp grunt of sex-hunger, and jerked rapidly towards Him. The only jarring note in this vast mutual admiration society was the fact that many of its members showed their fondness for their neighbour in an embarrassing way: that is they killed and ate them. But the weaker were so used to dying violent deaths and being eaten that they worried very little about it. – The West was gushing up a harmless volcano of fire, obviously intended as an immense dreamy nightcap.

Cantleman in the midst of his cogitation on surrounding life, surprised his faithless and unfriendly brain in the act of turning over an object which humiliated his meditation. He found that he was wondering whether at his return through the village lying between him and the Camp, he would see the girl he had passed there three hours before. At that time he had not begun his philosophizing, and without interference from conscience, he had noticed the redness of her cheeks, the animal fulness of the child-bearing hips, with an eye as innocent as the bird or the beast. He laughed without shame or pleasure, lit his pipe and turned back towards the village. – His fieldboots were covered with dust: his head was wet with perspiration and he carried his cap, in an unmilitary fashion, in his hand. In a week he was leaving for the Front, for the first time. So his thoughts and sensations all had, as a philosophic background, the prospect of death. The infantry, and his commission, implied death or mutilation unless he were very lucky. He had not a high opinion of his luck. He was pretty miserable at the thought, in a deliberate, unemotional way. But as he realized this he again laughed, a similar sound to that that the girl had caused. – For what was he unhappy about? He wanted to remain amongst his fellow insects and beasts, which were so beautiful, did he then: Well well! On the other hand, who was it that told him to do anything else? After all, supposing the values they attached to each other of 'beautiful,' 'interesting,' 'divine,' were unjustified in many cases on cooler observation; – nevertheless birds were more beautiful than pigs: and if pigs were absurd and ugly, rather than handsome, and possibly chivalrous, as they imagine themselves; then equally the odour of the violet was pleasant, and there was nothing offensive about most trees. The newspapers were the things that stank most on earth, and human beings anywhere were the most ugly and offensive of the brutes because of the confusion caused by their consciousness. Had it not been for that unmaterial gift that some bungling or wild hand had bestowed, our sisters and brothers would be no worse than dogs and sheep. That they could not reconcile their little meagre streams of sublimity with the needs of animal life should not be railed at. Well then, should not the sad amalgam, all it did, all it willed, all it demanded, be thrown over, for the fake and confusion that it was, and should not such as possessed a greater quantity of that wine of reason, retire, metaphorically, to the wilderness, and sit forever in a formal and gentle elation, refusing to be disturbed? – Should such allow himself to be disturbed by the quarrels of Jews, the desperate perplexities, resulting in desperate dice throws, of politicians, the crack-jaw and unreasoning tumult?

On the other hand, Cantleman had a more human, as well as a little more divine understanding, than those usually on his left and right, and he had had, not so long ago, conspicuous hopes that such a conjecture might produce a new human chemistry. But he must repudiate the human entirely, if that there were to be brought off. His present occupation, the trampling boots upon his feet, the belt that crossed his back and breast was his sacrifice, his compliment to the animal.

He then began dissecting his laugh, comparing it to the pig's grunt and the bird's cough. He laughed again several times in order to listen to it.

At the village he met the girl, this time with a second girl. He stared at her 'in such a funny way' that she laughed. He once more laughed the same sound as before, and bid her good evening. She immediately became civil. Inquiries about the village, and the best way back to the camp across the marsh, put in as nimble and at the same time rustic a form as he could contrive, lay the first tentative brick of what might become the dwelling of a friend, a sweetheart, a ghost, anything in the absurd world! He asked her to come and show him a short cut she had indicated.

'I couldn't. My mother's waiting for *me!*' In a rush of expostulation and semi-affected alarm. However, she concluded in a minute or two, that she could . . .

The young woman had, or had given herself, the unlikely name of Stella. In the narrow road where they got away from the village, Cantleman put his arm round Stella's waist and immediately experienced all the sensations that he had been divining in the creatures around him: the horse, the bird, the pig. The way in which Stella's hips stood out, the solid blood-heated expanse on which his hand lay, had the amplitude and flatness of a mare. Her lips had at once no practical significance, but only the aesthetic blandishments of a bull-like flower. With the gesture of a fabulous Faust he drew her against him, and kissed her with a crafty gentleness.

Cantleman turned up that evening in his quarters in a state of baffling good-humour. He took up *The Trumpet-Major* and was soon surrounded by the breathing and scratching of his room-mates, reading and writing. He chuckled somewhere where Hardy was funny. At this human noise the others fixed their eyes on him in sour alarm. He gave another, this time gratuitous, chuckle. They returned with disgust at his habits, his peculiarity, to what he considered their maid-servant's fiction and correspondence. Oh Christ, what abysms! Oh Christ, what abysms! Cantleman shook noisily in the wicker chair like a dog or a fly-blown old gentleman.

Once more on the following evening he was out in the fields, and once more his thoughts were engaged in recapitulations. – The miraculous camouflage of Nature did not deceive this observer. He saw everywhere the gun-pits and the 'nests of death.' Each puff of green leaves he knew was in some way as harmful as the burst of a shell. Decay and ruins, it is true, were soon covered up, but there was yet that parallel, and the sight of things smashed and corrupted. In the factory town ten miles away to the right, whose smoke could be seen, life was just as dangerous for the poor, and as uncomfortable, as for the soldier in his trench. The hypocrisy of Nature and the hypocrisy of War were the same. The only safety in life was for the man with the soft job. But that fellow was not conforming to life's conditions. He was life's paid man, and had the mark of the sneak. He was making too much of life, and too much out of it. He, Cantleman, did not want to owe anything to life, or enter into league or understanding with her. The thing was either to go out of existence: or, failing that, remain in it unreconciled, indifferent to Nature's threat, consorting openly with her enemies, making war within her war upon her servants. In short, the spectacle of the handsome English spring produced nothing but ideas of defiance in Cantleman's mind.

As to Stella, she was a sort of Whizzbang. With a treachery worthy of a Hun, Nature tempted him towards her. He was drugged with delicious appetites. Very well! He would hoist the Unseen Powers with his own petard. He could throw back Stella where she was discharged from (if it were allowable, now, to change her into a bomb) first having relieved himself of his humiliating gnawing and yearning in his blood.

As to Stella, considered as an unconscious agent, all women were contaminated with Nature's hostile power and might be treated as spies or enemies. The only time they could be trusted, or were likely to stand up to Nature and show their teeth, was as mothers. So he approached Stella with as much falsity as he could master.

At their third meeting he brought her a ring. Her melting gratitude was immediately ligotted with long arms, full of the contradictory and offending fire of Spring. On the warm earth consent flowed up into her body from all the veins of the landscape.

That night he spat out, in gushes of thick delicious rage, all the lust that had gathered in his body. The nightingale sang ceaselessly in the small wood at the top of the field where they lay. He grinned up towards it as he noticed it, and once more turned to the devouring of his mate. He bore down on her as though he wished to mix her body into the soil, and pour his seed into a more methodless matter, the brown phalanges of floury land. As their two bodies shook and melted together, he felt that he was raiding the bowels of Nature: he was proud that he could remain deliberately aloof, and gaze bravely, like a minute insect, up at the immense and melancholy night, with all its mad nightingales, piously folded small brown wings in a million nests, night-working stars, and misty useless watchmen. – They got up at last, she went furtively back to her home: Cantleman on his walk to camp, had a smile of severe satisfaction on his face. It did not occur to him that his action might be supremely unimportant as far as Stella was concerned. He had not even asked himself if, had he not been there that night, someone else might have been there in his place. He was also convinced that the laurels were his, and that Nature had come off badly. – He was still convinced of this when he received six weeks afterwards in France, a long appeal from Stella, telling him that she was going to have a child. She received no answer to that or any subsequent letter. Cantleman received [them] with

[107]

great regularity in the trenches, and read them all through from beginning to end, without comment of any sort. – And when he beat a German's brains out it was with the same impartial malignity that he had displayed in the English night with his Spring-mate. Only he considered there too that he was in some way outwitting Nature, and had no adequate realization of the extent to which evidently the death of a Hun was to the advantage of the world.

Thomas Middleton
1570?–1627

from Women Beware Women

Livia, a wealthy lady of Florence, has invited the recently-married newcomer, Bianca, to her home in the company of Bianca's mother-in-law. Guardiano, who is in collusion with Livia to corrupt Bianca, leads the young woman upstairs where the Duke of Florence awaits her. Livia distracts the mother-in-law with a game of chess where the moves mirror the seduction that is taking place upstairs.

LIV: Alas, poor widow, I shall be too hard for thee!
MOTH: You're cunning at the game, I'll be sworn, madam.
LIV: (*Aside*) It will be found so, ere I give you over. –
    She that can place her man well –
MOTH: As you do, madam.
LIV: As I shall, wench, can never lose her game:
    Nay, nay, the black king's mine.
MOTH: Cry you mercy, madam!
LIV: And this my queen.
MOTH: I see't now.
LIV: Here's a duke
    Will strike a sure stroke for the game anon;
    Your pawn cannot come back to relieve itself.
MOTH: I know that, madam.
LIV: You play well the whilst:
    How she belies her skill! I hold two ducats,
    I give you check and mate to your white king,
    Simplicity itself, your saintish king there.
MOTH: Well, ere now, lady,
    I've seen the fall of subtlety; jest on.
LIV: Ay, but simplicity receives two for one.
MOTH: What remedy but patience!
    (*Enter* GUARDIANO *and* BIANCA *above.*)

[109]

BIAN: Trust me, sir,
    Mine eye ne'er met with fairer ornaments.
GUAR: Nay, livelier, I'm persuaded, neither Florence
    Nor Venice can produce.
BIAN: Sir, my opinion
    Takes your part highly.
GUAR: There's a better piece
    Yet than all these.
BIAN: Not possible, sir!
GUAR: Believe it,
    You'll say so when you see't: turn but your eye now,
    You're upon't presently.
    (*Draws a curtain, and discovers the* DUKE; *then exit.*)
BIAN: O sir!
DUKE: He's gone, beauty:
    Pish, look not after him; he's but a vapour,
    That, when the sun appears, is seen no more.
BIAN: O, treachery to honour!
DUKE: Prithee, tremble not;
    I feel thy breast shake like a turtle panting
    Under a loving hand that makes much on't:
    Why art so fearful? as I'm friend to brightness,
    There's nothing but respect and honour near thee:
    You know me, you have seen me; here's a heart
    Can witness I have seen thee.
BIAN: The more's my danger.
DUKE: The more's thy happiness. Pish, strive not, sweet;
    This strength were excellent employ'd in love now,
    But here – 'tis spent amiss: strive not to seek
    Thy liberty, and keep me still in prison;
    I'faith, you shall not out till I'm releas'd now;
    We'll be both freed together, or stay still by't,
    So is captivity pleasant.
BIAN: O my lord!
DUKE: I am not here in vain; have but the leisure
    To think on that, and thou'lt be soon resolv'd:
    The lifting of thy voice is but like one
    That does exalt his enemy, who, proving high,
    Lays all the plots to confound him that rais'd him.

Take warning, I beseech thee; thou seem'st to me
A creature so compos'd of gentleness,
And delicate meekness – such as bless the faces
Of figures that are drawn for goddesses,
And makes art proud to look upon her work –
I should be sorry the least force should lay
An unkind touch upon thee.

BIAN: O my extremity!
    My lord, what seek you?

DUKE: Love.

BIAN: 'Tis gone already;
    I have a husband.

DUKE: That's a single comfort;
    Take a friend to him.

BIAN: That's a double mischief,
    Or else there's no religion.

DUKE: Do not tremble
    At fears of thine own making.

BIAN: Nor, great lord,
    Make me not bold with death and deeds of ruin,
Because they fear not you; me they must fright;
Then am I best in health: should thunder speak,
And none regard it, it had lost the name,
And were as good be still. I'm not like those
That take their soundest sleeps in greatest tempests;
Then wake I most, the weather fearfullest,
And call for strength to virtue.

DUKE: Sure, I think
Thou know'st the way to please me: I affect
A passionate pleading 'bove an easy yielding;
But never pitied any, – they deserve none –
That will not pity me. I can command,
Think upon that; yet if thou truly knewest
The infinite pleasure my affection takes
In gentle, fair entreatings, when love's businesses
Are carried courteously 'twixt heart and heart,
You'd make more haste to please me.

BIAN: Why should you seek, sir,
    To take away that you can never give?

DUKE: But I give better in exchange, – wealth, honour;
   She that is fortunate in a duke's favour
   'Lights on a tree that bears all women's wishes:
   If your own mother saw you pluck fruit there,
   She would commend your wit, and praise the time
   Of your nativity; take hold of glory.
   Do not I know you've cast away your life
   Upon necessities, means merely doubtful
   To keep you in indifferent health and fashion –
   A thing I heard too lately, and soon pitied –
   And can you be so much your beauty's enemy,
   To kiss away a month or two in wedlock,
   And weep whole years in wants for ever after?
   Come, play the wise wench, and provide for ever;
   Let storms come when they list, they find thee shelter'd.
   Should any doubt arise, let nothing trouble thee;
   Put trust in our love for the managing
   Of all to thy heart's peace: we'll walk together,
   And show a thankful joy for both our fortunes.
   (*Exeunt* DUKE *and* BIANCA *above*.)
LIV: Did not I say my duke would fetch you o'er, widow?
MOTH: I think you spoke in earnest when you said it, madam.
LIV: And my black king makes all the haste he can too.
MOTH: Well, madam, we may meet with him in time yet.
LIV: I've given thee blind mate twice.
MOTH: You may see, madam,
   My eyes begin to fail.
LIV: I'll swear they do, wench.

E. M. Forster
1879–1970

from Arthur Snatchfold

Sir Richard Conway is staying at the home of a boring business acquaintance,
Trevor Donaldson.

It was a silent sunless morning, and seemed earlier than it actually
was. The green of the garden and of the trees was filmed with grey,
as if it wanted wiping. Presently the electric pump started. He
looked at his watch again, slipped down the stairs, out of the
house, across the amphitheatre and through the yew hedge. He
did not run, in case he was seen and had to explain. He moved at
the maximum pace possible for a gentleman, known to be an
original, who fancies an early stroll in his pyjamas. 'I thought I'd
have a look at your formal garden, there wouldn't have been time
after breakfast' would have been the line. He had of course looked
at it the day before, also at the wood. The wood lay before him
now, and the sun was just tipping into it. There were two paths
through the bracken, a broad and a narrow. He waited until he
heard the milk-can approaching down the narrow path. Then he
moved quickly, and they met, well out of sight of the Donaldsonian
demesne.

'Hullo!' he called in his easy out-of-doors voice; he had several
voices, and knew by instinct which was wanted.

'Hullo! Somebody's out early!'

'You're early yourself.'

'Me? Whor'd the milk be if I worn't?' the milkman grinned,
throwing his head back and coming to a standstill. Seen at close
quarters he was coarse, very much of the people and of the thick-
fingered earth; a hundred years ago his type was trodden into the
mud, now it burst and flowered and didn't care a damn.

'You're the morning delivery, eh?'

'Looks like it.' He evidently proposed to be facetious – the clumsy fun which can be so delightful when it falls from the proper lips. 'I'm not the evening delivery anyway, and I'm not the butcher nor the grocer, nor'm I the coals.'

'Live around here?'

'Maybe. Maybe I don't. Maybe I flop about in them planes.'

'You live around here, I bet.'

'What if I do?'

'If you do you do. And if I don't I don't.'

This fatuous retort was a success, and was greeted with doubled-up laughter. 'If you don't you don't! Ho, you're a funny one! There's a thing to say! If you don't you don't! Walking about in yer night things, too, you'll ketch a cold you will, that'll be the end of you! Stopping back in the 'otel, I suppose?'

'No. Donaldson's. You saw me there yesterday.'

'Oh, Donaldson's, that's it. You was the old granfa' at the upstairs window.'

'Old granfa' indeed . . . I'll granfa' you,' and he tweaked at the impudent nose. It dodged, it seemed used to this sort of thing. There was probably nothing the lad wouldn't consent to if properly handled, partly out of mischief, partly to oblige. 'Oh, by the way . . .' and he felt the shirt as if interested in the quality of its material. 'What was I going to say?' and he gave the zip at the throat a downward pull. Much slid into view. 'Oh, I know – when's this round of yours over?'

''Bout eleven. Why?'

'Why not?'

''Bout eleven *at night*. Ha ha. Got yer there. Eleven at night. What you want to arst all them questions for? We're strangers, aren't we?'

'How old are you?'

'Ninety, same as yourself.'

'What's your address?'

'There you go on! Hi! I like that. Arstin questions after I tell you No.'

'Got a girl? Ever heard of a pint? Ever heard of two?'

'Go on. Get out.' But he suffered his forearm to be worked between massaging fingers, and he set down his milk-can. He was amused. He was charmed. He was hooked, and a touch would land him.

[114]

'You look like a boy who looks all right,' the elder man breathed.

'Oh, *stop* it . . . All right, I'll go with you.'

Conway was entranced. Thus, exactly thus, should the smaller pleasures of life be approached. They understood one another with a precision impossible for lovers. He laid his face on the warm skin over the clavicle, hands nudged him behind, and presently the sensation for which he had planned so cleverly was over. It was part of the past. It had fallen like a flower upon similar flowers.

He heard 'You all right?' It was over there too, part of a different past. They were lying deeper in the wood, where the fern was highest. He did not reply, for it was pleasant to lie stretched thus and to gaze up through bracken fronds at the distant treetops and the pale blue sky, and feel the exquisite pleasure fade.

'That was what you wanted, wasn't it?' Propped on his elbows the young man looked down anxiously. All his roughness and pertness had gone, and he only wanted to know whether he had been a success.

'Yes . . . Lovely.'

'Lovely? You say lovely?' he beamed, prodding gently with his stomach.

'Nice boy, nice shirt, nice everything.'

'That a fact?'

Conway guessed that he was vain, the better sort often are, and laid on the flattery thick to please him, praised his comeliness, his thrusting thrashing strength; there was plenty to praise. He liked to do this and to see the broad face grinning and feel the heavy body on him. There was no cynicism in the flattery, he was genuinely admiring and gratified.

'So you enjoyed that?'

'Who wouldn't?'

'Pity you didn't tell me yesterday.'

'I didn't know how to.'

'I'd a met you down where I have my swim. You could 'elped me strip, you'd like that. Still, we mustn't grumble.' He gave Conway a hand and pulled him up, and brushed and tidied the raincoat like an old friend. 'We could get seven years for this, couldn't we?'

'Not seven years, still we'd get something nasty. Madness, isn't it? What can it matter to anyone else if you and I don't mind?'

'Oh, I suppose they've to occupy themselves with somethink or other,' and he took up the milk-can to go on.

'Half a minute, boy – do take this and get yourself some trifle with it.' He produced a note which he had brought on the chance.

'I didn't do it fer that.'

'I know you didn't.'

'Naow, we was each as bad as the other . . . Naow . . . keep yer money.'

'I'd be pleased if you would take it. I expect I'm better off than you and it might come in useful. To take out your girl, say, or towards your next new suit. However, please yourself, of course.'

'Can you honestly afford it?'

'Honestly.'

'Well, I'll find a way to spend it, no doubt. People don't always behave as nice as you, you know.'

Conway could have returned the compliment. The affair had been trivial and crude, and yet they both had behaved perfectly. They would never meet again, and they did not exchange names. After a hearty handshake, the young man swung away down the path, the sunlight and shadow rushing over his back. He did not turn around, but his arm, jerking sideways to balance him, waved an acceptable farewell. The green flowed over his brightness, the path bent, he disappeared. Back he went to his own life, and through the quiet of the morning his laugh could be heard as he whooped at the maids.

Conway waited for a few moments, as arranged, and then he went back too. His luck held. He met no one, either in the amphitheatre garden or on the stairs, and after he had been in his room for a minute the maid arrived with his early tea. 'I'm sorry the milk was late again, sir,' she said. He enjoyed it, bathed and shaved and dressed himself for town. It was the figure of a superior city-man which was reflected in the mirror as he tripped downstairs. The car came round after breakfast to take him to the station, and he was completely sincere when he told the Trevor Donaldsons that he had had an out-of-the-way pleasant weekend.

They believed him, and their faces grew brighter. 'Come again then, come by all means again,' they cried as he slid off. In the train he read the papers rather less than usual and smiled to himself rather more. It was so pleasant to have been completely right over a stranger, even down to little details like the texture of the skin. It flattered his vanity. It increased his sense of power.

William Wycherley
1640?–1716

from The Country Wife

*In order to have free access to all the fashionable women of the town without
incurring either their dishonour or the suspicion of their husbands, Horner has
spread the rumour that he is impotent after a recent bout of venereal disease.
The success of his ploy is demonstrated here in the famous china scene, which
begins with Lady Fidget's visit to his lodgings.*

LADY FID: Well, Horner, am not I a woman of honour? you
see, I'm as good as my word.

HORN: And you shall see, madam, I'll not be behind-hand with
you in honour; and I'll be as good as my word too, if you
please but to withdraw into the next room.

LADY FID: But first, my dear sir, you must promise to have a
care of my dear honour.

HORN: If you talk a word more of your honour, you'll make me
incapable to wrong it. To talk of honour in the mysteries of
love, is like talking of Heaven or the Deity, in an operation
of witchcraft, just when you are employing the devil: it
makes the charm impotent.

LADY FID: Nay, fy! let us not be smutty. But you talk of
mysteries and bewitching to me; I don't understand you.

HORN: I tell you, madam, the word money in a mistress's
mouth, at such a nick of time, is not a more disheartening
sound to a younger brother, than that of honour to an
eager lover like myself.

LADY FID: But you can't blame a lady of my reputation to be
chary.

HORN: Chary! I have been chary of it already, by the report I
have caused of myself.

LADY FID: Ay, but if you should ever let other women know
that dear secret, it would come out. Nay, you must have a

great care of your conduct for my acquaintance are so censorious (oh, 'tis a wicked, censorious world, Mr Horner!), I say, are so censorious, and detracting, that perhaps they'll talk to the prejudice of my honour, though you should not let them know the dear secret.

HORN: Nay, madam, rather than they shall prejudice your honour, I'll prejudice theirs; and, to serve you, I'll lie with 'em all, make the secret their own, and then they'll keep it. I am a Machiavel in love, madam.

LADY FID: O, no, sir, not that way.

HORN: Nay, the devil take me, if censorious women are to be silenced any other way.

LADY FID: A secret is better kept, I hope, by a single person than a multitude; therefore pray do not trust anybody else with it, dear, dear Mr Horner. (*Embracing him*)
(*Enter* SIR JASPER FIDGET)

SIR JASP: How now!

LADY FID: (*Aside*) O my husband! – prevented – and what's almost as bad, found with my arms about another man – that will appear too much – what shall I say? – (*Aloud*) Sir Jasper, come hither: I am trying if Mr Horner were ticklish, and he's as ticklish as can be. I love to torment the confounded toad; let you and I tickle him.

SIR JASP: No, your ladyship will tickle him better without me, I suppose. But is this your buying china? I thought you had been at the china-house.

HORN: (*Aside*) China-house! that's my cue, I must take it. – (*Aloud*) A pox! can't you keep your impertinent wives at home? Some men are troubled with the husbands, but I with the wives; but I'd have you to know, since I cannot be your journeyman by night, I will not be your drudge by day, to squire your wife about, and be your man of straw, or scarecrow only to pies and jays, that would be nibbling at your forbidden fruit; I shall be shortly the hackney gentleman-usher of the town.

SIR JASP: (*Aside*) He! he! he! poor fellow, he's in the right on't, faith. To squire women about for other folks is as ungrateful an employment, as to tell money for other folks. – (*Aloud*) He! he! he! be'n't angry, Horner.

LADY FID: No, 'tis I have more reason to be angry, who am left by you, to go abroad indecently alone; or, what is more indecent, to pin myself upon such ill-bred people of your acquaintance as this is.

SIR JASP: Nay, prithee, what has he done?

LADY FID: Nay, he has done nothing.

SIR JASP: But what d'ye take ill, if he has done nothing?

LADY FID: Ha! ha! ha! faith, I can't but laugh however; why, d'ye think the unmannerly toad would come down to me to the coach? I was fain to come up to fetch him, or go without him, which I was resolved not to do; for he knows china very well, and has himself very good, but will not let me see it, lest I should beg some; but I will find it out, and have what I came for yet.

HORN: (*Apart to* LADY FIDGET, *as he follows her to the door*) Lock the door, madam (*Exit* LADY FIDGET, *and locks the door.*) (*Aloud*) So, she had got into my chamber and locked me out. Oh the impertinency of woman-kind! Well, Sir Jasper, plain-dealing is a jewel; if ever you suffer your wife to trouble me again here, she shall carry you home a pair of horns; by my lord mayor she shall; though I cannot furnish you myself, you are sure, yet I'll find a way.

SIR JASP: Ha! ha! he! (*Aside*) At my first coming in, and finding her arms about him, tickling him it seems, I was half jealous, but now I see my folly. (*Aloud*) He! he! he! poor Horner.

HORN: Nay, though you laugh now, 'twill be my turn ere long. Oh women, more impertinent, more cunning, and more mischievous than their monkeys, and to me almost as ugly – Now is she throwing my things about and rifling all I have; but I'll get in to her the back way, and so rifle her for it.

SIR JASP: Ha! ha! ha! poor angry Horner.

HORN: Stay here a little, I'll ferret her out to you presently I warrant. (*Exit at the other door*) (SIR JASPER *talks through the door to his Wife, she answers from within.*)

SIR JASP: Wife! my Lady Fidget! wife! he is coming in to you the back way.

LADY FID: Let him come, and welcome, which way he will.

SIR JASP: He'll catch you, and use you roughly, and be too strong for you.

LADY FID: Don't you trouble yourself, let him if he can.

QUACK: (*Aside*) This indeed I could not have believed from him, nor any but my own eyes.

(*Enter* MRS SQUEAMISH.)

MRS SQUEAM: Where's this woman-hater, this toad, this ugly, greasy, dirty sloven?

SIR JASP: (*Aside*) So, the women all will have him ugly: methinks he is a comely person, but his wants make his form contemptible to 'em; and 'tis e'en as my wife said yesterday, talking of him, that a proper handsome eunuch was as ridiculous a thing as a gigantic coward.

MRS SQUEAM: Sir Jasper, your servant: where is the odious beast?

SIR JASP: He's within in his chamber, with my wife; she's playing the wag with him.

MRS SQUEAM: Is she so? and he's a clownish beast, he'll give her no quarter, he'll play the wag with her again, let me tell you: come, let's go help her. – What, the door's locked?

SIR JASP: Ay, my wife locked it.

MRS SQUEAM: Did she so? let's break it open then.

SIR JASP: No, no, he'll do her no hurt.

MRS SQUEAM: (*Aside*) But is there no other way to get in to 'em? whither goes this? I will disturb 'em. (*Exit at another door*)

(*Enter* OLD LADY SQUEAMISH.)

LADY SQUEAM: Where is this harlotry, this impudent baggage, this rambling tomrigg? O Sir Jasper, I'm glad to see you here; did you not see my vile grandchild come in hither just now?

SIR JASP: Yes.

LADY SQUEAM: Ay, but where is she then? where is she? Lord, Sir Jasper, I have e'en rattled myself to pieces in pursuit of her: but can you tell what she makes here? they say below, no woman lodges here.

SIR JASP: No.

[121]

LADY SQUEAM: No! what does she here then? say, if it be not a woman's lodging, what makes she here? But are you sure no woman lodges here?

SIR JASP: No, nor no man either, this is Mr Horner's lodgings.

LADY SQUEAM: Is it so, are you sure?

SIR JASP: Yes, yes.

LADY SQUEAM: So; then there's no hurt in't, I hope. But where is he?

SIR JASP: He's in the next room with my wife.

LADY SQUEAM: Nay, if you trust him with your wife, I may with my Biddy. They say, he's a merry harmless man now, e'en as harmless a man as ever came out of Italy with a good voice, and as pretty, harmless company for a lady, as a snake without his teeth.

SIR JASP: Aye, ay, poor man.

(*Re-enter* MRS SQUEAMISH.)

MRS SQUEAM: I can't find 'em — Oh, are you here, grandmother? I followed, you must know, my Lady Fidget hither; 'tis the prettiest lodging, and I have been staring on the prettiest pictures —

(*Re-enter* LADY FIDGET *with a piece of china in her hand, and* HORNER *following.*)

LADY FID: And I have been toiling and moiling for the prettiest piece of china, my dear.

HORN: Nay, she has been too hard for me, do what I could.

MRS SQUEAM: Oh, lord, I'll have some china too. Good Mr Horner, don't think to give other people china, and me none; come in with me too.

HORN: Upon my honour, I have none left now.

MRS SQUEAM: Nay, nay, I have known you deny your china before now, but you shan't put me off so. Come.

HORN: This lady had the last there.

LADY FID: Yes indeed, madam, to my certain knowledge, he has no more left.

MRS SQUEAM: O, but it may be he may have some you could not find.

LADY FID: What, d'ye think if he had had any left, I would not have had it too? for we women of quality never think we have china enough.

HORN: Do not take it ill, I cannot make china for you all, but I will have a roll-waggon for you too, another time.

MRS SQUEAM: Thank you, dear toad.

LADY FID: (*Aside to* HORNER) What do you mean by that promise?

HORN: (*Aside to* LADY FIDGET) Alas, she has an innocent, literal understanding.

LADY SQUEAM: Poor Mr Horner! he has enough to do to please you all, I see.

HORN: Ay, madam, you see how they use me.

LADY SQUEAM: Poor gentleman, I pity you.

HORN: I thank you, madam: I could never find pity, but from such reverend ladies as you are; the young ones will never spare a man.

MRS SQUEAM: Come, come, beast, and go dine with us; for we shall want a man at ombre after dinner.

HORN: That's all their use of me, madam, you see.

MRS SQUEAM: Come, sloven, I'll lead you, to be sure of you. (*Pulls him by the cravat.*)

LADY SQUEAM: Alas, poor man, how she tugs him! Kiss, kiss her; that's the way to make such nice women quiet.

HORN: No, madam, that remedy is worse than the torment: they know I dare suffer anything rather than do it.

LADY SQUEAM: Prithee kiss her, and I'll give you her picture in little, that you admired so last night; prithee do.

HORN: Well, nothing but that could bribe me: I love a woman only in effigy, and good painting as much as I hate them – I'll do't, for I could adore the devil well painted. (*Kisses* MRS SQUEAMISH.)

MRS SQUEAM: Foh, you filthy toad! nay, now I've done jesting.

LADY SQUEAM: Ha! ha! ha! I told you so.

MRS SQUEAM: Foh! a kiss of his –

SIR JASP: Has no more hurt in't than one of my spaniel's.

MRS SQUEAM: Nor no more good neither.

❧

Henry Fielding
1707–54

from Joseph Andrews

Joseph Andrews, supposed brother of Samuel Richardson's Pamela Andrews, is a servant in the house of Lady Booby.

Now the rake Hesperus has called for his breeches, and, having well rubbed his drowsy eyes, prepared to dress himself for all night; by whose example his brother rakes on earth likewise leave those beds in which they had slept away the day. Now Thetis, the good housewife, began to put on the pot, in order to regale the good man Phœbus after his daily labours were over. In vulgar language, it was in the evening when Joseph attended his lady's orders.

But as it becomes us to preserve the character of this lady, who is the heroine of our tale; and as we have naturally a wonderful tenderness for that beautiful part of the human species called the fair sex; before we discover too much of her frailty to our reader, it will be proper to give him a lively idea of the vast temptation, which overcame all the efforts of a modest and virtuous mind; and then we humbly hope his good-nature will rather pity than condemn the imperfection of human virtue.

Nay, the ladies themselves will, we hope, be induced, by considering the uncommon variety of charms which united in this young man's person, to bridle their rampant passion for chastity, and be at least as mild as their violent modesty and virtue will permit them, in censuring the conduct of a woman, who, perhaps, was in her own disposition as chaste as those pure and sanctified virgins, who, after a life innocently spent in the gaieties of the town, begin about fifty to attend twice *per diem* at the polite churches and chapels, to return thanks for the grace which preserved them formerly amongst beaus from temptations perhaps less powerful than what now attacked the lady Booby.

Mr Joseph Andrews was now in the one-and-twentieth year of his age. He was of the highest degree of middle stature. His limbs were put together with great elegance, and no less strength. His legs and thighs were formed in the exactest proportion. His shoulders were broad and brawny; but yet his arms hung so easily, that he had all the symptoms of strength without the least clumsiness. His hair was of a nut-brown colour, and was displayed in wanton ringlets down his back. His forehead was high, his eyes dark, and as full of sweetness as of fire. His nose a little inclined to the Roman. His teeth white and even. His lips full, red, and soft. His beard was only rough on his chin and upper lip; but his cheeks, in which his blood glowed, were overspread with a thick down. His countenance had a tenderness joined with a sensibility inexpressible. Add to this the most perfect neatness in his dress, and an air which, to those who have not seen many noblemen, would give an idea of nobility.

Such was the person who now appeared before the lady. She viewed him some time in silence, and twice or thrice before she spoke changed her mind as to the manner in which she should begin. At length she said to him, 'Joseph, I am sorry to hear such complaints against you: I am told you behave so rudely to the maids, that they cannot do their business in quiet; I mean those who are not wicked enough to hearken to your solicitations. As to others, they may, perhaps, not call you rude; for there are wicked sluts, who make one ashamed of one's own sex, and are as ready to admit any nauseous familiarity, as fellows to offer it: nay, there are such in my family; but they shall not stay in it; that impudent trollop who is with child by you, is discharged by this time.'

As a person who is struck through the heart with a thunderbolt, looks extremely surprised, nay, and perhaps is so too – thus the poor Joseph received the false accusation of his mistress; he blushed and looked confounded, which she misinterpreted to be symptoms of his guilt, and thus went on:

'Come hither, Joseph: another mistress might discard you for these offences; but I have a compassion for your youth, and if I could be certain you would be no more guilty – Consider, child,' (laying her hand carelessly upon his) 'you are a handsome young fellow, and might do better; you might make your fortune.' – 'Madam,' said Joseph, 'I do assure your ladyship, I don't know whether any maid in the house is man or woman.' – 'O fie! Joseph,' answered the lady, 'don't commit another crime in denying the truth. I could pardon the first; but I hate a liar.' – 'Madam,' cries Joseph, 'I hope your ladyship will not be offended at my asserting my innocence; for by all that is sacred, I have never offered more than kissing.' 'Kissing!' said the lady, with great discomposure of countenance, and more redness in her cheeks, than anger in her eyes; 'Do you call that no crime? Kissing, Joseph, is as a prologue to a play. Can I believe a young fellow of your age and complexion will be content with kissing? No, Joseph, there is no woman who grants that, but will grant more; and I am deceived greatly in you, if you would not put her closely to it. What would you think, Joseph, if I admitted you to kiss me?' Joseph replied, He would sooner die than have any such thought. 'And yet, Joseph,' returned she, 'ladies have admitted their footmen to such familiarities; and footmen, I confess to you, much less deserving them; fellows without half your charms, – for such might almost excuse the crime. Tell me therefore, Joseph, if I should admit you to such freedom, what would you think of me? – tell me freely.' – 'Madam,' said Joseph, 'I should think your ladyship condescended a great deal below yourself.' – 'Pugh!' said she, 'that I am to answer to myself: but would not you insist on more? Would you be contented with a kiss? Would not your inclinations be all on fire rather by such a favour?' – 'Madam,' said Joseph, 'if they were, I hope I should be able to controul them, without suffering them to get the better of my virtue.' – You have heard, reader, poets talk of the statue of Surprise; you have heard likewise, or else you have heard very little, how surprise made one of the sons of Crœsus speak, though he was dumb. You have seen the faces, in the eighteen-penny gallery, when, through the trap-door, to soft or no music, Mr Bridgwater, Mr William Mills, or some other of ghostly appearance, hath ascended, with a face all pale with powder, and a shirt all bloody with ribands; – but from none of these, nor from Phidias or Praxiteles, if they should return to life – no, not from the inimitable pencil of my friend Hogarth, could you receive such an idea of surprise, as would have entered in at your eyes had they beheld the lady Booby, when those last words issued out from the lips of Joseph. – 'Your virtue!' said the lady, recovering after a silence of two minutes, 'I shall never survive it. Your virtue! – intolerable confidence! Have you the assurance to pretend, that when a lady demeans herself to throw aside the rules of decency, in order to honour you with the highest favour in her power, your virtue should resist her inclination? that when she had conquered her own virtue, she should find an obstruction in yours?' – 'Madam,' said Joseph, 'I can't see why her having no virtue should be a reason against my having any: or why, because I am a man, or because I am poor, my virtue must be subservient to her pleasures.' – 'I am out of patience,' cries the lady: 'Did ever mortal hear of a man's virtue! Did ever the greatest, or the gravest, men pretend to any of this kind! Will magistrates who punish lewdness, or parsons who preach against it, make any scruple of committing it? And can a boy, a stripling, have the confidence to talk of his virtue?' – 'Madam,' says Joseph, 'that boy is the brother of Pamela, and would be ashamed that the chastity of his family, which is preserved in her, should be stained in him. If there are such men as your ladyship mentions, I am sorry for it; and I wish they had an opportunity of reading over those letters, which my father hath sent me of my sister Pamela's; nor do I doubt but such an example would amend them.' – 'You impudent villain!' cries the lady in a rage, 'do you insult me with the follies of my relation, who hath exposed himself all over the country upon your sister's account? a little vixen, whom I have always wondered my late lady Booby ever kept in her house. Sirrah! get out of my sight, and prepare to set out this night; for I will order you your wages immediately, and you shall be stripped and turned away.' – 'Madam,' says Joseph, 'I am sorry I have offended your ladyship, I am sure I never intended it.' – 'Yes, sirrah,' cries she, 'you have had the vanity to misconstrue the little innocent freedom I took, in order to try whether what I had heard was true. O' my conscience, you have had the assurance to imagine I was fond of you myself.' Joseph answered, he had only spoke out of tenderness for his virtue; at which words she flew into a violent passion, and, refusing to hear more, ordered him instantly to leave the room.

He was no sooner gone, than she burst forth into the following exclamation: – 'Whither doth this violent passion hurry us! What meannesses do we submit to from its impulse! Wisely we resist its first and least approaches; for it is then only we can assure ourselves the victory. No woman could ever safely say, so far only will I go. Have I not exposed myself to the refusal of my footman? – I cannot bear the reflexion.' Upon which she applied herself to the bell, and rung it with infinite more violence than was necessary, – the faithful Slipslop attending near at hand: To say the truth, she had conceived a suspicion at her last interview with her mistress; and had waited ever since in the antechamber, having carefully applied her ears to the keyhole during the whole time that the preceding conversation passed between Joseph and the lady.

❧

Thomas Middleton
1570?–1627 and

William Rowley
1585?–1642?

from The Changeling

Beatrice mistakenly believed that she could bribe her father's steward, De Flores – who is passionately attracted to her – to rid her of an unwelcome suitor, so that she can marry Alsemero, whom she loves. This is the scene where De Flores returns to claim from Beatrice his reward after murdering Piracquo.

DE F: (*Aside*) My thoughts are at a banquet; for the deed,
 I feel no weight in't; 'tis but light and cheap
 For the sweet recompense that I set down for't.
BEAT: De Flores!
DE F: Lady?
BEAT: Thy looks promise cheerfully.
DE F: All things are answerable, time, circumstance,
 Your wishes, and my service.
BEAT: Is it done, then?
DE F: Piracquo is no more.
BEAT: My joys start at mine eyes; our sweet'st delights
 Are evermore born weeping.
DE F: I've a token for you.
BEAT: For me?
DE F: But it was sent somewhat unwillingly;
 I could not get the ring without the finger.
 (*Producing the ring and the finger.*)
BEAT: Bless me, what hast thou done?
DE F: Why, is that more
 Than killing the whole man? I cut his heart-strings:
 A greedy hand thrust in a dish at court,
 In a mistake hath had as much as this.

[129]

BEAT: 'Tis the first token my father made me send him.

DE F: And I have made him send it back again
For his last token; I was loath to leave it,
And I'm sure dead men have no use of jewels;
He was as loath to part with't, for it stuck
As if the flesh and it were both one substance.

BEAT: At the stag's fall, the keeper has his fees;
'Tis soon applied, all dead men's fees are yours, sir:
I pray, bury the finger, but the stone
You may make use on shortly; the true value,
Tak't of my truth, is near three hundred ducats.

DE F: 'Twill hardly buy a capcase for one's conscience though,
To keep it from the worm, as fine as 'tis:
Well, being my fees, I'll take it;
Great men have taught me that, or else my merit
Would scorn the way on't.

BEAT: It might justly, sir;
Why, thou mistak'st, De Flores, 'tis not given
In state of recompense.

DE F: No, I hope so, lady;
You should soon witness my contempt to't then.

BEAT: Prithee, – thou look'st as if thou wert offended.

DE F: That were strange, lady; 'tis not possible
My service should draw such a cause from you:
Offended! could you think so? that were much
For one of my performance, and so warm
Yet in my service.

BEAT: 'Twere misery in me to give you cause, sir.

DE F: I know so much, it were so; misery
In her most sharp condition.

BEAT: 'Tis resolv'd then;
Look you, sir, here's three thousand golden florens;
I have not meanly thought upon thy merit.

DE F: What! salary? now you move me.

BEAT: How, De Flores?

DE F: Do you place me in the rank of verminous fellows,
To destroy things for wages? offer gold
[For] the life-blood of man? is anything
Valued too precious for my recompense?

[130]

BEAT: I understand thee not.

DE F: I could ha' hir'd
    A journeyman in murder at this rate,
    And mine own conscience might have [slept at ease],
    And have had the work brought home.

BEAT: (*Aside*) I'm in a labyrinth;
    What will content him? I'd fain be rid of him.
    I'll double the sum, sir.

DE F: You take a course
    To double my vexation, that's the good you do.

BEAT: (*Aside*) Bless me, I'm now in worse plight than I was;
    I know not what will please him. For my fear's sake.
    I prithee, make away with all speed possible;
    And if thou be'st so modest not to name
    The sum that will content thee, paper blushes not,
    Send thy demand in writing, it shall follow thee;
    But, prithee, take thy flight.

DE F: You must fly too then.

BEAT: I?

DE F: I'll not stir a foot else.

BEAT: What's your meaning?

DE F: Why, are not you as guilty? in, I'm sure,
    As deep as I; and we should stick together:
    Come, your fears counsel you but ill; my absence
    Would draw suspect upon you instantly,
    There were no rescue for you.

BEAT: (*Aside*) He speaks home!

DE F: Nor is it fit we two, engag'd so jointly,
    Should part and live asunder.

BEAT: How now, sir?
    This shows not well.

DE F: What makes your lip so strange?
    This must not be betwixt us.

BEAT: The man talks wildly!

DE F: Come, kiss me with a zeal now.

BEAT: (*Aside*) Heaven, I doubt him!

DE F: I will not stand so long to beg 'em shortly.

BEAT: Take heed, De Flores, of forgetfulness,
    'Twill soon betray us.

DE F: Take you heed first;
    Faith, you're grown much forgetful, you're to blame in't.
BEAT: (*Aside*) He's bold, and I am blam'd for't.
DE F: I have eas'd you
    Of your trouble, think on it; I am in pain,
    And must be eas'd of you; 'tis a charity,
    Justice invites your blood to understand me.
BEAT: I dare not.
DE F: Quickly!
BEAT: O, I never shall!
    Speak it yet further off, that I may lose
    What has been spoken, and no sound remain on't;
    I would not hear so much offence again
    For such another deed.
DE F: Soft, lady, soft!
    The last is not yet paid for: O, this act
    Has put me into spirit; I was as greedy on't
    As the parch'd earth of moisture, when the clouds weep:
    Did you not mark, I wrought myself into't,
    Nay, sued and kneel'd for't? why was all that pains took?
    You see I've thrown contempt upon your gold;
    Not that I want it [not], for I do piteously,
    In order I'll come unto't, and make use on't,
    But 'twas not held so precious to begin with,
    For I place wealth after the heels of pleasure;
    And were not I resolv'd in my belief
    That thy virginity were perfect in thee,
    I should but take my recompense with grudging,
    As if I had but half my hopes I agreed for.
BEAT: Why, 'tis impossible thou canst be so wicked,
    Or shelter such a cunning cruelty,
    To make his death the murderer of my honour!
    Thy language is so bold and vicious,
    I cannot see which way I can forgive it
    With any modesty.
DE F: Push! you forget yourself;
    A woman dipp'd in blood, and talk of modesty!
BEAT: O misery of sin! would I'd been bound
    Perpetually unto my living hate

[132]

In that Piracquo, than to hear these words!
Think but upon the distance that creation
Set 'twixt thy blood and mine, and keep thee there.
DE F: Look but into your conscience, read me there;
'Tis a true book, you'll find me there your equal:
Push! fly not to your birth, but settle you
In what the act has made you; you're no more now.
You must forget your parentage to me;
You are the deed's creature; by that name
You lost your first condition, and I challenge you,
As peace and innocency has turn'd you out,
And made you one with me.
BEAT: With thee, foul villain!
DE F: Yes, my fair murderess; do you urge me?
Though thou writ'st maid, thou whore in thy affection?
'Twas chang'd from thy first love, and that's a kind
Of whoredom in the heart; and he's chang'd now
To bring thy second on, thy Alsemero,
Whom, by all sweets that ever darkness tasted,
If I enjoy thee not, thou ne'er enjoyest!
I'll blast the hopes and joys of marriage,
I'll confess all; my life I rate at nothing.
BEAT: De Flores!
DE F: I shall rest from all love's plagues then;
I live in pain now; that shooting eye
Will burn my heart to cinders.
BEAT: O sir, hear me!
DE F: She that in life and love refuses me,
In death and shame my partner she shall be.
BEAT: (*Kneeling*) Stay, hear me once for all; I make thee master
Of all the wealth I have in gold and jewels;
Let me go poor unto my bed with honour,
And I am rich in all things!
DE F: Let this silence thee;
The wealth of all Valencia shall not buy
My pleasure from me;
Can you weep Fate from its determin'd purpose?
So soon may you weep me.
BEAT: Vengeance begins;

Murder, I see, is follow'd by more sins:
Was my creation in the womb so curst,
It must engender with a viper first?

DE F: (*Raising her*) Come, rise and shroud your blushes in my
    bosom;
Silence is one of pleasure's best receipts:
Thy peace is wrought for ever in this yielding.
'Las! how the turtle pants! thou'lt love anon
What thou so fear'st and faint'st to venture on.
(*Exeunt.*)

🜲

Molly Keane
1904–

from Time after Time

*Jasper and Leda are both old, and Leda has gone blind in the years following
their transitory adolescent romance, which was on Leda's only previous visit to
Jasper's Irish country house.*

Jasper was sitting up in bed – rather a little-boy-home-from-
school look about his austere pyjama jacket. His eyepatch was off
and his hair was turned freakishly upwards by the pillows in their
valued habitual arrangement. His mind was concerned absolutely
and entirely with the propagation of azaleas; a manual on the
subject was in one hand and the violet-patterned cup of Complan,
with its powdering of nutmeg and its bottlecap of whiskey, was in
the other. He was absorbed in the pleasures of reading about
things he would never do, when his door opened and Leda came
in. She waited, standing with her back to the dim white door, a
dark figure from a dream.

'Speak to me,' she said in a very ordinary tone of voice, 'say
something, so that I know where your bed is.'

Jasper put down his Complan and reached for his eyepatch,
determined on an immediate evacuation of his bed. But she had
located him. She was coming across the room, her head forward-
seeking: a blind earthworm.

'Do sit. Have some eiderdown,' was all he could think of to say.

'I couldn't sleep, Jasper.'

'So I see, dear. What a bother.'

'Jasper,' she said, 'I'm sorry I ruined our cake.'

'Don't let that worry you. I thought my failure rather an
improvement. Less goo-some. What did you think?'

'Awful. Awful.'

'Perhaps you're right. We must try again.'

He felt her hand on his knee, above the blankets and the electric blanket. He thought again of the knitted gloves and the blue face-cloth carriage rug. He thought of an evening's unhappiness by the river, and he thought of a mushroom field. He wished he was back in total forgetfulness. He was glad that he was no longer young, or suffering. Even as a good tease for the girls he did not want Leda in, or even on, his bed. It fidgeted him to think of her weight on the electric blanket. He leaned forward, the battery was on the floor, to click off its switch.

Very quietly Leda slid along the bed to where she thought his arms waited for her. There were no arms waiting. Jasper's hands were clasped, embarrassed and protective, over the somnolence of his private person.

'Dearest girl,' he said, 'let me offer you half a Mogadon. It's all I have.'

'Oh, thank you. That will be a help.'

When he put the half tablet on to the fat palm of her hand and the tooth-glass of water into the other hand, he congratulated himself on his diplomacy and felt grateful for her tactful acceptance of a non-event.

'Thank you so much. I'm sure I'll get to sleep now. Awful of me to disturb you, but May was asleep and I couldn't wake April and June's not one for pills. So there was only you.' She stilled her voice on the last words. She waited another moment.

'I should get back to bed before the Mog wears off. It was a rather small half,' Jasper said uneasily.

'Yes. So it was. Night-night.'

Jasper felt he should get up and help her downstairs. But he wasn't wearing his patch, and only the top half of his pyjamas, so what if they should meet one of the girls? . . . No. It was better to leave well alone. Not that it was very well either – a miserable distraction from his reading; and the Complan, disgustingly cool now, was less soothing than usual.

Wise and Foolish Virgins

Sylvia Plath
1932–63

from The Bell Jar

The narrator, Esther Greenwood, is at the end of her stay in a psychiatric hospital. She has decided that she wants to lose her virginity.

'I suppose you have lots and lots of affairs in Cambridge,' I told Irwin cheerily, as I stuck a snail with a pin in one of Cambridge's determinedly French restaurants.

'I seem,' Irwin admitted with a small, modest smile, 'to get on with the ladies.'

I picked up my empty snail shell and drank the herb-green juice. I had no idea if this was proper, but after months of wholesome, dull asylum diet, I was greedy for butter.

I had called Doctor Nolan from a pay phone at the restaurant and asked for permission to stay overnight in Cambridge with Joan. Of course, I had no idea whether Irwin would invite me back to his apartment after dinner or not, but I thought his dismissal of the Slavic lady – another professor's wife – looked promising.

I tipped back my head and poured down a glass of Nuits St George.

'You do like wine,' Irwin observed.

'Only Nuits St George. I imagine him . . . with the dragon . . .'

Irwin reached for my hand.

I felt the first man I slept with must be intelligent, so I would respect him. Irwin was a full professor at twenty-six and had the pale, hairless skin of a boy genius. I also needed somebody quite experienced to make up for my lack of it, and Irwin's ladies reassured me on this head. Then, to be on the safe side, I wanted somebody I didn't know and wouldn't go on knowing – a kind of impersonal, priestlike official, as in the tales of tribal rites.

By the end of the evening I had no doubts about Irwin whatsoever.

Ever since I'd learned about the corruption of Buddy Willard my virginity weighed like a millstone around my neck. It had been of such enormous importance to me for so long that my habit was to defend it at all costs. I had been defending it for five years and I was sick of it.

It was only as Irwin swung me into his arms, back at the apartment, and carried me, wine-dazed and limp, into the pitch-black bedroom, that I murmured, 'You know, Irwin, I think I ought to tell you, I'm a virgin.'

Irwin laughed and flung me down on the bed.

A few minutes later an exclamation of surprise revealed that Irwin hadn't really believed me. I thought how lucky it was I had started practising birth control during the day, because in my winey state that night I would never have bothered to perform the delicate and necessary operation. I lay, rapt and naked, on Irwin's rough blanket, waiting for the miraculous change to make itself felt.

But all I felt was a sharp, startlingly bad pain.

'It hurts,' I said. 'Is it supposed to hurt?'

Irwin didn't say anything. Then he said, 'Sometimes it hurts.'

After a little while Irwin got up and went into the bathroom, and I heard the rushing of shower water. I wasn't sure if Irwin had done what he planned to do, or if my virginity had obstructed him in some way. I wanted to ask him if I was still a virgin, but I felt too unsettled. A warm liquid was seeping out between my legs. Tentatively, I reached down and touched it.

When I held my hand up to the light streaming in from the bathroom, my fingertips looked black.

'Irwin,' I said nervously, 'bring me a towel.'

Irwin strolled back, a bathtowel knotted around his waist, and tossed me a second, smaller towel. I pushed the towel between my legs and pulled it away almost immediately. It was half black with blood.

'I'm bleeding!' I announced, sitting up with a start.

'Oh, that often happens,' Irwin reassured me. 'You'll be all right.'

Then the stories of blood-stained bridal sheets and capsules of red ink bestowed on already deflowered brides floated back to me. I wondered how much I would bleed, and lay down, nursing the towel. It occurred to me that the blood was my answer. I couldn't possibly be a virgin any more. I smiled into the dark. I felt part of a great tradition.

Surreptitiously, I applied a fresh section of white towel to my wound, thinking that as soon as the bleeding stopped, I would take the late trolley back to the asylum. I wanted to brood over my new condition in perfect peace. But the towel came away black and dripping.

'I . . . think I better go home,' I said faintly.

'Surely not so soon.'

'Yes, I think I better.'

I asked if I could borrow Irwin's towel and packed it between my thighs as a bandage. Then I pulled on my sweaty clothes. Irwin offered to drive me home, but I didn't see how I could let him drive me to the asylum, so I dug in my pocketbook for Joan's address. Irwin knew the street and went out to start the car. I was too worried to tell him I was still bleeding. I kept hoping every minute that it would stop.

But as Irwin drove me through the barren, snow-banked streets I felt the warm seepage let itself through the dam of the towel and my skirt and on to the car seat.

As we slowed, cruising by house after lit house, I thought how fortunate it was I had not discarded my virginity while living at college or at home, where such concealment would have been impossible.

Joan opened the door with an expression of glad surprise. Irwin kissed my hand and told Joan to take good care of me.

I shut the door and leaned back against it, feeling the blood drain from my face in one spectacular flush.

'Why, Esther,' Joan said, 'what on earth's the matter?'

I wondered when Joan would notice the blood trickling down my legs and oozing, stickily, into each black patent leather shoe. I thought I could be dying from a bullet wound and Joan would still stare through me with her blank eyes, expecting me to ask for a cup of coffee and a sandwich.

'Is that nurse here?'

'No, she's on night duty at Caplan . . .'

'Good.' I made a little bitter grin as another soak of blood let itself through the drenched padding and started the tedious journey into my shoes. 'I mean . . . bad.'

'You look funny,' Joan said.

'You better get a doctor.'

'Why?'

'Quick.'

'But . . .'

Still she hadn't noticed anything.

I bent down, with a brief grunt, and slipped off one of my winter-cracked black Bloomingdale shoes. I held the shoe up, before Joan's enlarged, pebbly eyes, tilted it, and watched her take in the stream of blood that cascaded on to the beige rug.

'My God! What is it?'

'I'm hæmorrhaging.'

Joan half-led, half-dragged me to the sofa and made me lie down. Then she propped some pillows under my bloodstained feet. Then she stood back and demanded, 'Who was that man?'

For one crazy minute I thought Joan would refuse to call a doctor until I confessed the whole story of my evening with Irwin and that after my confession she would still refuse, as a sort of punishment. But then I realized that she honestly took my explanation at face value, that my going to bed with Irwin was utterly incomprehensible to her, and his appearance a mere prick to her pleasure at my arrival.

'Oh somebody,' I said, with a flabby gesture of dismissal. Another pulse of blood released itself and I contracted my stomach muscles in alarm. 'Get a towel.'

Joan went out and came back almost immediately with a pile of towels and sheets. Like a prompt nurse, she peeled back my blood-wet clothes, drew a quick breath as she arrived at the original royal red towel, and applied a fresh bandage. I lay, trying to slow the beating of my heart, as every beat pushed forth another gush of blood.

I remembered a worrisome course in the Victorian novel where woman after woman died, palely and nobly, in torrents of blood, after a difficult childbirth. Perhaps Irwin had injured me in some awful, obscure way, and all the while I lay there on Joan's sofa I was really dying.

Joan pulled up an Indian hassock and began to dial down the long list of Cambridge doctors. The first number didn't answer. Joan began to explain my case to the second number, which did answer, but then broke off and said 'I see' and hung up.

'What's the trouble?'

'He'll only come for regular customers or emergencies. It's Sunday.'

I tried to lift my arm and look at my watch, but my hand was a rock at my side and wouldn't budge. Sunday – the doctor's paradise! Doctors at country clubs, doctors at the seaside, doctors with mistresses, doctors with wives, doctors in church, doctors in yachts, doctors everywhere resolutely being people, not doctors.

'For God's sake,' I said, 'tell them I'm an emergency.'

The third number didn't answer and, at the fourth, the party hung up the minute Joan mentioned it was about a period. Joan began to cry.

'Look, Joan,' I said painstakingly, 'call up the local hospital. Tell them it's an emergency. They'll have to take me.'

Joan brightened and dialled a fifth number. The Emergency Service promised her a staff doctor would attend to me if I could come in to the ward. Then Joan called a taxi.

Joan insisted on riding with me. I clasped my fresh padding of towels with a sort of desperation as the cabby, impressed by the address Joan gave him, cut corner after corner in the dawn-pale streets and drew up with a great squeal of tyres at the Emergency Ward entrance.

I left Joan to pay the driver and hurried into the empty, glaringly lit room. A nurse bustled out from behind a white screen. In a few swift words, I managed to tell her the truth about my predicament before Joan came in the door, blinking and wide-eyed as a myopic owl.

The Emergency Ward doctor strolled out then, and I climbed, with the nurse's help, on to the examining table. The nurse whispered to the doctor, and the doctor nodded and began unpacking the bloody towelling. I felt his fingers start to probe, and Joan stood, rigid as a soldier, at my side, holding my hand, for my sake or hers I couldn't tell.

'Ouch!' I winced at a particularly bad jab.

The doctor whistled.

'You're one in a million.'

'What do you mean?'

'I mean it's one in a million it happens to like this.'

The doctor spoke in a low, curt voice to the nurse, and she hurried to a side table and brought back some rolls of gauze and silver instruments. 'I can see,' the doctor bent down, 'exactly where the trouble is coming from.'

'But can you fix it?'

The doctor laughed. 'Oh, I can fix it, all right.'

George Gordon, Lord Byron
1788–1824

from Don Juan

'Twas on the sixth of June, about the hour
   Of half-past six – perhaps still nearer seven –
When Julia sate within as pretty a bower
   As e'er held houri in that heathenish heaven
Described by Mahomet, and Anacreon Moore,
   To whom the lyre and laurels have been given,
With all the trophies of triumphant song –
He won them well, and may he wear them long!

She sate, but not alone; I know not well
   How this same interview had taken place,
And even if I knew, I should not tell –
   People should hold their tongues in any case;
No matter how or why the thing befell,
   But there were she and Juan, face to face –
When two such faces are so, 'twould be wise,
But very difficult, to shut their eyes.

How beautiful she look'd! her conscious heart
   Glow'd in her cheek, and yet she felt no wrong.
Oh Love! how perfect is thy mystic art,
   Strengthening the weak, and trampling on the strong,
How self-deceitful is the sagest part
   Of mortals whom thy lure hath led along –
The precipice she stood on was immense,
So was her creed in her own innocence.

She thought of her own strength, and Juan's youth,
  And of the folly of all prudish fears,
Victorious virtue, and domestic truth,
  And then of Don Alfonso's fifty years:
I wish these last had not occurr'd, in sooth,
  Because that number rarely much endears,
And through all climes, the snowy and the sunny,
Sounds ill in love, whate'er it may in money.

When people say, 'I've told you *fifty* times,'
  They mean to scold, and very often do;
When poets say, 'I've written *fifty* rhymes,'
  They make you dread that they'll recite them too;
In gangs of *fifty*, thieves commit their crimes;
  At *fifty* love for love is rare, 'tis true,
But then, no doubt, it equally as true is,
A good deal may be bought for *fifty* Louis.

Julia had honour, virtue, truth, and love
  For Don Alfonso; and she inly swore,
By all the vows below to powers above,
  She never would disgrace the ring she wore,
Nor leave a wish which wisdom might reprove;
  And while she ponder'd this, besides much more,
One hand on Juan's carelessly was thrown,
Quite by mistake – she thought it was her own;

Unconsciously she lean'd upon the other,
  Which play'd within the tangles of her hair;
And to contend with thoughts she could not smother
  She seem'd, by the distraction of her air.
'Twas surely very wrong in Juan's mother
  To leave together this imprudent pair,
She who for many years had watch'd her son so –
I'm very certain *mine* would not have done so.

The hand which still held Juan's, by degrees
　　Gently, but palpably confirm'd its grasp,
As if it said, 'Detain me, if you please;'
　　Yet there's no doubt she only meant to clasp
His fingers with a pure Platonic squeeze;
　　She would have shrunk as from a toad, or asp,
Had she imagined such a thing could rouse
A feeling dangerous to a prudent spouse.

I cannot know what Juan thought of this,
　　But what he did, is much what you would do;
His young lip thank'd it with a grateful kiss,
　　And then, abash'd at its own joy, withdrew
In deep despair, lest he had done amiss, –
　　Love is so very timid when 'tis new:
She blush'd, and frown'd not, but she strove to speak,
And held her tongue, her voice was grown so weak.

The sun set, and up rose the yellow moon:
　　The devil's in the moon for mischief; they
Who call'd her CHASTE, methinks, began too soon
　　Their nomenclature; there is not a day,
The longest, not the twenty-first of June,
　　Sees half the business in a wicked way,
On which three single hours of moonshine smile –
And then she looks so modest all the while.

There is a dangerous silence in that hour,
　　A stillness, which leaves room for the full soul
To open all itself, without the power
　　Of calling wholly back its self-control;
The silver light which, hallowing tree and tower,
　　Sheds beauty and deep softness o'er the whole,
Breathes also to the heart, and o'er it throws
A loving languor, which is not repose.

And Julia sate with Juan, half embraced
    And half retiring from the glowing arm,
Which trembled like the bosom where 'twas placed;
    Yet still she must have thought there was no harm,
Or else 'twere easy to withdraw her waist;
    But then the situation had its charm,
And then – God knows what next – I can't go on;
I'm almost sorry that I e'er begun.

Oh Plato! Plato! you have paved the way,
    With your confounded fantasies, to more
Immoral conduct by the fancied sway
    Your system feigns o'er the controulless core
Of human hearts, than all the long array
    Of poets and romancers: – You're a bore,
A charlatan, a coxcomb – and have been,
At best, no better than a go-between.

And Julia's voice was lost, except in sighs,
    Until too late for useful conversation;
The tears were gushing from her gentle eyes,
    I wish, indeed, they had not had occasion;
But who, alas! can love, and then be wise?
    Not that remorse did not oppose temptation;
A little still she strove, and much repented,
And whispering 'I will ne'er consent' – consented.

D. H. Lawrence
1885–1930

from Sons and Lovers

There was a great crop of cherries at the farm. The trees at the back of the house, very large and tall, hung thick with scarlet and crimson drops, under the dark leaves. Paul and Edgar were gathering the fruit one evening. It had been a hot day, and now the clouds were rolling in the sky, dark and warm. Paul climbed high in the tree, above the scarlet roofs of the buildings. The wind, moaning steadily, made the whole tree rock with a subtle, thrilling motion that stirred the blood. The young man, perched insecurely in the slender branches, rocked till he felt slightly drunk, reached down the boughs where the scarlet beady cherries hung thick underneath, and tore off handful after handful of the sleek, cool-fleshed fruit. Cherries touched his ears and his neck as he stretched forward, their chill finger-tips sending a flash down his blood. All shades of red, from a golden vermilion to a rich crimson, glowed and met his eyes under a darkness of leaves.

The sun, going down, suddenly caught the broken clouds. Immense piles of gold flared out of the south-east, heaped in soft, glowing yellow right up the sky. The world, till now dusk and grey, reflected the gold glow, astonished. Everywhere the trees, and the grass, and the far-off water, seemed roused from the twilight and shining.

Miriam came out wondering.

'Oh!' Paul heard her mellow voice call, 'isn't it wonderful?'

He looked down. There was a faint gold glimmer on her face, that looked very soft, turned up at him.

'How high you are!' she said.

Beside her, on the rhubarb leaves, were four dead birds, thieves that had been shot. Paul saw some cherry-stones hanging quite bleached, like skeletons, picked clear of flesh. He looked down again to Miriam.

'Clouds are on fire,' he said.

'Beautiful!' she cried.

She seemed so small, so soft, so tender, down there. He threw a handful of cherries at her. She was startled and frightened. He laughed with a low, chuckling sound, and pelted her. She ran for shelter, picking up some cherries. Two fine pairs she hung over her ears; then she looked up again.

'Haven't you got enough?' she asked.

'Nearly. It is like being on a ship up here.'

'And how long will you stay?'

'While the sunset lasts.'

She went to the fence and sat there, watching the gold clouds fall to pieces, and go in immense, rose-coloured ruin towards the darkness. Gold flamed to scarlet, like pain in its intense brightness. Then the scarlet sank to rose, and rose to crimson, and quickly the passion went out of the sky. All the world was dark grey. Paul scrambled quickly down with his basket, tearing his shirt-sleeve as he did so.

'They are lovely,' said Miriam, fingering the cherries.

'I've torn my sleeve,' he answered.

She took the three-cornered rip, saying:

'I shall have to mend it.' It was near the shoulder. She put her fingers through the tear. 'How warm!' she said.

He laughed. There was a new strange note in his voice, one that made her pant.

'Shall we stay out?' he said.

'Won't it rain?' she asked.

'No, let us walk a little way.'

They went down the fields and into the thick plantation of fir-trees and pines.

'Shall we go in among the trees?' he asked.

'Do you want to?'

'Yes.'

It was very dark among the firs, and the sharp spines pricked her face. She was afraid. Paul was silent and strange.

'I like the darkness,' he said. 'I wish it were thicker – good, thick darkness.'

He seemed to be almost unaware of her as a person: she was only to him then a woman. She was afraid. He stood against a pine-tree trunk and took her in his arms. She relinquished herself to him, but it was a sacrifice in which she felt something of horror. This thick-voiced, oblivious man was a stranger to her.

Later it began to rain. The pine-trees smelled very strong. Paul lay with his head on the ground, on the dead pine-needles, listening to the sharp hiss of the rain – a steady, keen noise. His heart was down, very heavy. Now he realized that she had not been with him all the time, that her soul had stood apart, in a sort of horror. He was physically at rest, but no more. Very dreary at heart, very sad, and very tender, his fingers wandered over her face pitifully. Now again she loved him deeply. He was tender and beautiful.

'The rain!' he said.

'Yes – it is coming on you?'

She put her hands over him, on his hair, on his shoulders, to feel if the raindrops fell on him. She loved him dearly. He, as he lay with his face on the dead pine-leaves, felt extraordinarily quiet. He did not mind if the raindrops came on him; he would have lain and got wet through; he felt as if nothing mattered, as if his living were smeared away into the beyond, near and quite lovable. This strange, gentle reaching-out to death was new to him.

Aphra Behn
1640–89

The Willing Mistriss

Amyntas led me to a Grove,
　　Where all the Trees did shade us;
The Sun it self, though it had Strove,
　　It could not have betray'd us:
The place secur'd from humane Eyes,
　　No other fear allows,
But when the Winds that gently rise,
　　Doe Kiss the yeilding Boughs.

Down there we satt upon the Moss,
　　And did begin to play
A Thousand Amorous Tricks, to pass
　　The heat of all the day.
A many Kisses he did give:
　　And I return'd the same
Which made me willing to receive
　　That which I dare not name.

His Charming Eyes no Aid requir'd
　　To tell their softning Tale;
On her that was already fir'd,
　　'Twas Easy to prevaile.
He did but Kiss and Clasp me round,
　　Whilst those his thoughts Exprest:
And lay'd me gently on the Ground;
　　Ah who can guess the rest?

Angela Carter
1940–

from Heroes and Villains

Marianne is the wife of Jewel, the leader of the barbarian tribe which has captured her. The half-witted boy is the son of its powerful shaman.

She sat on the bank and paddled her hand in the standing water. The setting sun beamed red darts through the brown stems of hazel and dyed the still stream with henna. The hazels were covered with nuts. She listened to the soft plop of water through her fingers. She was moist with sweat and had scarcely taken off her clothes for weeks, had slept, walked, ridden, attended a burial, killed a man/not-man and gone to a public execution of justice in the same shirt and trousers; it was a wonder she was not yet overwhelmed with lice, though she often trapped a flea. She put her burning cheek flat down against the cool face of the water and, when she raised her head, the half-witted boy was squatting on the bank beside her, as if they had made a secret assignation for this place but had forgotten to mention it to one another. Some trick of the amber light turned his bare shoulders a healthier colour than usual. He picked his nose with the finger that wore Jewel's ruby ring, if it were a real ruby and not glass. She saw the mark of his collar round his neck.

'Why does your father keep you chained up so much?' she asked him.

'He's afraid of me because I have better fits than he does,' said the boy. 'Watch me.'

He rolled his eyes, foamed at the mouth and threshed about on the grass so vigorously she was afraid he would hurt himself.

'Stop it,' she said firmly. He shuddered to a standstill and fixed her with white, astonished eyes. His foam-flecked tongue lolled over his pale, cracked, swollen lips.

[153]

'Of course, you're Jewel's woman, aren't you,' he said as though this explained everything.

'I'm his wife,' she said.

'Same thing.'

'No, it isn't. There's no choice in being a wife. It is entirely out of one's hands.'

He wagged his dirty brown head; he did not understand her.

'It's the same thing,' he insisted.

'No.'

''Tis.'

'No.'

''Tis! 'Tis! 'Tis!' Again he rolled over and over shouting ''Tis!' in a cracked, imperious voice until Marianne said firmly: 'You're making a fool of yourself.'

He started up, gazing at her with something like wonder because she stopped him.

'What do you mean?'

He was panting. The serpents on his breast writhed in and out and curled round the old bruises on his ribs. He raised his hands and hid behind them, squinting through his fingers at her; his movements were sinuous but erratic, if he had known how to be graceful it would have been delightful to watch him. He rocked back and forth on his heels until, without the shadow of a warning, he jumped on her. He was weightless as a hollow-boned bird or an insect that carries its structure on its outside without a cargo within. She could have pushed him away maybe with one finger, even have thrown him into the stream had she wished to defend herself but she realized this was the first opportunity she had had to betray her husband and instantly she took advantage of it.

The gaunt, crazy, shameless child rolled her among the roots for a while as he probed underneath her clothes with fingers amazingly long and delicate but, it would seem, moved more by curiosity than desire and she wondered if he were too young to do it so she unbuttoned her shirt and rubbed his wet mouth against her breasts for him. The tips of her breasts were so tender she whined under her breath and he became very excited. He began to mutter incomprehensible snatches of his father's prayers and maxims and she roughly seized hold of him and crushed him inside her with her hand for she had not sufficient patience to rely

[154]

on instinct. He made two or three huge thrusts and came with such a terrible cry it seemed the loss of his virginity caused him as much anguish or, at least, consternation as the loss of her own had done. He slid weakly out of her, shivering, but she retained him in her arms and kissed the tangles of his hair. She was unsatisfied but full of pleasure because she had done something irreparable, though she was not yet quite sure what it was. So they lay there for a while in the inexpressible stillness and sombre colours of evening.

🌹

attributed to John Wilmot, Earl of Rochester
1648–80

---

from Sodom

(*Enter* PRICKET *and* SWIVIA *embracing him.*)
SWIVIA: Twelve months must pass ere you can yet arrive
    To be a perfect man, that is to swive,
    As Pockenello doth ———————————————
    Your age to fifteen does but yet incline.
PRICKET: You know I could have stript my Prick at nine. (*He*
    shows.)
SWIVIA: By h—en's a neat one, now we are alone
    I'll shut the door and you shall see my thing. (*She shows.*)
PRICKET: Strange how it looks, me thinks it smells of ling
    It has a beard too, and the mouth's all raw.
    The strangest Creature that I ever saw:
    Are these the Beards that keep men in such aw?
SWIVIA: 't Was such as these Philosophers have taught
    That all mankind into the world have brought.
    t' Was such a thing the King our Sire bestir'd
    Out of whose whomb we came, ———————————
PRICKET: ———————————————— the Devil we did.
SWIVIA: This is the ware house of the world's chief Trade,
    On this soft anvil all mankind was made.
    Come 't is a harmless thing, draw near and try
    You will desire no other Death to dye.
PRICKET: Is 't death then?
SWIVIA: Ay, but with such plaisant pain,
    That it will tickle you to live again.
PRICKET: I feel my spirits in an agony.
SWIVIA: These are the symptoms of young Letchery
    Does not your Prick stand, and your Pulse beat fast?
    Don't you desire some unknown bliss to taste?
PRICKET: My heart invites me to some new desire,

My blood boils over. ————————————————————

SWIVIA: ———————————————— I can allay the fire.
Come little Rogue and on my belly lie (*Lies on her.*)
A little lower, yet, now, dearest, try.

PRICKET: I am a stranger to these unknown parts
And never vers'd in Loves obliging arts:
Pray, guide me, I was ne'er this way before.

SWIVIA: There, can't you enter? Now you've found the door.

PRICKET: Now I am in, and 't is as soft as wool.

SWIVIA: Then move it up and down, you little fool.

PRICKET: I do, o he—ens, I am at my wits' end.

SWIVIA: Is 't not such pleasure as I did commend?

PRICKET: Yes. I find Cunt a most obliging friend
Speak to me sister ere my soul depart.

SWIVIA: I cannot speak, you've stabb'd me to the heart.

PRICKET: I faint, I can't one moment more survive,
I am dead ——————————————————————————

SWIVIA: Oh, Brother, but . . . Alive
And why should you lie dead, to increase my pain,
Kiss me, dear rogue, and thou shalt live again.

❦

Mary de la Riviere Manley
1663–1724

from The New Atalantis

The Duke has conceived a sudden passion for Charlot, his young ward, whom he had intended to marry his son. He plans to seduce her.

The Duke had observed that Charlot had been, but with disgust, denied the gay part of reading. It is natural for young people to choose the diverting before the instructive. He sent for her into the gallery, where was a noble library in all languages, a collection of the most valuable authors, with a mixture of the most amorous. He told her that now her understanding was increased, with her stature, he resolved to make her mistress of her own conduct; and as the first thing that he intended to oblige her in, that *Governante* who had hitherto had the care of her actions should be dismissed; because he had observed the severity of her temper had sometimes been displeasing to her. That she should henceforward have none above her that she should need to stand in awe of; and to confirm to her that good opinion that he seemed to have, he presented to her the key of that gallery, to improve her mind and seek her diversion among those authors he had formerly forbid her the use of.

Charlot made him a very low curtsey and, with a blushing grace, returned him thanks for the two favours he bestowed upon her. She assured him that no action of hers should make him repent the distinction; that her whole endeavour should be to walk in that path he had made familiar to her; and that virtue should ever be her only guide. Though this was not what the Duke wanted, it was nothing but what he expected. He observed formerly that she was a great lover of poetry, especially when it was forbid her. He took down an Ovid, and opening it just at the love of Myrra for her father, conscious red overspread his face. He

[158]

gave it her to read, she obeyed him with a visible delight. Nothing is more pleasing to young girls than in being first considered as women. Charlot saw the Duke entertained her with an air of consideration more than usual, passionate and respectful. This taught her to refuge in the native pride and cunning of her sex; she assumed an air more haughty, the leavings of a girl just beginning to believe herself capable of attaining that empire over mankind which they are all born and taught by instinct to expect.

She took the book and placed herself by the Duke. His eyes feasted themselves upon her face, thence wandered over her snowy bosom, and saw the young swelling breasts just beginning to distinguish themselves, and which were gently heaved at the impression of Myrra's sufferings made upon her heart. By this dangerous reading he pretended to show her that there were pleasures her sex were born for, and which she might consequently long to taste! Curiosity is an early and dangerous enemy to virtue. The young Charlot, who had by a noble inclination of gratitude a strong propension of affection for the Duke, whom she called and esteemed her papa, being a girl of wonderful reflection, and consequently application, wrought her imagination up to such a lively height at the father's anger after the possession of his daughter, which she judged highly unkind and unnatural, that she dropped her book, tears filled her eyes, sobs rose to oppress her, and she pulled out her handkerchief to cover the disorder.

The Duke, who was master of all mankind, could trace them in all the meanders of dissimulation and cunning, was not at a loss how to interpret the agitation of a girl who knew no hypocrisy; all was artless, the beautiful product of innocence and nature. He drew her gently to him, drank her tears with his kisses, sucked her sighs, and gave her by that dangerous commerce (her soul before prepared to softness) new and unfelt desires. Her virtue was becalmed, or rather unapprehensive of him for an invader. He pressed her lips with his, the nimble beatings of his heart, apparently seen and felt through his open breast! the glowings! the trembling of his limbs! the glorious sparkles from his guilty eyes! his shortness of breath, and eminent disorder were all things new to her that had never seen, heard or read before of those powerful operations struck from the fire of the two meeting sex. Nor had she leisure to examine his disorders, possessed by greater of her own!

Greater! because that modesty opposing nature forced a struggle of dissimulation. But the Duke's pursuing kisses overcame the very thoughts of anything; but that new and lazy poison stealing to her heart, and spreading swiftly and imperceptibly through all her veins, she closed her eyes with languishing delight! Delivered up the possession of her lips and breath to the amorous invader; returned his eager grasps and, in a word, gave her whole person into his arms in meltings full of delight!

The Duke, by that lovely ecstasy carried beyond himself, sunk over the expiring fair in raptures too powerful for description! calling her his admirable Charlot! his charming Angel! his adorable Goddess! But all was so far modest that he attempted not beyond her lips and breast, but cried that she should never be another's. The empire of his soul was hers; enchanted by inexplicable, irresistible magic! she had power beyond the gods themselves! Charlot, returned from that amiable disorder, was anew charmed at the Duke's words. Words that set her so far above what was mortal, the woman assumed in her, and she would have no notice taken of the transports she had shown. He saw and favoured her modesty, secure of that fatal sting he had fixed within her breast, that taste of delight, which powerful love and nature would call upon her to repeat. He owned he loved her; that he never could love any other; that 'twas impossible for him to live a day, an hour, without seeing her; that in her absence he had felt more than ever had been felt by mortal. He begged her to have pity on him, to return his love, or else he should be the most lost, undone thing alive. Charlot, amazed and charmed, felt all those dangerous perturbations of nature that arise from an amorous constitution. With pride and pleasure she saw herself necessary to the happiness of one that she had hitherto esteemed so much above her, ignorant of the power of love, that leveller of mankind; that blender of distinction and hearts. Her soft answer was that she was indeed reciprocally charmed, she knew not how; all he had said and done was wonderful and pleasing to her; and if he would still more please her (if there was a more) it should be never to be parted from her. The Duke had one of those violent passions where, to heighten it, resistance was not at all necessary; it had already reached the ultimate, it could not be more ardent; yet was he loth to rush upon the possession of the fair, lest the too early pretension might disgust her. He would steal himself into her soul, he would make himself necessary to her quiet, as she was to his.

From the library he led her to his cabinet. From forth his strong box he took a set of jewels that had been her mother's; he told her she was now of an age to expect the ornaments as well as pleasures of a woman. He was pleased to see her look down with a seeming contempt upon what most other girls would have been transported with. He had taught her other joys, those of the mind and body. She sighed, she raved to herself, she was all charmed and uneasy! The Duke, casting over the rest of his jewels, made a collection of such as were much more valuable than her mother's; he presented her with, and would force her to accept them. But Charlot, tender and gallant as the Duke, seeing his picture in little, set round with diamonds, begged that he would only honour her with that mark of his esteem. The ravished Duke consented, conditionally, that she would give him hers in return.

After this tender, dangerous commerce, Charlot found everything insipid, nothing but the Duke's kisses could relish with her; all those conversations she had formerly delighted in were insupportable. He was obliged to return to court, and had recommended to her reading the most dangerous books of love, Ovid, Petrarch, Tibullus, those moving tragedies that so powerfully expose the force of love and corrupt the mind. He went even farther, and left her such as explained the nature, manner and raptures of enjoyment. Thus he infused poison into the ears of the lovely virgin. She easily (from those emotions she had found in herself) believed as highly of those delights as was imaginable; her waking thoughts, her golden slumber ran all of a bliss only imagined but never proved. She even forgot, as one that wakes from sleep and visions of the night, all those precepts of airy virtue which she found had nothing to do with nature. She longed again to renew those dangerous delights. The Duke was an age absent from her, she could only in imagination possess what she believed so pleasing. Her memory was prodigious, she was indefatigable in reading. The Duke had left orders she should not be controlled in anything. Whole nights were wasted by her in the gallery; she had too well informed herself of the speculative joys of love. There are books dangerous to the community of mankind; abominable for virgins and destructive to youth; such as explain the mysteries of nature, the congregated pleasures of Venus, the full delights of mutual lovers, and which rather ought to pass the fire than the press. The Duke had laid in her way such as made no mention of Virtue or Hymen, but only advanced native, generous and undissembled love. She was become so great a proficient that nothing of the theory was a stranger to her.

While Charlot was thus employed the Duke was not idle; he had prepared her a post at court with Henriquez's Queen. The young lady was sent for; neither art, money nor industry was wanting to make her appearance glorious. The Duke, awed and trembling with his passion, approached her as a goddess; conscious of his and her own desires, the mantling blood would smile upon her cheeks, sometimes glowing with delight, then afterwards, by a feeble recollection of virtue sink apace, to make room for a guilty succeeding paleness. The Duke knew all the motions of her heart. He debated with himself whether it were best to attempt the possession of her whilst so young, or permit her time to know and set a value upon what she granted. His love was highly impatient, but respectful. He longed to be happy but he dreaded to displease her. The ascendant she had over him was wonderful; he had let slip those first impressions which strike deepest in the hearts of women, to be successful. *One ought never to allow them time to think, their vivacity being prodigious and their foresight exceeding short and limited. The first hurry of their passions, if they are but vigorously followed, is what is generally most favourable to lovers.* Charlot by this time had informed herself that there were such terrible things as perfidy and inconstancy in mankind; that even the very favours they received often disgusted; and that to be entirely happy one ought never to think of the faithless sex. This brought her back to those precepts of virtue that had embellished her dawn of life; but alas! these admonitions were too feeble. The Duke was all submissive, passionate, eager to obey and to oblige. He watched her uprisings, scarce could eat without her; she was mistress of his heart and fortune; his own family and the whole court imagined that he resolved her for his Duchess; they almost looked upon her as such. She went often to his palace, where all were devoted to her service; the very glance of her eyes commanded their attention; at her least request, as soon as her mouth was opened to speak, before her words were half-formed, they started to obey her.

She had learnt to manage the Duke and to distrust herself. She would no more permit of kisses, that sweet and dangerous commerce. The Duke had made her wise at his own cost, and vainly languished for a repetition of delight. He guessed at the interest he had in her heart, and proved the warmth of her constitution, and was resolved he would no more be wanting to his own happiness. He omitted no occasion by which he might express his love, pressing her to crown his longings. Her courage did not reach to ask him that honourable proof of his passion, which it is believed he would not have refused if she had but insisted on it. The treaty was still depending, he might marry the Princess Dowager. Charlot tenderly dropped a word that spoke her apprehensions of it. He assured her there was nothing in it. All he aimed at was to purchase the succession, that he might make her a princess, as she deserved. Indeed, the hopes his agent had given the lady, of becoming her husband, was not the smallest inducement to the treaty. Therefore he delayed his marriage with Charlot; for if that were but once confirmed, the Princess (by resenting, as she ought, the abuse that had been laid upon her) would put an end to it, infinitely to his prejudice.

Charlot, very well satisfied with these reasons, and unwilling to do anything against the interest of a man whom she tenderly loved, accustomed herself to hear his eager solicitations. He could no longer contend with a fire that consumed him, he must be gratified or die. She languished under the same disquiets. The season of the year was come that he must make the campaign with the King; he could not resolve to depart unblessed; Charlot still refused him that last proof of her love. He took a tender and passionate farewell. Charlot, drowned in tears, told him it was impossible she should support his absence; all the court would ridicule her melancholy. This was what he wanted; he bid her take care of that. A maid was but an ill figure that brought herself to be sport of laughters; but since her sorrow (so pleasing and glorious to him) was like to be visible, he advised her to pass some days at his villa, till the height of melancholy should be over, under the pretence of indisposition. He would take care that the Queen should be satisfied of the necessity of her absence; he advised her even to depart that hour. Since the King was already on his journey he must be gone that moment and endeavour to overtake him. He assured her he would write by every courier, and begged her not to admit of another lover, though he was sensible there were many (taking advantage of his absence, would endeavour to please her.) To all this she answered so as to disquiet his distrust and fears; her tears drowned her sighs, her words were lost in sobs and groans! The Duke did not show less concern, but led her all trembling to put her in a coach that was to convey her to his villa; where he had often wished to have her, but she distrusted herself and would not go with him; nor had she ventured now, but that she thought he was to follow the King, who could not be without him.

Charlot no sooner arrived, but the weather being very hot, she ordered a bath to be prepared for her. Soon as she was refreshed with that, she threw herself down upon a bed with only one thin petticoat and a loose nightgown, the bosom of her gown and shift open; her nightclothes tied carelessly with a cherry-coloured ribbon which answered well to the yellow and silver stuff of her gown. She lay uncovered in a melancholy careless posture, her head resting upon one of her hands. The other held a handkerchief, that she employed to dry those tears that sometimes fell from her eyes; when raising herself a little at a gentle noise she heard from the opening of a door that answered to the bedside, she was quite astonished to see enter the amorous Duke. Her first emotions were all joy; but in a minute she recollected herself, thinking he was not come there for nothing. She was going to rise but he prevented her by flying to her arms where, as we may call it, he nailed her down to the bed with kisses. His love and resolution gave him a double vigour, he would not stay a moment to capitulate with her; whilst yet her surprise made her doubtful of his designs, he took advantage of her constitution to accomplish them; neither her prayers, tears, nor strugglings could prevent him, but in her arms he made himself a full amends for all those pains he had suffered for her.

Thus was Charlot undone! thus ruined by him that ought to have been her protector! It was very long before he could appease her; but so artful, so amorous, so submissive was his address, so violent his assurances, he told her that he must have died without the happiness. Charlot espoused his crime by sealing his forgiveness. He passed the whole night in her arms, pleased, transported and out of himself; whilst the ravished maid was not at all behindhand in ecstasies and guilty transports. He stayed a whole week with Charlot in a surfeit of love and joy! that week more inestimable than all the pleasures of his life before! whilst the court believed him with the King, posting to the army. He neglected Mars to devote himself wholly to Venus; abstracted from all business, that happy week sublimed him almost to an immortal. Charlot was formed to give and take all those raptures necessary to accomplish the lover's happiness; none were ever more amorous! none were ever more happy!

Philip Larkin
1922–86

Deceptions

'Of course I was drugged, and so heavily I did not regain my consciousness till the next morning. I was horrified to discover that I had been ruined, and for some days I was inconsolable, and cried like a child to be killed or sent back to my aunt.'

Mayhew, *London Labour and the London Poor*

Even so distant, I can taste the grief,
Bitter and sharp with stalks, he made you gulp.
The sun's occasional print, the brisk brief
Worry of wheels along the street outside
Where bridal London bows the other way,
And light, unanswerable and tall and wide,
Forbids the scar to heal, and drives
Shame out of hiding. All the unhurried day
Your mind lay open like a drawer of knives.

Slums, years, have buried you. I would not dare
Console you if I could. What can be said,
Except that suffering is exact, but where
Desire takes charge, readings will grow erratic?
For you would hardly care
That you were less deceived, out on that bed,
Than he was, stumbling up the breathless stair
To burst into fulfilment's desolate attic.

from Moll Flanders

I had all the advantages of education that I could have had if I had been as much a gentlewoman as they were with whom I lived; and in some things I had the advantage of my ladies, though they were my superiors, viz., that mine were all the gifts of nature, and which all their fortunes could not furnish. First, I was apparently handsomer than any of them, secondly, I was better shaped, and, thirdly, I sang better, by which I mean, I had a better voice; in all which you will, I hope, allow me to say, I do not speak my own conceit, but the opinion of all that knew the family.

I had, with all these, the common vanity of my sex, viz., that being really taken for very handsome, or, if you please, for a great beauty, I very well knew it, and had as good an opinion of myself as anybody else could have of me, and particularly I loved to hear anybody speak of it, which happened often, and was a great satisfaction to me.

Thus far I have had a smooth story to tell of myself, and in all this part of my life I not only had the reputation of living in a very good family, and a family noted and respected everywhere for virtue and sobriety, and for every valuable thing, but I had the character too of a very sober, modest, and virtuous young woman, and such I had always been; neither had I yet any occasion to think of anything else, or to know what a temptation to wickedness meant.

But that which I was too vain of, was my ruin, or rather my vanity was the cause of it. The lady in the house where I was had two sons, young gentlemen of extraordinary parts and behaviour, and it was my misfortune to be very well with them both, but they managed themselves with me in a quite different manner.

The eldest, a gay gentleman, that knew the town as well as the country, and, though he had levity enough to do an ill-natured thing, yet had too much judgment of things to pay too dear for his pleasures; he began with that unhappy snare to all women, viz. taking notice upon all occasions how pretty I was, as he called it, how agreeable, how well-carriaged, and the like; and this he contrived so subtly, as if he had known as well how to catch a woman in his net as a partridge when he went a-setting, for he would contrive to be talking this to his sisters, when, though I was not by, yet he knew I was not so far off but that I should be sure to hear him. His sisters would return softly to him, 'Hush, brother, she will hear you, she is but in the next room.' Then he would put it off and talk softlier, as if he had not known it, and begin to acknowledge he was wrong; and then, as if he had forgot himself, he would speak aloud again, and I, that was so well pleased to hear it, was sure to listen for it upon all occasions.

After he had thus baited his hook, and found easily enough the method how to lay it in my way, he played an open game; and one day, going by his sister's chamber when I was there, he comes in with an air of gaiety. 'Oh, Mrs Betty,' said he to me, 'how do you do, Mrs Betty? Don't your cheeks burn, Mrs Betty?' I made a curtsey and blushed, but said nothing. 'What makes you talk so, brother?' said the lady. 'Why,' says he, 'we have been talking of her below-stairs this half-hour.' 'Well,' says his sister, 'you can say no harm of her, that I am sure, so 'tis no matter what you have been talking about.' 'Nay,' says he, ''tis so far from talking harm of her, that we have been talking a great deal of good and a great many fine things have been said of Mrs Betty, I assure you; and particularly, that she is the handsomest young woman in Colchester; and, in short, they begin to toast her health in the town.'

'I wonder at you, brother,' says the sister. 'Betty wants but one thing, but she had as good want everything, for the market is against our sex just now; and if a young woman has beauty, birth, breeding, wit, sense, manners, modesty, and all to an extreme, yet if she has not money she's nobody, she had as good want them all; nothing but money now recommends a woman; the men play the game all into their own hands.'

Her younger brother, who was by, cried, 'Hold, sister, you run too fast; I am an exception to your rule. I assure you, if I find a woman so accomplished as you talk of, I won't trouble myself about the money.' 'Oh,' says the sister, 'but you will take care not to fancy one then without the money.'

'You don't know that neither,' says the brother.

'But why, sister,' says the elder brother, 'why do you exclaim so about the fortune? You are none of them that want a fortune, whatever else you want.'

'I understand you, brother,' replies the lady very smartly; 'you suppose I have the money, and want the beauty; but as times go now, the first will do, so I have the better of my neighbours.'

'Well,' says the younger brother, 'but your neighbours may be even with you, for beauty will steal a husband sometimes in spite of money, and, when the maid chances to be handsomer than the mistress, she oftentimes makes as good a market, and rides in a coach before her.'

I thought it was time for me to withdraw, and I did so, but not so far but that I heard all their discourse, in which I heard abundance of fine things said of myself, which prompted my vanity, but, as I soon found, was not the way to increase my interest in the family, for the sister and the younger brother fell grievously out about it; and as he said some very disobliging things to her, upon my account, so I could easily see that she resented them by her future conduct to me, which indeed was very unjust, for I had never had the least thought of what she suspected as to her younger brother; indeed, the elder brother, in his distant, remote way, had said a great many things as in jest, which I had the folly to believe were in earnest, or to flatter myself with the hopes of what I ought to have supposed he never intended.

It happened one day that he came running upstairs, towards the room where his sisters used to sit and work, as he often used to do; and calling to them before he came in, as was his way too, I being there alone, stepped to the door, and said 'Sir, the ladies are not here; they are walked down the garden.' As I stepped forward to say this, he was just got to the door, and, clasping me in his arms, as if it had been by chance, 'Oh, Mrs Betty,' says he, 'are you here? That's better still; I want to speak with you more than I do with them'; and then, having me in his arms, he kissed me three or four times.

I struggled to get away, and yet did it but faintly neither, and he

[169]

held me fast, and still kissed me, till he was out of breath, and, sitting down, says he, 'Dear Betty, I am in love with you.'

His words, I must confess, fired my blood; all my spirits flew about my heart, and put me into disorder enough. He repeated it afterwards several times, that he was in love with me, and my heart spoke as plain as a voice that I liked it; nay, whenever he said 'I am in love with you,' my blushes plainly replied 'Would you were, sir.' However, nothing else passed at the time; it was but a surprise, and I soon recovered myself. He had stayed longer with me, but he happened to look out at the window and see his sisters coming up the garden, so he took his leave, kissed me again, told me he was very serious, and I should hear more of him very quickly, and away he went infinitely pleased; and had there not been one misfortune in it, I had been in the right, but the mistake lay here, that Mrs Betty was in earnest, and the gentleman was not.

From this time my head ran upon strange things, and I may truly say I was not myself, to have such a gentleman talk to me of being in love with me, and of my being such a charming creature, as he told me I was. These were things I knew not how to bear; my vanity was elevated to the last degree. It is true I had my head full of pride, but, knowing nothing of the wickedness of the times, I had not one thought of my virtue about me; and, had my young master offered it at first sight, he might have taken any liberty he thought fit with me; but he did not see his advantage, which was my happiness for that time.

It was not long but he found an opportunity to catch me again, and almost in the same posture; indeed, it had more of design in it on his part, though not on my part. It was thus: the young ladies were gone a-visiting with their mother; his brother was out of town; and, as for his father, he had been at London for a week before. He had so well watched me that he knew where I was, though I did not so much as know that he was in the house, and he briskly comes up the stairs, and seeing me at work, comes into the room to me directly, and began just as he did before, with taking me in his arms, and kissing me for almost a quarter of an hour together.

It was his younger sister's chamber that I was in, and, as there was nobody in the house but the maid below-stairs, he was, it may be, the ruder; in short, he began to be in earnest with me indeed. Perhaps he found me a little too easy, for I made no resistance to him while he only held me in his arms and kissed me; indeed, I was too well pleased with it to resist him much.

Well, tired with that kind of work, we sat down, and there he talked with me a great while; he said he was charmed with me, and that he could not rest till he had told me how he was in love with me, and, if I could love him again and would make him happy, I should be the saving of his life, and many such fine things. I said little to him again, but easily discovered that I was a fool, and that I did not in the least perceive what he meant.

Then he walked about the room, and, taking me by the hand, I walked with him; and by-and-by, taking his advantage, he threw me down upon the bed, and kissed me there most violently; but, to give him his due, offered no manner of rudeness to me – only kissed me a great while. After this he thought he had heard somebody come upstairs, so he got off from the bed, lifted me up, professing a great deal of love for me; but told me it was all an honest affection, and that he meant no ill to me, and with that put five guineas into my hand, and went downstairs.

I was more confounded with the money that I was before with the love, and began to be so elevated that I scarce knew the ground I stood on. I am the more particular in this, that, if it comes to be read by any innocent young body, they may learn from it to guard themselves against the mischiefs which attend an early knowledge of their own beauty. If a young woman once thinks herself handsome, she never doubts the truth of any man that tells her he is in love with her; for if she believes herself charming enough to captivate him, 'tis natural to expect the effects of it.

This gentleman had now fired his inclination as much as he had my vanity, and, as if he had found that he had an opportunity, and was sorry he did not take hold of it, he comes up again in about half-an-hour, and falls to work with me again just as he did before, only with a little less introduction.

And first, when he entered the room, he turned about and shut the door. 'Mrs Betty,' said he, 'I fancied before somebody was coming upstairs, but it was not so; however,' adds he, 'if they find me in the room with you, they shan't catch me a-kissing of you.' I told him I did not know who should be coming upstairs, for I believed there was nobody in the house but the cook and the other maid, and they never came up those stairs. 'Well, my dear,' says he, ''tis good to be sure, however'; and so he sits down, and we began to talk. And now, though I was still on fire with his first visit, and said little, he did as it were put words in my mouth, telling me how passionately he loved me, and that, though he could not till he came to his estate, yet he was resolved to make me happy then, and himself too; that is to say, to marry me, and abundance of such things, which I, poor fool, did not understand the drift of, but acted as if there was no kind of love but that which tended to matrimony; and if he had spoken of that, I had no room, as well as no power, to have said no; but we were not come to that length yet.

We had not sat long, but he got up, and, stopping my very breath with kisses, threw me upon the bed again; but then he went further with me than decency permits me to mention, nor had it been in my power to have denied him at that moment had he offered much more than he did.

However, though he took these freedoms with me, it did not go to that which they call the last favour, which, to do him justice, he did not attempt; and he made that self-denial of his a plea for all his freedoms with me upon other occasions after this. When this was over he stayed but a little while, but he put almost a handful of gold in my hand, and left me a thousand protestations of his passion for me, and of his loving me above all the women in the world.

It will not be strange if I now began to think; but, alas! it was but with very little solid reflection. I had a most unbounded stock of vanity and pride, and but a very little stock of virtue. I did indeed cast sometimes with myself what my young master aimed at, but thought of nothing but the fine words and the gold; whether he intended to marry me or not seemed a matter of no great consequence to me; nor did I so much as think of making any capitulation for myself till he made a kind of formal proposal to me, as you shall hear presently.

Thus I gave up myself to ruin without the least concern, and am a fair memento to all young women whose vanity prevails over their virtue. Nothing was ever so stupid on both sides. Had I acted as became me, and resisted as virtue and honour required, he had either desisted his attacks, finding no room to expect the end of his design, or had made fair and honourable proposals of marriage; in which case, whoever blamed him, nobody could have blamed me. In short, if he had known me, and how easy the trifle he aimed at was to be had, he would have troubled his head no further, but have given me four or five guineas, and have lain with me the next time he had come at me. On the other hand, if I had known his thoughts, and how hard he supposed I would be to be gained, I might have made my own terms, and, if I had not capitulated for an immediate marriage, I might for a maintenance till marriage, and might have had what I would; for he was rich to excess, besides what he had in expectation; but I had wholly abandoned all such thoughts, and was taken up only with the pride of my beauty, and of being beloved by such a gentleman. As for the gold, I spent whole hours in looking upon it; I told the guineas over a thousand times a day. Never poor vain creature was so wrapt up with every part of the story as I was, not considering what was before me, and how near my ruin was at the door; and indeed I think I rather wished for that ruin than studied to avoid it.

In the meantime, however, I was cunning enough not to give the least room to any in the family to imagine that I had the least correspondence with him, I scarce ever looked towards him in public, or answered if he spoke to me; when, but for all that, we had every now and then a little encounter, where we had room for a word or two, and now and then a kiss, but no fair opportunity for the mischief intended; and especially considering that he made more circumlocution than he had occasion for; and the work appearing difficult to him, he really made it so.

But as the devil is an unwearied tempter, so he never fails to find an opportunity for the wickedness he invites to. It was one evening that I was in the garden, with his two younger sisters and himself, when he found means to convey a note into my hand, by which he told me that he would to-morrow desire me publicly to go of an errand for him, and that I should see him somewhere by the way.

Accordingly, after dinner, he very gravely says to me, his sisters being all by, 'Mrs Betty, I must ask a favour of you.' 'What's that?' says the second sister. 'Nay, sister,' says he very gravely, 'if you can't spare Mrs Betty to-day, any other time will do.' Yes, they said, they could spare her well enough; and the sister begged pardon for asking. 'Well, but,' says the eldest sister, 'you must tell Mrs Betty what it is; if it be any private business that we must not hear, you may call her out. There she is.' 'Why, sister,' says the gentleman very gravely, 'what do you mean? I only desire her to go into the High Street (and then he pulls out a turnover) to such a shop'; and then he tells them a long story of two fine neckcloths he had bid money for, and he wanted to have me go and make an errand to buy a neck to that turnover that he showed, and if they would not take my money for the neckcloths, to bid a shilling more, and haggle with them; and then he made more errands, and so continued to have such petty business to do that I should be sure to stay a good while.

When he had given me my errands, he told them a long story of a visit he was going to make to a family they all knew, and where was to be such-and-such gentlemen, and very formally asked his sisters to go with him, and they as formally excused themselves, because of company that they had notice was to come and visit them that afternoon; all which, by the way, he had contrived on purpose.

He had scarce done speaking but his man came up to tell him that Sir W— H—'s coach stopped at the door; so he runs down, and comes up again immediately. 'Alas!' says he aloud, 'there's all my mirth spoiled at once; Sir W— has sent his coach for me, and desires to speak with me.' It seems this Sir W— was a gentleman who lived about three miles off, to whom he had spoke on purpose to lend him his chariot for a particular occasion, and had appointed it to call for him, as it did – about three o'clock.

Immediately he calls for his best wig, hat, and sword, and, ordering his man to go to the other place to make his excuse – that was to say, he made an excuse to send his man away – he prepares to go into the coach. As he was going, he stopped awhile, and speaks mightily earnestly to me about his business, and finds an opportunity to say very softly 'Come away, my dear, as soon as ever you can.' I said nothing, but made a curtsey, as if I had done so to what he said in public. In about a quarter of an hour I went out too; I had no dress other than before, except that I had a hood, a mask, a fan, and a pair of gloves in my pocket; so that there was not the least suspicion in the house. He waited for me in

[174]

a back-lane which he knew I must pass by, and the coachman knew whither to go, which was to a certain place, called Mile End, where lived a confidant of his, where we went in, and where was all the convenience in the world to be as wicked as we pleased.

When we were together he began to talk very gravely to me, and to tell me he did not bring me there to betray me; that his passion for me would not suffer him to abuse me; that he resolved to marry me as soon as he came to his estate; that in the meantime, if I would grant his request, he would maintain me very honourably; and made me a thousand protestations of his sincerity and of his affection to me; and that he would never abandon me, and, as I may say, made a thousand more preambles than he need to have done.

However, as he pressed me to speak, I told him I had no reason to question the sincerity of his love to me after so many protestations, but – , and there I stopped, as if I left him to guess the rest. 'But what, my dear?' says he. 'I guess what you mean: what if you should be with child? Is not that it? Why, then,' says he, 'I'll take care of you, and provide for you, and the child too; and that you may see I am not in jest', says he, 'here's an earnest for you,' and with that he pulls out a silk purse with a hundred guineas in it, and gave it me; 'and I'll give you such another,' says he, 'every year till I marry you.'

My colour came and went at the sight of the purse, and with the fire of his proposal together, so that I could not say a word, and he easily perceived it; so, putting the purse into my bosom, I made no more resistance to him, but let him do just what he pleased, and as often as he pleased; and thus I finished my own destruction at once, for from this day, being forsaken of my virtue and my modesty, I had nothing of value left to recommend me, either to God's blessing or man's assistance.

But things did not end here. I went back to the town, did the business he directed me to, and was at home before anybody thought me long. As for my gentleman, he stayed out till late at night, and there was not the least suspicion in the family either on his account or on mine.

We had after this frequent opportunities to repeat our crime, and especially at home, when his mother and the young ladies went abroad a-visiting, which he watched so narrowly as never to miss; knowing always beforehand when they went out, and then failed not to catch me all alone, and securely enough; so that we took our fill of our wicked pleasures for near half-a-year; and yet, which was the most to my satisfaction, I was not with child.

William Blake
1757–1827

The Sick Rose

O Rose, thou art sick!
The invisible worm
That flies in the night,
In the howling storm,

Has found out thy bed
Of crimson joy,
And his dark secret love
Does thy life destroy.

Samuel Richardson
1689–1761

from Clarissa

Clarissa has been tricked into running away from home by the aristocratic Lovelace, as part of his sustained attempt to seduce her. This letter from the heroine to her friend and confidante, Anna, describes the methods he finally uses once Clarissa is under his supposed protection. With the help of two female accomplices masquerading as his aunt and cousin, Lady Betty and Miss Montague, he succeeds in inveigling Clarissa back into the brothel where he lodged her earlier. Under pretence of giving her restoratives, the brothel-keeper Mrs Sinclair and her assistant Dorcas administer incapacitating drugs.

In the midst of these agreeablenesses, the coach came to the door. The pretended Lady Betty besought me to give them my company to their cousin Leeson's. I desired to be excused: yet suspected nothing. She would not be denied. How happy would a visit so condescending make her cousin Leeson! – Her cousin Leeson was not unworthy of my acquaintance: and would take it for the greatest favour in the world.

I objected my dress. But the objection was not admitted. She bespoke a supper of Mrs Moore to be ready at nine.

Mr Lovelace, vile hypocrite, and wicked deceiver! seeing, as he said, my dislike to go, desired her ladyship not to insist upon it.

Fondness for my company was pleaded. She begged me to oblige her: made a motion to help me to my fan herself: and, in short, was so very urgent, that my feet complied against my speech and my mind: and being, in a manner, led to the coach by her, and made to step in first, she followed me: and her pretended niece, and the wretch followed her: and away it drove.

Nothing but the height of affectionate complaisance passed all the way: over and over, what a joy would this unexpected visit give her cousin Leeson! What a pleasure must it be to such a mind as mine, to be able to give so much joy to everybody I came near!

The cruel, the savage seducer (as I have since recollected) was in rapture all the way; but yet such a sort of rapture, as he took visible pains to check.

Hateful villain! how I abhor him! – What mischief must be then in his plotting heart! – What a devoted victim must I be in all their eyes!

Though not pleased, I was nevertheless just then thoughtless of danger; they endeavouring thus to lift me up above all apprehensions of that, and above myself too.

But think, my dear, what a dreadful turn all had upon me, when, through several streets and ways I knew nothing of, the coach slackening its pace, came within sight of the dreadful house of the dreadfullest woman in the world; as she proved to me.

Lord be good unto me! cried the poor fool, looking out of the coach – Mr Lovelace! – Madam! turning to the pretended Lady Betty! – Madam! turning to the niece, my hands and eyes lifted up – Lord be good unto me!

What! What! What! my dear.

He pulled the string – What need to have come this way? said he – But since we are, I will but ask a question – My dearest life, *why* this apprehension?

The coachman stopped: *his* servant, who, with one of hers was behind, alighted – Ask, said he, if I have any letters? Who knows, my dearest creature, turning to me, but we may already have one from the Captain? – We will not go out of the coach! – Fear nothing. – Why so apprehensive? – Oh! these fine spirits! – cried the execrable insulter.

Dreadfully did my heart then misgive me: I was ready to faint. Why this terror, my life? you shall not stir out of the coach – but one question, now the fellow has drove us this way.

Your lady will faint, cried the execrable Lady Betty, turning to him – My dearest Niece! (niece I *will* call you, taking my hand) – we must alight, if you are so ill. – Let us alight – only for a glass of water and hartshorn – indeed we must alight.

No, no, no – I am well – quite well – Won't the man drive on? – I am well – quite well – indeed I am. – *Man*, drive on, putting my head out of the coach – *Man*, drive on! – though my voice was too low to be heard.

The coach stopt at the door. How I trembled!

Dorcas came to the door, on its stopping.

My dearest creature, said the vile man, gasping, as it were for breath, you shall *not* alight – any letters for me, Dorcas?

There are two, sir. And there is a gentleman, Mr Belton, sir, waits for your honour; and has done so above an hour.

I'll just speak to him. Open the door – You sha'n't step out, my dear – a letter perhaps from the Captain already! – You shan't step out, my dear.

I sighed as if my heart would burst.

But we *must* step out, nephew: your lady will faint. Maid, a glass of hartshorn and water! – My dear, you *must* step out – You will faint, child. – We must cut your laces. – (I believe my complexion was all manner of colours by turns.) – Indeed, you must step out, my dear.

He knew, he said, I should be well, the moment the coach drove from the door. I should *not* alight. By his soul, I should not.

Lord, Lord, nephew, Lord, Lord, cousin, both women in a breath, what ado you make about nothing! You *persuade* your lady to be afraid of alighting. – See you not that she is just fainting?

Indeed, Madam, said the vile seducer, my dearest love must not be moved in this point against her will. I beg it may not be insisted upon.

Fiddle-faddle, foolish man – What a pother is here! I guess how it is: you are ashamed to let us see what sort of people you carried your lady among – but do you go out, and speak to your friend, and take your letters.

He stept out; but shut the coach door after him, to oblige me.

The coach may go on, Madam, said I.

The coach *shall* go on, my dear life, said he. – But he gave not, nor intended to give, orders that it should.

Let the coach go on! said I – Mr Lovelace may come after us.

Indeed, my dear, you are ill! – Indeed you must alight – alight but for one quarter of an hour. – Alight but to give orders yourself about your things. Whom can you be afraid of in my company,

[180]

and my niece's; these people must have behaved shockingly to you! Please the Lord, I'll inquire into it! – I'll see what sort of people they are!

Immediately came the old creature to the door. A thousand pardons, dear Madam, stepping to the coach-side, if we have any way offended you – Be pleased, ladies (to the other two), to alight.

Well, my dear, whispered *the* Lady Betty, I now find that a hideous description of a person we never saw is an advantage to them. I thought the woman was a monster – but really she seems tolerable.

I was afraid I should have fallen into fits: but still refused to go out – Man! – Man! – Man! – cried I, gaspingly, my head out of the coach and in, by turns, half a dozen times running, drive on! – Let us go!

My heart misgave me beyond the power of my own accounting for it; for still I did not suspect these women. But the antipathy I had taken to the vile house, and to find myself so near it, when I expected no such matter, with the sight of the old creature, all together made me behave like a distracted person.

The hartshorn and water was brought. The pretended Lady Betty made me drink it. Heaven knows if there were anything else in it!

Besides, said she, whisperingly, I must see what sort of creatures the *nieces* are. Want of delicacy cannot be hid from me. You could not surely, my dear, have this aversion to re-enter a house, for a few minutes, in our company, in which you lodged and boarded several weeks, unless these women could be so presumptuously vile, as my nephew ought not to know.

Out stept the pretended lady; the servant, at her command, having opened the door.

Dearest Madam, said the other to me, let me follow you (for I was next the door). Fear nothing: I will not stir from your presence.

Come, my dear, said the pretended lady, give me your hand; holding out hers. Oblige me this once.

I will bless your footsteps, said the old creature, if once more you honour my house with your presence.

A crowd by this time was gathered about us; but I was too much affected to mind that.

Again the pretended Miss Montague urged me; standing up as ready to go out if I would give her room. – Lord, my dear, said she, who can bear this crowd? – What will people think?

The pretended lady again pressed me, with both her hands held out – Only, my dear, to give orders about your things.

And thus pressed, and gazed at (for then I looked about me), the women so richly dressed, people whispering; in an evil moment, out stepped I, trembling, forced to lean with both my hands (frighted too much for ceremony) on the pretended Lady Betty's arm – Oh! that I had dropped down dead upon the guilty threshold!

We shall stay but a few minutes, my dear! – but a few minutes! said the same specious jilt – out of breath with her joy, as I have since thought, that they had thus triumphed over the unhappy victim!

Come, Mrs Sinclair, I think your name is, show us the way – following her, and leading me. I am very thirsty. You have frighted me, my dear, with your strange fears. I must have tea made, if it can be done in a moment. We have farther to go, Mrs Sinclair, and must return to Hampstead this night.

It shall be ready in a moment, cried the wretch. We have water boiling.

Hasten, then – Come, my dear, to me, as she led me through the passage to the fatal inner house – lean upon me – how you tremble! – how you falter in your steps! – Dearest niece Lovelace (the old wretch being in hearing), why these hurries upon your spirits? – We'll be gone in a minute.

And thus she led the poor sacrifice into the old wretch's too well known parlour.

Never was anybody so gentle, so meek, so low voiced, as the odious woman; drawling out, in a puling accent, all the obliging things she could say: awed, I then thought, by the conscious dignity of a woman of quality; glittering with jewels.

The called-for tea was ready presently.

There was no Mr Belton, I believe: for the wretch went not to anybody, unless it were while we were parleying in the coach. No such person, however, appeared at the tea-table.

I was made to drink two dishes, with milk, complaisantly urged by the pretended ladies helping me each to one. I was stupid to their hands; and when I took the tea, almost choked with vapours; and could hardly swallow.

I thought, *transiently* thought, that the tea, the last dish particularly, had an odd taste. They, on my palating it, observed that the milk was *London milk*; far short in goodness of what they were accustomed to from their own dairies.

I have no doubt that my two dishes, and perhaps my hartshorn, were prepared for me; in which case it was more proper for their purpose, that *they* should help me, than that I should help *myself*. Ill before, I found myself still more and more disordered in my head; a heavy torpid pain increasing fast upon me. But I imputed it to my terror.

Nevertheless, at the pretended lady's motion, I went upstairs, attended by Dorcas; who affected to weep for joy, that she once more saw my *blessed* face; that was the vile creature's word: and immediately I set about taking out some of my clothes, ordering what should be put up, and what sent after me.

While I was thus employed, up came the pretended Lady Betty, in a hurrying way – My dear, you won't be long before you are ready. My nephew is very busy in writing answers to his letters: so, I'll just whip away, and change my dress, and call upon you in an instant.

O Madam! – I *am* ready! I am *now* ready! – You must not leave me here. And down I sunk, affrighted, into a chair.

This instant, this instant, I will return – before you can be ready – before you can have packed up your things – we would not be late – the robbers we have heard of may be out – don't let us be late.

And away she hurried before I could say another word. Her pretended niece went with her, without taking notice to me of her going.

I had no suspicion yet that these women were not indeed the ladies they personated; and I blamed myself for my weak fears. – It cannot *be*, thought I, that *such* ladies will abet treachery against a poor creature they are so fond of. They must undoubtedly *be* the persons they *appear* to be – what folly to doubt it! The air, the dress, the dignity of women of quality. How unworthy of them, and of my charity, concluded I, is this ungenerous shadow of suspicion!

So, recovering my stupefied spirits, as well as they could be recovered (for I was heavier and heavier! and wondered to Dorcas what ailed me, rubbing my eyes, and taking some of her snuff, pinch after pinch, to very little purpose), I pursued my employment: but when that was over, all packed up that I designed to be packed up; and I had nothing to do but to *think*; and found them tarry so long; I thought I should have gone distracted. I shut myself into the chamber that had been mine; I kneeled, I prayed; yet knew not what I prayed for: then ran out again: it was almost dark night, I said: where, where, where was Mr Lovelace?

He came to me, taking no notice at first of my consternation and wildness (what they had given me made me incoherent and wild): All goes well, said he, my dear! – A line from Captain Tomlinson!

All indeed did go well for the villainous project of the most cruel and most villainous of men!

I *demanded* his aunt! – I *demanded* his cousin! – The evening, I said, was closing! – My head was very, *very* bad, I remember I said – and it grew worse and worse.

Terror, however, as yet kept up my spirits; and I insisted upon his going himself to hasten them.

He called his servant. He raved at the *sex* for *their* delay: 'twas well that business of consequence seldom depended upon such parading, unpunctual triflers!

His servant came.

He ordered him to fly to his cousin Leeson's, and to let Lady Betty and his cousin know how uneasy we both were at their delay: adding, of his own accord, desire them, if they don't come instantly, to send their coach, and we will go without them. Tell them I wonder they'll serve me so!

I thought this was considerately and fairly put. But now, indifferent as my head was, I had a little time to consider the man and his behaviour. He terrified me with his looks, and with his violent emotions, as he gazed upon me. Evident *joy-suppressed* emotions, as I have since recollected. His sentences short, and pronounced as if his breath were touched. Never saw I his abominable eyes look as then they looked – Triumph in them! – fierce and wild; and more disagreeable than the women's at the vile house appeared to me when I first saw them: and at times, such a leering, mischief-boding cast! – I would have given the world to have been a hundred miles from him. Yet his behaviour was decent – a decency, however, that I might have seen to be struggled for – for he snatched my hand two or three times, with a vehemence in his grasp that hurt me; speaking words of tenderness through his shut teeth, as it seemed; and let it go with a beggar-voiced humbled accent, like the vile woman's just before; half-inward; yet his words and manner carrying the appearance of strong and almost convulsed passion! – Oh my dear! what mischief was he not then meditating!

I complained once or twice of thirst. My mouth seemed parched. At the time, I supposed that it was my terror (gasping often as I did for breath) that parched up the roof of my mouth. I called for water: some table-beer was brought me: beer, I suppose was a better vehicle (if I were not dosed enough before) for their potions. I told the maid that she knew I seldom tasted malt liquor: yet suspecting nothing of this nature, being extremely thirsty, I drank it, as what came next: and instantly, as it were, found myself much worse than before: as if inebriated, I should fancy: I know not how.

IIis servant was gone twice as long as he needed; and just before his return, came one of the pretended Lady Betty's with a letter for Mr Lovelace.

He sent it up to me. I read it: and then it was that I thought myself a lost creature; it being to put off her going to Hampstead that night, on account of violent fits which Miss Montague was pretended to be seized with; for then immediately came into my head his vile attempt upon me in this house; the revenge that my flight might too probably inspire him with on that occasion, and because of the difficulty I made to forgive him, and to be reconciled to him; his very looks wild and dreadful to me; and the women of the house such as I had more reason than ever, even from the pretended Lady Betty's hint, to be afraid of: all these crowding together in my apprehensive mind, I fell into a kind of phrensy.

I have not remembrance how I was for the time it lasted: but I know that, in my first agitations, I pulled off my head-dress, and tore my ruffles in twenty tatters, and ran to find him out.

When a little recovered, I insisted upon the hint he had given of their coach. But the messenger, he said, had told him that it was sent to fetch a physician, lest his chariot should be put up, or not ready.

I then insisted upon going directly to Lady Betty's lodgings.

Mrs Leeson's was now a crowded house, he said: and as my earnestness could be owing to nothing but groundless apprehension (and oh! what vows, what protestations of his honour, did he then make!) he hoped I would not add to their present concern. Charlotte, indeed, was used to fits, he said, upon any great surprises, whether of joy or grief; and they would hold her for a week together, if not got off in a few hours.

You are an *observer of eyes*, my dear, said the villain; perhaps in secret insult: Saw you not in Miss Montague's, now and then at Hampstead, something wildish? I was afraid for her then. Silence and quiet only do her good: your concern for *her*, and her love for *you*, will but augment the poor girl's disorder, if you should go.

All impatient with grief and apprehension, I still declared myself resolved not to stay in that house till morning. All I had in the world, my rings, my watch, my little money, for a coach; or, if one were not to be got, I would go on foot to Hampstead that night, though I walked it by myself.

A coach was hereupon sent for, or pretended to be sent for. Any price, he said, he would give to oblige me, late as it was; and he would attend me with all his soul. But no coach was to be got.

Let me cut short the rest. I grew worse and worse in my head! now stupid, now raving, now senseless. The vilest of vile women was brought to frighten me. Never was there so horrible a creature as she appeared to me at this time.

I remember I pleaded for mercy. I remember that I said *I would be his* – indeed *I would be his* – to obtain his mercy. But no mercy found I! My strength, my intellects failed me – And then such scenes followed – Oh, my dear, such dreadful scenes! – fits upon fits (faintly indeed and imperfectly remembered) procuring me no compassion – But death was withheld from me. That would have been too great a mercy!

Thus was I tricked and deluded back by blacker hearts of my own sex than I thought there were in the world; who appeared to me to be persons of honour: and, when in his power, thus barbarously was I treated by this villainous man!

I was so senseless, that I dare not aver, that the horrid creatures of the house were personally aiding and abetting: but some visionary remembrances I have of female figures, flitting, as I may say, before my sight: the wretched woman's particularly. But as these confused ideas might be owing to the terror I had conceived of the worse than masculine violence she had been permitted to assume to me, for expressing my abhorrence of her house; and as what I suffered from his barbarity wants not that aggravation; I will say no more on the subject so shocking as this must ever be to my remembrance.

I never saw the personating wretches afterwards. He persisted to the last (dreadfully invoking Heaven as a witness to the truth of his assertion) that they were really and truly the ladies they pretended to be; declaring that they could not take leave of me when they left town, because of the state of senselessness and phrensy I was in. For their intoxicating, or rather stupefying potions, had almost deleterious effects upon my intellects, as I have hinted; insomuch that, for several days together, I was under a strange delirium; now moping, now dozing, now weeping, now raving, now scribbling, tearing what I scribbled as fast as I wrote it: *most* miserable when now and then a ray of reason brought confusedly to my remembrance what I had suffered.

William Shakespeare
1564–1616

---

from Measure for Measure

A room in ANGELO'*s house*

ANG: When I would pray and think, I think and pray
    To several subjects. Heaven hath my empty words;
    Whilst my invention, hearing not my tongue,
    Anchors on Isabel: Heaven in my mouth,
    As if I did but only chew his name;
    And in my heart the strong and swelling evil
    Of my conception. The state, whereon I studied,
    Is like a good thing, being often read,
    Grown fear'd and tedious; yea, my gravity,
    Wherein – let no man hear me – I take pride,
    Could I with boot change for an idle plume,
    Which the air beats for vain. O place, O form,
    How often dost thou with thy case, thy habit,
    Wrench awe from fools, and tie the wiser souls
    To thy false seeming! Blood, thou art blood:
    Let's write good angel on the devil's horn;
    'Tis not the devil's crest.
    (*Enter a* SERVANT.)
                       How now! who's there?
SERV: One Isabel, a sister, desires access to you.
ANG: Teach her the way. O heavens!
    Why does my blood thus muster to my heart,
    Making both it unable for itself,
    And dispossessing all my other parts
    Of necessary fitness?
    So play the foolish throngs with one that swoons;
    Come all to help him, and so stop the air
    By which he should revive: and even so

The general subject to a well-wish'd king
Quit their own part, and in obsequious fondness
Crowd to his presence, where their untaught love
Must needs appear offence.
(*Enter* ISABELLA.)
                                    How now, fair maid?

ISAB: I am come to know your pleasure.

ANG: That you might know it, would much better please me
Than to demand what 'tis. Your brother cannot live.

ISAB: Even so. – Heaven keep your honour!

ANG: Yet may he live awhile; and, it may be,
As long as you or I: yet he must die.

ISAB: Under your sentence?

ANG: Yea.

ISAB: When, I beseech you? that in his reprieve,
Longer or shorter, he may be so fitted
That his soul sicken not.

ANG: Ha! fie, these filthy vices! It were as good
To pardon him that hath from nature stolen
A man already made, as to remit
Their saucy sweetness that do coin heaven's image
In stamps that are forbid: 'tis all as easy
Falsely to take away a life true made,
As to put metal in restrained means
To make a false one.

ISAB: 'Tis set down so in heaven, but not in earth.

ANG: Say you so? then I shall pose you quickly.
Which had you rather, – that the most just law
Now took your brother's life; or, to redeem him,
Give up your body to such sweet uncleanness
As she that he hath stain'd?

ISAB: Sir, believe this,
I had rather give my body than my soul.

ANG: I talk not of your soul: our compell'd sins
Stand more for number than for accompt.

ISAB: How say you?

ANG: Nay, I'll not warrant that; for I can speak
Against the thing I say. Answer to this: –
I, now the voice of the recorded law,

Pronounce a sentence on your brother's life:
Might there not be a charity in sin
To save this brother's life?
ISAB: Please, you to do't,
        I'll take it as a peril to my soul,
        It is no sin at all, but charity.
ANG: Pleased you to do't at peril of your soul,
        Were equal poise of sin and charity.
ISAB: That I do beg his life, if it be sin,
        Heaven let me bear it! you granting of my suit,
        If that be sin, I'll make it my morn prayer
        To have it added to the faults of mine,
        And nothing of your answer.
ANG: Nay, but hear me.
        Your sense pursues not mine: either you are ignorant,
        Or seem so, craftily; and that's not good.
ISAB: Let me be ignorant, and in nothing good,
        But graciously to know I am no better.
ANG: Thus wisdom wishes to appear most bright
        When it doth tax itself; as these black masks
        Proclaim an enshield beauty ten times louder
        Than beauty could, display'd. But mark me;
        To be received plain, I'll speak more gross:
        Your brother is to die.
ISAB: So.
ANG: And his offence is so, as it appears,
        Accountant to the law upon that pain.
ISAB: True
ANG: Admit no other way to save his life, –
        As I subscribe not that, nor any other,
        But in the loss of question, – that you, his sister,
        Finding yourself desired of such a person,
        Whose credit with the judge, or own great place,
        Could fetch your brother from the manacles
        Of the all-building law; and that there were
        No earthly mean to save him, but that either
        You must lay down the treasures of your body
        To this supposed, or else to let him suffer;
        What would you do?

ISAB: As much for my poor brother as myself:
    That is, were I under the terms of death,
    The impression of keen whips I'ld wear as rubies,
    And strip myself to death, as to a bed
    That longing have been sick for, ere I'ld yield
    My body up to shame.
ANG: Then must your brother die.
ISAB: And 'twere the cheaper way:
    Better it were a brother died at once,
    Than that a sister, by redeeming him,
    Should die for ever.
ANG: Were not you, then, as cruel as the sentence
    That you have slander'd so?
ISAB: Ignomy in ransom and free pardon
    Are of two houses: lawful mercy
    Is nothing kin to foul redemption.
ANG: You seem'd of late to make the law a tyrant:
    And rather proved the sliding of your brother
    A merriment than a vice.
ISAB: O, pardon me, my lord; it oft falls out,
    To have what we would have, we speak not what we mean:
    I something do excuse the thing I hate,
    For his advantage that I dearly love.
ANG: We are all frail.
ISAB: Else let my brother die,
    If not a feodary, but only he
    Owe and succeed thy weakness.
ANG: Nay, women are frail too.
ISAB: Ay, as the glasses where they view themselves:
    Which are as easy broke as they make forms.
    Women! – Help Heaven! men their creation mar
    In profiting by them. Nay, call us ten times frail;
    For we are soft as our complexions are,
    And credulous to false prints.
ANG: I think it well:
    And from this testimony of your own sex, –
    Since, I suppose, we are made to be no stronger
    Than faults may shake our frames, – let me be bold; –
    I do arrest your words. Be that you are,

That is, a woman; if you be more, you're none;
If you be one, – as you are well express'd
By all external warrants, – show it now,
By putting on the destined livery.

ISAB: I have no tongue but one: gentle my lord,
Let me entreat you speak the former language.

ANG: Plainly conceive, I love you.

ISAB: My brother did love Juliet,
And you tell me that he shall die for it.

ANG: He shall not, Isabel, if you give me love.

ISAB: I know your virtue hath a license in't,
Which seems a little fouler than it is,
To pluck on others.

ANG: Believe me, on mine honour,
My words express my purpose.

ISAB: Ha! little honour to be much believed,
And most pernicious purpose! – Seeming, seeming! –
I will proclaim thee, Angelo; look for't:
Sign me a present pardon for my brother,
Or with an outstretch'd throat I'll tell the world aloud
What man thou art.

ANG: Who will believe thee, Isabel?
My unsoil'd name, the austereness of my life,
My vouch against you, and my place i' the state,
Will so your accusation overweigh,
That you shall stifle in your own report,
And smell of calumny. I have begun;
And now I give my sensual race the rein:
Fit thy consent to my sharp appetite;
Lay by all nicety and prolixious blushes,
That banish what they sue for; redeem thy brother
By yielding up thy body to my will;
Or else he must not only die the death,
But thy unkindness shall his death draw out
To lingering sufferance. Answer me to-morrow,
Or, by the affection that now guides me most,
I'll prove a tyrant to him. As for you,
Say what you can, my false o'erweighs your true. (*Exit.*)

ISAB: To whom should I complain? Did I tell this.

Who would believe me? O perilous mouths,
That bear in them one and the self-same tongue,
Either of condemnation or approof;
Bidding the law make court'sy to their will;
Hooking both right and wrong to the appetite,
To follow as it draws! I'll to my brother:
Though he hath fall'n by prompture of the blood,
Yet hath he in him such a mind of honour,
That, had he twenty heads to tender down
On twenty bloody blocks, he'ld yield them up,
Before his sister should her body stoop
To such abhorr'd pollution.
Then, Isabel, live chaste, and, brother, die:
More than our brother is our chastity.
I'll tell him yet of Angelo's request,
And fit his mind to death, for his soul's rest. (*Exit.*)

Matthew G. Lewis
1775–1818

from The Monk

Ambrosio is a Capuchin abbot who is reputed to be a saint. Matilda has gained access to his abbey by disguising herself as the novice, Rosario.

Ambrosio did not find himself inclined to sleep; he opened his casement, and gazed upon the moon-beams as they played upon the small stream whose waters bathed the walls of the monastery. The coolness of the night breeze, and tranquillity of the hour, inspired the friar's mind with sadness; he thought upon Matilda's beauty and affection; upon the pleasures which he might have shared with her, had he not been restrained by monastic fetters. He reflected that, unsustained by hope, her love for him could not long exist; that doubtless she would succeed in extinguishing her passion, and seek for happiness in the arms of one more fortunate. He shuddered at the void which her absence would leave in his bosom; he looked with disgust on the monotony of a convent, and breathed a sigh towards that world from which he was for ever separated. Such were the reflections which a loud knocking at his door interrupted. The bell of the church had already struck two. The abbot hastened to enquire the cause of this disturbance. He opened the door of his cell, and a lay-brother entered, whose looks declared his hurry and confusion.

'Hasten, reverend father!' said he, 'hasten to the young Rosario: he earnestly requests to see you; he lies at the point of death.'

'Gracious God! where is father Pablos? Why is he not with him? Oh! I fear, I fear – '

'Father Pablos has seen him, but his art can do nothing. He says that he suspects the youth to be poisoned.'

'Poisoned? Oh! the unfortunate! It is then as I suspected! But let me not lose a moment; perhaps it may yet be time to save her.'

He said, and flew towards the cell of the novice. Several monks were already in the chamber; father Pablos was one of them, and held a medicine in his hand, which he was endeavouring to persuade Rosario to swallow. The others were employed in admiring the patient's divine countenance, which they now saw for the first time. She looked lovelier than ever; she was no longer pale or languid; a bright glow had spread itself over her cheeks; her eyes sparkled with a serene delight, and her countenance was expressive of confidence and resignation.

'Oh! torment me no more!' was she saying to Pablos, when the terrified abbot rushed hastily into the cell; 'my disease is far beyond the reach of your skill, and I wish not to be cured of it.' Then perceiving Ambrosio – 'Ah, 'tis he!' she cried; 'I see him once again before we part for ever! Leave me, my brethren; much have I to tell this holy man in private.'

The monks retired immediately, and Matilda and the abbot remained together.

'What have you done, imprudent woman?' exclaimed the latter, as soon as they were left alone: 'tell me; are my suspicions just? Am I indeed to lose you? Has your own hand been the instrument of your destruction?'

She smiled, and grasped his hand.

'In what have I been imprudent, father? I have sacrificed a pebble, and saved a diamond. My death preserves a life valuable to the world, and more dear to me than my own. – Yes, father, I am poisoned; but know, that the poison once circulated in your veins.'

'Matilda!'

'What I tell you I resolved never to discover to you but on the bed of death; that moment is now arrived. You cannot have forgotten the day already, when your life was endangered by the bite of a cientipedoro. The physician gave you over, declaring himself ignorant how to extract the venom. I knew but of one means, and hesitated not a moment to employ it. I was left alone with you; you slept; I loosened the bandage from your hand; I kissed the wound, and drew out the poison with my lips. The effect has been more sudden than I expected. I feel death at my heart; yet an hour, and I shall be in a better world.'

'Almighty God!' exclaimed the abbot, and sunk almost lifeless upon the bed.

After a few minutes he again raised himself up suddenly, and gazed upon Matilda with all the wildness of despair.

'And you have sacrificed yourself for me! You die, and die to preserve Ambrosio! And is there indeed no remedy, Matilda? And is there indeed no hope? Speak to me, oh! speak to me! Tell me that you have still the means of life!'

'Be comforted, my only friend! Yes, I have still the means of life in my power; but it is a means which I dare not employ; it is dangerous; it is dreadful! Life would be purchased at too dear a rate, – unless it were permitted me to live for you.'

'Then live for me, Matilda; for me and gratitude!' – (He caught her hand, and pressed it rapturously to his lips.) – 'Remember our late conversations; I now consent to every thing. Remember in what lively colours you described the union of souls; be it ours to realize those ideas. Let us forget the distinctions of sex, despise the world's prejudices, and only consider each other as brother and friend. Live then, Matilda, oh! live for me!'

'Ambrosio, it must not be. When I thought thus, I deceived both you and myself: either I must die at present, or expire by the lingering torments of unsatisfied desire. Oh! since we last conversed together, a dreadful veil has been rent from before my eyes. I love you no longer with the devotion which is paid to a saint; I prize you no more for the virtues of your soul; I lust for the enjoyment of your person. The woman reigns in my bosom, and I am become a prey to the wildest of passions. Away with friendship! 'tis a cold unfeeling word: my bosom burns with love, with unutterable love, and love must be its return. Tremble then, Ambrosio, tremble to succeed in your prayers. If I live, your truth, your reputation, your reward of a life past in sufferings, all that you value, is irretrievably lost. I shall no longer be able to combat my passions, shall seize every opportunity to excite your desires, and labour to effect your dishonour and my own. No, no, Ambrosio, I must not live; I am convinced with every moment that I have but one alternative; I feel with every heart-throb, that I must enjoy you or die.'

'Amazement! Matilda! Can it be you who speak to me?'

He made a movement as if to quit his seat. She uttered a loud shriek, and, raising herself half out of the bed, threw her arms round the friar to detain him.

'Oh! do not leave me! Listen to my errors with compassion: in a few hours I shall be no more: yet a little, and I am free from this disgraceful passion.'

'Wretched woman, what can I say to you? I cannot – I must not – But live, Matilda! oh, live!'

'You do not reflect on what you ask. What? live to plunge myself in infamy? to become the agent of hell? to work the destruction both of you and of myself? Feel this heart, father.'

She took his hand. Confused, embarrassed, and fascinated, he withdrew it not, and felt her heart throb under it.

'Feel this heart, father! It is yet the seat of honour, truth, and chastity: if it beats tomorrow, it must fall a prey to the blackest crimes. Oh, let me then die today! Let me die while I yet deserve the tears of the virtuous. Thus will I expire!' – (She reclined her head upon his shoulder; her golden hair poured itself over his chest.) – 'Folded in your arms, I shall sink to sleep; your hand shall close my eyes for ever, and your lips receive my dying breath. And will you not sometimes think of me? Will you not sometimes shed a tear upon my tomb? Oh, yes, yes, yes! that kiss is my assurance.'

The hour was night. All was silence around. The faint beams of a solitary lamp darted upon Matilda's figure, and shed through the chamber a dim, mysterious light. No prying eye or curious ear was near the lovers: nothing was heard but Matilda's melodious accents. Ambrosio was in the full vigour of manhood; he saw before him a young and beautiful woman, the preserver of his life, the adorer of his person; and whom affection for him had reduced to the brink of the grave. He sat upon her bed; his hand rested upon her bosom; her head reclined voluptuously upon his breast. Who then can wonder if he yielded to the temptation? Drunk with desire, he pressed his lips to those which sought them; his kisses vied with Matilda's in warmth and passion: he clasped her rapturously in his arms; he forgot his vows, his sanctity, and his fame; he remembered nothing but the pleasure and opportunity.

'Ambrosio! Oh, my Ambrosio!' sighed Matilda.

'Thine, ever thine,' murmured the friar, and sunk upon her bosom.

Sara Maitland
1949–

from Virgin Territory

Karen is a lesbian and a feminist who lives in a communal house with several other women, including Sybil, whose car she has borrowed for the outing described here. She has fallen in love with Anna – as yet unaware of Karen's feelings – an American nun who has come from South America to London to test her vocation.

On the motorway there was little conversation, Sybil's car too engine-noisy for comfort, but fat white clouds bounced along beside them and the downs as they approached them seemed clean and curvaceous. Anna thought it innocent country, neither claustrophobic nor threatening. She was at ease suddenly in the brightness and placed a new faith in Karen who would know the way, tell her what to see and instruct her in its meaning. Avebury itself was too full of tourists to be personal but the presence of the monument was undeniable; a strange dark magic from too far away to be imagined. The ancient standing stones and laborious ditchings were baffling and demanded too much thought, too much imaginative effort to make sense of. They were touched and interested, but in their heads alone. Karen felt disappointed, as though her spell had not worked somehow; but then she realized that she was relaxed. Her disproportionate expectations for the day were evaporated and she felt comfortable and pleased.

Silbury Hill was better, rising beside the main road with that abrupt authority. Breast and belly and so much extraordinary work for so apparently little purpose. Karen wanted to climb to the top and was furious with the barbed wire prevention; furious that other people's desires should so match hers that she could not be allowed to fulfil them. But then they drove on and had lunch in a pub, and everything became lovely, happy, carefree, sweet, fun. After lunch they drove on through Swindon and out on to the tiny road to Uffington. There was no hurry, the summer afternoon long long and lazy, forever, endless and easy. They walked from the car park across the timeless hill fort and the wind curling over the distant sunlit fields caught them playfully and they felt free. They broke out of the circle and the valley lay below them, serene and stunning. Tranquil, amazing, a free gift. Karen led them so that they came upon the chalk horse from above, directly over its face, and there was no way to make sense of the stencilled shapes. It took a proper time, walking round, backing off, speculating and calculating; an effort of imagination commensurate with the reward.

And then suddenly the horse was whole and galloping free across the hillside and of course the stencil was the true way to make it move so and so freely. It was a gift but not free like the valley below, a gift from Karen to Anna, a gift they had both worked into fullness. They were moved by the horse and sat above its ears on the crisp grass. Now the valley was changed by their poise over it: the drop foreshortened, the unexpected humped shape of St George's Hill flattened off by the angle, and it was too easy to believe that here he had fought the great white dragon and conquered it. Further below them the steep-sided rough hill-face met the upreaching cultivated curves of the field below at the point that was exactly beautiful. They sat in peace and thought their thoughts. Looking down from there Anna entered into a silence that she had not known for a very long time; her head was swept clean. She heard no voices and wrestled with no shadows, except the distant moving ones of the friendly clouds. The roads and the railway line ran neatly horizontal across the landscape and were there for balance not intrusion. Karen noticed that all her impatience was gone; she would wait forever if the waiting was like this; there was no hurry, there was no driving need, just sun and wind and Anna near her, clear and calm. Further away they could hear voices, the area was not empty of people, but they felt not isolated but uninterrupted. And miraculously, without warning or expectation, there was a hang-glider sailing underneath them, wings like a bird but magically below them.

'God, I would like to do that,' Karen said, delighted, as though it were something laid on just for her and Anna, a treat from the heavens. Now there was one there were more than one; in differing patterns four or five garish giant birds moving through the air somehow lazily. Flying, not free but visibly dependent on the invisible winds. They watched for at least an hour, wishing joyful flying and soft landings on each of the strange graceful craft. When they finally stood up to leave they were holding hands and neither of them had noticed when or how it had happened. They were as innocent as children and they ran like children across the steep side of the hill and back to the car, laughing, panting, racing and competing.

They drove back through the gently folding evening and were at peace, relaxing their bodies in the noisy car. Karen stole a glance at Anna on the motorway and saw a sweetness in her face which reminded her of that first smile which had been the basis of their friendship. Sod it, she thought, what does it matter? We're friends and that is good. Not all she had wanted, not the whole; but so much, so good and so comfortable. She would never be free of her, she thought; Anna had called out a tender passion in her that would never be dissipated, never abandoned. Everything before had been half; and this was the other half. All it needed was patience. Sybil simply had not understood. No one but she could understand what Anna needed: time to find a way back to herself. She could wait for ever and be happy while she waited; she was strong and tough and solid and she could wait out Anna's fears, Anna's doubts, Anna's slowness.

Anna barely thought at all. Her head was soothed and sleepy from the sunshine and the wind. She saw Kate now flying free, floating on the shoulder of the wind. She saw Karen as a friend. She saw the curved movement of the white horse, a muscle from the beginning of history, linked somehow to all those other ancient reminders that people thought in other ways and of other Gods, joined to the lost cathedrals of the jungle, and the strange harsh temples of the Andes' Indians. She saw Mary lean into Elizabeth's arms and the two women empowered by each other singing the songs of freedom. Visual images were enough. She was locked inside the car, the outside could not reach her, a lazy easy movement. She would have liked the journey to go on forever, never to have to move from this noisy peaceful silence, the rumbling of the motor simpler than any other rhythm, and Karen, dear Karen, her hands long and eager, fine-boned on the steering wheel. And Karen had given her this day as a joy gift. She owed Karen so much, loved her so much, and the spaces which would be destitute without her were full and running over with sweet oil and delight.

It was dark by the time they got back. Karen drove beyond the convent doors, looking for a parking space, a place to say goodnight, to part without haste, to bring the day to a gentle end. They sat for a moment or two as though waiting for an excuse to present itself, some reason to prolong the pleasure of the day. Then Anna turned to thank Karen for the whole loveliness of it all. Moved by gratitude and by something in Karen's face she leaned forward to give her a kiss, casual, affectionate. When their cheeks touched something exploded, the trumpets sounded and the wall in Anna came tumbling down. Without conspiracy or forethought they were wrapped around each other and Anna knew blindingly what she had been waiting for. She felt no surprise and without consciousness she moved into the embrace; unthinking, unquestioning, her lips sought Karen's greedily. Then they were kissing, tongues both tentative and eager; lips and faces and ears and eyes, eyes especially thought Anna with delight who had never imagined such a thing; and her tongue curled delicately along Karen's eyelids, and how could she not have known the unbelievable excitement and sweetness and need to be nearer, closer, inner. And desire, exploding desire and greed and driving wants. She could not stop now, did not want to stop and did not need to think where this was going. She was perfectly and uniquely in the present, there was no point of reference outside, nor anything but enormous melting and longing and demanding, which had no name or description except Karen, and to kiss and kiss and be closer.

Karen felt more control; she was intensely suprised; but there was no reason, she knew no reason to hesitate or to hold back. She had known always that they would come to this place and it was not necessary to know the times and the seasons. She had a tiny regret, a little hovering sorrow, because she had wanted to take this initiative, she had fantasized that it would be she who would have the power and she would surrender it to make things tender and sweet and easy for Anna. But now she knew that there was little careful tenderness here; she tasted Anna's lust and her own swelled to meet it. Delicately, ready to make more space if Anna seemed to need it she reached for Anna's breast; it was firm and pleased through the shirt and she, with the skill of practice, undid enough buttons and reached for Anna's skin. She found her nipple; she was not gentle now, the time for gentleness and withdrawal had suddenly passed. How had she ever imagined that Anna was not sexually responsive. Her own desire, disciplined and controlled for too long, leapt out of its hiding place and devoured the two of them. (Sybil was right she thought, they could have done this weeks ago, and it would have been more convenient somewhere else though the car was adequate.) And she knew that she was physically stronger than Anna and that delighted some part of her. She was here with Anna and Anna desired her, and desired her desire. She wanted her. Her head was filled with glory and triumph, with joy, with joy, with the joy of being wanted so hungrily. The hunger of twenty years and all given to her now with passion and enthusiasm. And indeed skill. That might have surprised her, and later was to surprise her very much, but then it was just a part of the explosion and the victory.

Anna was lost. She had plunged too far, too fast; it was too like the great fall that she had feared for too long; this was the dreaded falling into the depths of chasm where she would be smashed and destroyed. She was panicked suddenly and pulled her head away. But then the air was too cold and the distance unbearable and she had to go back. The wave of terror subsided, but she knew that it was there. She needed, she had to, she must get nearer, nearer to Karen, to be enclosed there in her, lost within her before the terror could find her out. But that was too near and too much and too much, and between the terror of loss and distance and the terror of need and openness she was battered. Her hands discovered new places and those places in herself cried out for Karen. She tried to find something, something to say, and she attempted to laugh and said, 'It is the jungle, it's the great jungle swamp.' But she ought not to have spoken, because words were the possession of the Fathers, and in using them she was dragged back into their power. They crashed in on the sides of the car. She could not. Too dangerous. She could not. Too wonderful. It was all too much. If she went any further here she would never get back again: they would eat her, destroy her, break her, no she was already broken, but they would smash her bones and grind them between the thighs of the high mountains. The storms that had threatened the Mother House when she was there before had been held at bay by the ghosts of dead virgins. But now there were no virgins and no death, no propitiation to offer them.

They will kill her.

Karen experienced her fear as excitement, and as mounting towards somewhere else. She said, 'For God's sake, dearest, let's go home. Let's go somewhere we can have a bed.'

The fear took over. Anna jolted from her arms as though struck by an electric current. Quite deliberately, although she did not know why, she banged her forehead ferociously, dangerously hard against the windscreen of the car. Karen reached for her, confused, alarmed. The pain devoured all of Anna. She banged her head again. Then she did not need to repeat it; the Fathers took her by the scruff of the neck and pounded her against the glass until her teeth shook. The Fathers took over her physical coordination and they took over her voice. She was their victim.

'I have to go in now. Thank you for the day.'

Even Anna knew it was unforgivable. It was not acceptable. But she did not know what else to do; trapped between the two terrors, the terror of the fury of the Fathers and the terror of the delight of her desire.

Karen was pale with shock. 'You can't.'

'I can. I don't have to make love to you. It's not obligatory.'

'No, it isn't, you're right, it fucking isn't. But you do have to follow it through. You can't set up something like this, you can't want it as much as you want it, and set up that wanting in me, and then just walk out. You bloody can't.'

She tried to calm down, tried to put a brake on her anger, 'Look Anna please, please just come home. You don't have to do anything. Just don't leave me, don't walk out on me like this. Come home and talk to me, be with me please.'

Anna said, 'They'll kill me.' She was pleading with Karen, but Karen could not hear her now, it was too late to ask for Karen's tenderness. And she could not understand what Anna was talking about; she assumed that she meant the nuns behind the convent door, so she said, 'Oh don't be silly; they can't hurt you.'

But Anna knew that this was not true. There was no escape. If she gave even a tiny inch to Karen now, if she consented to Karen, if she consented to herself, they would kill her, they would carry her off to their dungeons and torture her. She was a witch and she knew what they did to witches, the Fathers. They tortured witches until they were unable to stand, to talk, to think, and then, when all that was left was the reality of pain, they took them out into a public square and burned them alive. Alive she would smell her own cooking flesh and her soul would be damned for all eternity to that burning, burning, burning. For if she gave herself to Karen she would not be able to repent; that she knew.

She could not even speak, locked into her fear, her pain and the physical effort of moving her heavy body away from Karen. It would break her, that effort to move away. She would have cried out from the strain except that the Fathers might think she was asking Karen to help her. The desire and the fear, the sex and the violence were too close, too near each other. She could not have one without the other, it was not permitted. She would have to do without. She might not even look at Karen, she must drag her broken body away from the only waterhole and crawl out into the desert to die like all sick animals. She had no choice.

But she knew that this was not true. She had a choice; she could defy the Fathers and she would be free of them forever, but there would be nothing left. She would always have to live without their rewards and their comforts. She could not live without the power that could control her, could discipline her, make her behave. She did not dare; she did not dare take the risk, make the leap. She held her body so rigid that to Karen it looked hard, uncaring. She must not even let Karen see how painful the choices were; she must not see the confusion and the melting longing. The Fathers would not tolerate even that.

Pleading, begging, needing, Karen said, 'Anna please. Please don't go. I love you.' She had not said that for fifteen years; she had never said it as one adult to another. Anna could not bear it. Karen's needs and submerged angers were yet another threat, another force that would destroy her. If she listened to them she would die. She opened the car door and stood up. The effort made her walk as though with decision. Karen exploded with wrath. She switched on the car engine. For one delightful moment, in colours of scarlet and purple, she thought that she would drive up on to the pavement and run Anna down and kill her. In fear she saw her own fist swinging back to hit Sybil; this bloody nun had broken her, had stolen her fine high courage, and all her self-respect. She had been reduced to violence and pathetic passivity. As Anna moved towards the door of the convent, Karen rolled down the window of the car and shouted, deafening the blank windows of the night-time street, 'Go fuck yourself, you stupid bitch. It's all you want to do anyway.' She gunned the engine and drove off towards Hackney ferociously. At least she would be the one to do the leaving.

Anna collapsed, hanging against the door, weak and battered.

The Fathers found her there, their fangs tore into her. The soft damp place between her legs, marinated and ready for Karen, gave their teeth a sweet meal. Her skin was all open and vulnerable for their whips to scourge. They no longer wasted breath on speech. She stumbled into the still, virginal house where the prim and holy sisters slept undisturbed. She cringed past the chapel which she did not dare to enter and sought the privacy of her burrow. But there, with their lone prisoner kept so long in this isolation cell, weakened by sensory deprivation, she was at their mercy. They were not grateful that she had stopped and left Karen to her own misery; in their opinion she had already gone too far in her desire. They would break her and punish her and she would thank them for the pain and the humiliation. She was to be grateful for the punishment and adore them for the pain. They laughed at her without amusement and without pity as she took Karen's parting advice and hated herself and Karen for it. She submitted herself to their rigours; all alone she learned just how closely the sweetness of orgasm and the violence of self-disgust could entangle themselves, and she fell not so much into sleep as into unconsciousness, her body wracked by pain, electrocuted by lust, whipped and pierced and penetrated by the Fathers, flagellated by her own guilt.

Anon
1828

---

from The Lustful Turk

The narrator Emily Barlow, on a voyage from Portsmouth to Gibraltar with her maid Eliza, has been captured by Moorish pirates and sold into the harem of the Dey of Algiers.

No sooner were the Captain and Eliza withdrawn than the Dey rose from the couch, walking leisurely towards me, and laid hold of my hand which trembled in his grasp. After considering a few moments, he chucked me under the chin, and said in good English, that Mahomet had been kind in blessing him with so fair a slave as myself. I was not much surprised to hear the Dey speak English, the Captain having spoken it so well, but the terror his address gave me cannot be described, and indeed good reason I had for my apprehensions. Directly he had spoken, he was leading me towards the couch, but I instantaneously drew back, on which without further ceremony he caught me round the waist, and spite of the resistance I made, forced me to it; then seating himself he drew me to him, and forced me to seat myself upon his knees. If it had been in my power to have resisted, the excess of my confusion alone would have prevented my throwing any effectual obstacle in the way of his proceedings. Directly he had got me thus he threw one of his arms round my neck, and drew my lips to his, closing my mouth with his audacious kisses. Whilst his lips were as it were glued to mine, he forced his tongue into my mouth in a manner which created a sensation it is quite impossible to describe. It was the first liberty of the kind I ever sustained. You may guess the shock it at first gave me, but you will scarcely credit it when I own that my indignation was not of long continuance. Nature, too powerful nature, had become alarmed and assisted his lascivious proceedings, conveying his kisses, brutal as they were, to the inmost recesses of my heart. On a sudden new and wild sensations blended with my shame and rage, which exerted themselves but faintly; in fact, Silvia, in a few short moments his kisses and his tongue threw my senses into a complete tumult; an unknown fire rushed through every part of me, hurried on by a strange pleasure; all my loud cries dwindled into gentle sighs, and spite of my inward rage and grief, I could not resist. So wanting strength for self-defence, I could only bewail my situation. I told you he had me on his knees, with one of his arms round my neck – finding how little I resisted, and having me thus with our lips joined, his other hand he suddenly thrust under my petticoats. Aroused by this vital insult, I strove to break from his arms, but it was of no use, he held me firm, my cries and reproaches he heeded not! If by my struggles I contrived to free my lips, they were quickly regained again; thus with his hand and lips he kept me in the greatest disorder, whilst in proportion as it increased I felt my fury and strength diminish; at last a dizzy sensation seized on every sense. I felt his hand rapidly divide my thighs, and quickly one of his fingers penetrated that place which God knows, no male hand had ever before touched. If anything was wanting to complete my confusion, it was the thrilling sensation I felt, caused by the touches of his finger. What a dreadful moment was this for my virtue! With all the highest notions of the charms of that dear innocence which I was doomed to be so soon deprived of, dreading how strange then it was that pleasure should overcome with such fear about me. Why did this not instantly snatch me from the pleasure? I wished some help would come to save me from the danger, but had no sooner formed the wish, than a kiss, and his finger created a contrary emotion, and each following kiss grew more and more pleasing, till at last I almost wished nothing might oppose my absolute defeat. In blushing at what I felt, I blush to write, I longed to feel more. Without an idea what I panted for could be, I eagerly awaited the instruction until the impetuous ardour began to be too powerful for the senses.

Finding that I made no attempt to withdraw my lips from his thrilling pleasure, his arm which was around my neck he removed to my waist. Being thus drawn by it more strongly to his bosom, his right arm became closely confined between his body and mine, my hand being placed and held firmly between his thighs. Whilst in this position, I felt something beneath his clothes gradually enlarging and moving against my hand; from the length I felt against my arm, I judged it to be very long and thick also. If I had wished to remove my hand from its position I could not; and so wonderful was the fascination I felt from the mere touch of this unknown object, I think I could not have removed my hand had it been perfectly at liberty. Without knowing what it was, every throb created in me a tremor unaccountable. I little dreamed the dreadful anguish I was doomed to experience by that which my hand was warming and raising to life.

By this time the Dey had satisfied himself of my being a virgin. Sunk as I was in every soft idea, still I had not been able to silence the unfortunate monitor within my breast, who though hitherto unsuccessful was yet reproaching me for my weakness. The Dey fully perceiving the impression he had made, resolved to take immediate advantage of it. But how shall I describe what I still blush to think of – but it must be done – he withdrew his hand from between my thighs, forced me on my back on the couch, and in an instant turned up my clothes above my navel. Thus all my secret charms became exposed to his view. Exhausted as I was and lost in desire, I could make no further resistance; his hands quickly divided my thighs and he got between them. During my struggles my neckerchief had become loose and disordered; he now entirely removed it, leaving my neck and breast quite bare.

Although I could scarcely keep my eyes open from the tumult of my senses, still I could not help observing as he was on his knees between my thighs that he was divesting himself of his lower garments before he laid on me. For the first time in my life I caught a view of that terrible instrument, that fatal foe to virginity. With unutterable sensations I felt his naked glowing body join mine, again my lips were glued to his, softening me to ruin with his inflamed suctions. In a delirium little short of pleasure, panting with desire I waited my coming fate. I really think if at this moment he had committed my seduction, I should not have regretted my loss of virtue – but no, it was decreed on being deprived of my innocence I should be entirely free of all those soft desires he had so powerfully excited, and that I should suffer during my defloration every anguish a maid can feel, personal as well as mental. But to my unfortunate tale. The Dey had properly fixed himself to do that which I ought but most certainly at the moment did not dread. No, not even as I felt his daring hand fixing the head of his terrible instrument where his lascivious fingers had so potently assisted in reducing me to my then passive state, I own I felt it even with pleasure stiffly distending my until that moment untouched modesty. But on the very instant when I had willingly resigned everything to what I then considered my fixed destiny, his eyes, whose lustre and expression I could scarcely sustain the sight of, on a sudden were filled with languor. He seemed as it were abashed, and kissing me with less violence, he grew by degrees even weaker than myself: suddenly I felt my thighs overflowed by something warm that spurted in torrents from his instrument, and at last he sunk in my arms in a kind of trance.

William Wordsworth
1770–1850

The Thorn

'There is a Thorn – it looks so old,
In truth, you'd find it hard to say
How it could ever have been young,
It looks so old and grey.
Not higher than a two years' child
It stands erect, this aged Thorn;
No leaves it has, no prickly points;
It is a mass of knotted joints,
A wretched thing forlorn.
It stands erect, and like a stone
With lichens is it overgrown.

'Like rock or stone, it is o'ergrown,
With lichens to the very top,
And hung with heavy tufts of moss,
A melancholy crop:
Up from the earth these mosses creep,
And this poor Thorn they clasp it round
So close, you'd say that they are bent
With plain and manifest intent
To drag it to the ground;
And all have joined in one endeavour
To bury this poor Thorn for ever.

'High on a mountain's highest ridge,
Where oft the stormy winter gale
Cuts like a scythe, while through the clouds
It sweeps from vale to vale;
Not five yards from the mountain path,
This Thorn you on your left espy;
And to the left, three yards beyond,
You see a little muddy pond
Of water – never dry,
Though but of compass small, and bare
To thirsty suns and parching air.

'And, close beside this aged Thorn,
There is a fresh and lovely sight,
A beauteous heap, a hill of moss,
Just half a foot in height.
All lovely colours there you see,
All colours that were ever seen;
And mossy network too is there,
As if by hand of lady fair
The work had woven been;
And cups, the darlings of the eye,
So deep is their vermilion dye.

'Ah me! what lovely tints are there
Of olive green and scarlet bright,
In spikes, in branches, and in stars,
Green, red, and pearly white!
This heap of earth o'ergrown with moss,
Which close beside the Thorn you see,
So fresh in all its beauteous dyes,
Is like an infant's grave in size,
As like as like can be:
But never, never any where,
An infant's grave was half so fair.

'Now would you see this aged Thorn,
This pond, and beauteous hill of moss,
You must take care and choose your time
The mountain when to cross.
For oft there sits between the heap,
So like an infant's grave in size,
And that same pond of which I spoke,
A Woman in a scarlet cloak,
And to herself she cries,
"Oh misery! oh misery!
Oh woe is me! oh misery!"

'At all times of the day and night
This wretched Woman thither goes;
And she is known to every star,
And every wind that blows;
And there, beside the Thorn, she sits
When the blue daylight's in the skies,
And when the whirlwind's on the hill,
Or frosty air is keen and still,
And to herself she cries,
"Oh misery! oh misery!
Oh woe is me! oh misery!" '

'Now wherefore, thus, by day and night,
In rain, in tempest, and in snow,
Thus to the dreary mountain-top
Does this poor Woman go?
And why sits she beside the Thorn
When the blue daylight's in the sky
Or when the whirlwind's on the hill,
Or frosty air is keen and still,
And wherefore does she cry? —
O wherefore? wherefore? tell me why
Does she repeat that doleful cry?'

'I cannot tell; I wish I could;
For the true reason no one knows:
But would you gladly view the spot,
The spot to which she goes;
The hillock like an infant's grave,
The pond – and Thorn, so old and grey;
Pass by her door – 'tis seldom shut –
And if you see her in her hut –
Then to the spot away!
I never heard of such as dare
Approach the spot when she is there.'

'But wherefore to the mountain-top
Can this unhappy Woman go,
Whatever star is in the skies,
Whatever wind may blow?'
'Full twenty years are past and gone
Since she (her name is Martha Ray)
Gave with a maiden's true good-will
Her company to Stephen Hill;
And she was blithe and gay,
While friends and kindred all approved
Of him whom tenderly she loved.

'And they had fixed the wedding day,
The morning that must wed them both;
But Stephen to another Maid
Had sworn another oath;
And, with this other Maid, to church
Unthinking Stephen went –
Poor Martha! on that woeful day
A pang of pitiless dismay
Into her soul was sent;
A fire was kindled in her breast,
Which might not burn itself to rest.

'They say, full six months after this,
While yet the summer leaves were green,
She to the mountain-top would go,
And there was often seen.
What could she seek? – or wish to hide?
Her state to any eye was plain;
She was with child, and she was mad;
Yet often was she sober sad
From her exceeding pain.
O guilty Father – would that death
Had saved him from that breach of faith!

'Sad case for such a brain to hold
Communion with a stirring child!
Sad case, as you may think, for one
Who had a brain so wild!
Last Christmas-eve we talked of this,
And grey-haired Wilfred of the glen
Held that the unborn infant wrought
About its mother's heart, and brought
Her senses back again:
And, when at last her time drew near,
Her looks were calm, her senses clear.

'More know I not, I wish I did,
And it should all be told to you;
For what became of this poor child
No mortal ever knew;
Nay – if a child to her was born
No earthly tongue could ever tell;
And if 'twas born alive or dead,
Far less could this with proof be said;
But some remember well
That Martha Ray about this time
Would up the mountain often climb.

'And all that winter, when at night
The wind blew from the mountain-peak,
'Twas worth your while, though in the dark,
The churchyard path to seek:
For many a time and oft were heard
Cries coming from the mountain head:
Some plainly living voices were;
And others, I've heard many swear,
Were voices of the dead:
I cannot think, whate'er they say,
They had to do with Martha Ray.

'But that she goes to this old Thorn,
The Thorn which I described to you,
And there sits in a scarlet cloak,
I will be sworn is true.
For one day with my telescope,
To view the ocean wide and bright,
When to this country first I came,
Ere I had heard of Martha's name,
I climbed the mountain's height: –
A storm came on, and I could see
No object higher than my knee.

''Twas mist and rain, and storm and rain:
No screen, no fence could I discover;
And then the wind! in sooth, it was
A wind full ten times over.
I looked around, I thought I saw
A jutting crag, – and off I ran,
Head-foremost, through the driving rain,
The shelter of the crag to gain;
And, as I am a man,
Instead of jutting crag I found
A Woman seated on the ground.

'I did not speak – I saw her face;
Her face! – it was enough for me;
I turned about and heard her cry,
"Oh misery! oh misery!"
And there she sits, until the moon
Through half the clear blue sky will go;
And when the little breezes make
The waters of the pond to shake,
As all the country know,
She shudders, and you hear her cry,
"Oh misery! oh misery!" '

'But what's the Thorn? and what the pond?
And what the hill of moss to her?
And what the creeping breeze that comes
The little pond to stir?'
'I cannot tell; but some will say
She hanged her baby on the tree;
Some say she drowned it in the pond,
Which is a little step beyond:
But all and each agree,
The little Babe was buried there,
Beneath that hill of moss so fair.

'I've heard, the moss is spotted red
With drops of that poor infant's blood;
But kill a new-born infant thus,
I do not think she could!
Some say if to the pond you go,
And fix on it a steady view,
The shadow of a babe you trace,
A baby and a baby's face,
And that it looks at you;
Whene'er you look on it, 'tis plain
The baby looks at you again.

'And some had sworn an oath that she
Should be to public justice brought;
And for the little infant's bones
With spades they would have sought.
But instantly the hill of moss
Before their eyes began to stir!
And, for full fifty yards around,
The grass – it shook upon the ground!
Yet all do still aver
The little Babe lies buried there,
Beneath that hill of moss so fair.

'I cannot tell how this may be,
But plain it is the Thorn is bound
With heavy tufts of moss that strive
To drag it to the ground;
And this I know, full many a time,
When she was on the mountain high,
By day, and in the silent night,
When all the stars shone clear and bright,
That I have heard her cry,
"Oh misery! oh misery!
Oh woe is me! oh misery!" '

Jennifer Dawson
1929–

from The Ha-Ha

Alasdair and the narrator, Josephine, are inmates of a psychiatric hospital, both nearing release. Together they make a day's excursion to a hill that Josephine has often seen in the distance from the window of her ward.

I could hear the whisper of water behind us; the tiny waterfall rolling over the log into the river. The fire smoked. The future was there, all round us.

'The future,' I embraced it with my arms, 'on this side of the hill. Here.'

'That's right,' Alasdair whispered. 'The future's nothing to be afraid of.' He rolled over the fire to my side and slid his arms underneath me.

The smoke from the fire fluttered and faded and merged in the pale sky. A pheasant squawked in a wood. I prodded the potato. It was soft. I picked it out lovingly, broke it in half, and gave half to Alasdair. I took a bite and was amazed at the grand gesture I had made. I had never made a gesture like that before, breaking food in half and handing half to a man to share. It was a grand, worldly gesture. The potato rested in my palm.

Alasdair took a bite of his and chucked it out towards the river. 'So much for Farmer Tingewick's potatoes.' He snatched my half and threw it in the other direction. 'We'll go to The Bull when we get back, so there is no need to stuff yourself with vegetable.'

He was close beside me, breathing heavily, with his hands on my wrists. I could feel his leg running down mine, and his face hovering over me. The draught from his nostrils tickled my face; his lips twitched like butterflies.

'You are so real,' he whispered. 'I'm afraid of the other ones, the people who possess the earth.'

He stretched farther over and pushed his face closer until I could only see the whites of his eyes, and hear his breathing, heavy and close, and feel hot sheets of air pouring down my throat.

The feel of solid things is very good; the feel of the hard sand by the river; the feel of the stone wall of the settlement, the feel of water when you are thirsty, the cold of a glass after a nightmare, and the sound of another voice that is not your own talking.

The water flowed noisily over the jutting-out wood; the fire fell to powder in its hearth, and we lay there.

'No one was unkind at Oxford,' I said softly, dreamily, almost to myself. 'They were very friendly as they passed, it was just that I did not have the knack of existing.'

I was gazing at my past. I was clutching at Alasdair as though it were a matter of life and death, as though my salvation lay in holding on there.

'You exist for me, at any rate,' he whispered urgently. 'Too much so in fact! Come on, nice thing. Come on, let's get ready.'

He was moving slowly about, stooping over with his back to me, fumbling with his jacket, patting his pockets, and untying his shoe-laces.

As he stooped or stood erect, bent or fumbled, the world seemed to close in till it was like a room with walls and ceilings. It was because of that that I obeyed the summons to share what reality there was with someone else. It put a floor under your feet, and even though it was odd, inappropriate; even though it was painful, that seemed part of the mysterious instructions to use any means you have to cling to that which is real because it may establish something further.

I felt nothing more, though, only the discomfort of this initiation ceremony and his heavy breathing and clutching, for life or death. At last Alasdair was lying on his side apart and breathing deeply and peacefully. I felt slightly sick, and the hill and everything seemed a long way away. Even Alasdair seemed distant.

He got up after a bit and wiped his face and went down to the river and stooped over the dark grey and drank. He came back wiping himself and smiling.

'All right?' he asked. It seemed as though he were calling over a distance. 'It's always a bit odd the first time.'

I nodded numbly.

'A matter of adjustment,' he went on, 'like a new screw that's stiff, if you'll excuse the delicate metaphor.' He smiled contentedly, and licked the river water from round his mouth. 'Just a matter of adjustment.' He looked sleek and satisfied like a cat.

'You mean next time we come here. . . ?'

He was bending over his shoe-laces. Perhaps he did not hear. I could see him smiling as he put himself together.

It was a new and strange experience to me, and it did not surprise me that I did not enjoy it. I had not expected pleasure, only some contact with the real world, and that I had found. Only my head felt odd, as though it were not mine, and the world seemed farther, not nearer.

Alasdair saw me leaning on my shoulder staring down at the river. He caught my hand and lay back staring at the wide sky.

'Hungry?' he asked.

'Now that we are . . . are lovers,' I supposed that was the word, '. . . will we come here often and light a fire and cook and eat? We could make a kind of camp here.' Strange music was running in my head. 'We could make a kind of retreat from the settlement. You said you hated it there.'

'Hey! Ho!' he carolled. 'Hey ho the holly, this life is so jolly.'

We left the river without saying goodbye – I thought we should return there tomorrow or the day after or at the weekend, every weekend – and Alasdair talked and laughed all the way back to the road. When we got to where the bus had dropped us, the first lorry that he thumbed stopped. We climbed up into the high cabin, and Alasdair and the driver starting talking about the new motorway, and generally exchanging motorists' experiences till we arrived back at the town.

🌹

Thomas Hardy
1840–1928

---

from Tess of the d'Urbervilles

Alec d'Urberville has rescued Tess, employed on his estate, from her drunken and resentful workmates on their way home from a dance late one night.

The twain cantered along for some time without speech, Tess as she clung to him still panting in her triumph, yet in other respects dubious. She had perceived that the horse was not the spirited one he sometimes rode, and felt no alarm on that score, though her seat was precarious enough despite her tight hold of him. She begged him to slow the animal to a walk, which Alec accordingly did.

'Neatly done, was it not, dear Tess?' he said by and by.

'Yes!' said she. 'I am sure I ought to be much obliged to you.'

'And are you?'

She did not reply.

'Tess, why do you always dislike my kissing you?'

'I suppose – because I don't love you.'

'You are quite sure?'

'I am angry with you sometimes!'

'Ah, I half feared as much.' Nevertheless, Alec did not object to that confession. He knew that anything was better than frigidity. 'Why haven't you told me when I have made you angry?'

'You know very well why. Because I cannot help myself here.'

'I haven't offended you often by love-making?'

'You have sometimes.'

'How many times?'

'You know as well as I – too many times.'

'Every time I have tried?'

She was silent, and the horse ambled along for a considerable distance, till a faint luminous fog, which had hung in the hollows all the evening, became general and enveloped them. It seemed to hold the moonlight in suspension, rendering it more pervasive than in clear air. Whether on this account, or from absent-mindedness, or from sleepiness, she did not perceive that they had long ago passed the point at which the lane to Trantridge branched from the highway, and that her conductor had not taken the Trantridge track.

She was inexpressibly weary. She had risen at five o'clock every morning of that week, had been on foot the whole of each day, and on this evening had in addition walked the three miles to Chaseborough, waited three hours for her neighbours without eating or drinking, her impatience to start them preventing either; she had then walked a mile of the way home, and had undergone the excitement of the quarrel, till, with the slow progress of their steed, it was now nearly one o'clock. Only once, however, was she overcome by actual drowsiness. In that moment of oblivion her head sank gently against him.

D'Urberville stopped the horse, withdrew his feet from the stirrups, turned sideways on the saddle, and enclosed her waist with his arm to support her.

This immediately put her on the defensive, and with one of those sudden impulses of reprisal to which she was liable she gave him a little push from her. In his ticklish position he nearly lost his balance and only just avoided rolling over into the road, the horse, though a powerful one, being fortunately the quietest he rode.

'That is devilish unkind!' he said. 'I mean no harm – only to keep you from falling.'

She pondered suspiciously; till, thinking that this might after all be true, she relented, and said quite humbly, 'I beg your pardon, sir.'

'I won't pardon you unless you show some confidence in me. Good God!' he burst out, 'what am I, to be repulsed so by a mere chit like you? For near three mortal months have you trifled with my feelings, eluded me, and snubbed me; and I won't stand it!'

'I'll leave you tomorrow, sir.'

'No, you will not leave me tomorrow! Will you, I ask once more, show your belief in me by letting me clasp you with my arm? Come, between us two and nobody else, now. We know each other well; and you know that I love you, and think you the prettiest girl in the world, which you are. Mayn't I treat you as a lover?'

She drew a quick pettish breath of objection, writhing uneasily on her seat, looked far ahead, and murmured, 'I don't know – I wish – how can I say yes or no when – '

He settled the matter by clasping his arm round her as he desired, and Tess expressed no further negative. Thus they sidled slowly onward till it struck her they had been advancing for an unconscionable time – far longer than was usually occupied by the short journey from Chaseborough, even at this walking pace, and that they were no longer on hard road, but in a mere trackway.

'Why, where be we?' she exclaimed.

'Passing by a wood.'

'A wood – what wood? Surely we are quite out of the road?'

'A bit of The Chase – the oldest wood in England. It is a lovely night, and why should we not prolong our ride a little?'

'How could you be so treacherous!' said Tess, between archness and real dismay, and getting rid of his arm by pulling open his fingers one by one, though at the risk of slipping off herself. 'Just when I've been putting such trust in you, and obliging you to please you, because I thought I had wronged you by that push! Please set me down, and let me walk home.'

'You cannot walk home, darling, even if the air were clear. We are miles away from Trantridge, if I must tell you, and in this growing fog you might wander for hours among these trees.'

'Never mind that,' she coaxed. 'Put me down, I beg you. I don't mind where it is; only let me get down, sir, please!'

'Very well, then, I will – on one condition. Having brought you here to this out-of-the-way place, I feel myself responsible for your safe-conduct home, whatever you may yourself feel about it. As to your getting to Trantridge without assistance, it is quite imposs-ible; for, to tell the truth, dear, owing to this fog, which so disguises everything, I don't quite know where we are myself. Now, if you will promise to wait beside the horse while I walk through the bushes till I come to some road or house and ascertain exactly our whereabouts, I'll deposit you here willingly. When I come back I'll give you full directions, and if you insist upon walking you may; or you may ride – at your pleasure.'

She accepted these terms, and slid off on the near side, though not till he had stolen a cursory kiss. He sprang down on the other side.

'I suppose I must hold the horse?' said she.

'Oh no; it's not necessary,' replied Alec, patting the panting creature. 'He's had enough of it for tonight.'

He turned the horse's head into the bushes, hitched him on to a bough, and made a sort of couch or nest for her in the deep mass of dead leaves.

'Now, you sit there,' he said. 'The leaves have not got damp as yet. Just give an eye to the horse – it will be quite sufficient.'

He took a few steps away from her, but, returning, said, 'By the bye, Tess, your father has a new cob today. Somebody gave it to him.'

'Somebody? You!'

D'Urberville nodded.

'O how very good of you that is!' she exclaimed, with a painful sense of the awkwardness of having to thank him just then.

'And the children have some toys.'

'I didn't know – you ever sent them anything!' she murmured, much moved. 'I almost wish you had not – yes, I almost wish it!'

'Why, dear?'

'It – hampers me so.'

'Tessy – don't you love me ever so little now?'

'I'm grateful,' she reluctantly admitted. 'But I fear I do not – ' The sudden vision of his passion for herself as a factor in this result so distressed her that, beginning with one slow tear, and then following with another, she wept outright.

'Don't cry, dear, dear one! Now sit down here, and wait till I come.' She passively sat down amid the leaves he had heaped, and shivered slightly. 'Are you cold?' he asked.

'Not very – a little.'

He touched her with his fingers, which sank into her as into down. 'You have only that puffy muslin dress on – how's that?'

'It's my best summer one. 'Twas very warm when I started, and I didn't know I was going to ride, and that it would be night.'

'Nights grow chilly in September. Let me see.' He pulled off a light overcoat that he had worn, and put it round her tenderly. 'That's it – now you'll feel warmer,' he continued. 'Now, my pretty, rest there; I shall soon be back again.'

Having buttoned the overcoat round her shoulders he plunged into the webs of vapour which by this time formed veils between the trees. She could hear the rustling of the branches as he ascended the adjoining slope, till his movements were no louder than the hopping of a bird, and finally died away. With the setting of the moon the pale light lessened, and Tess became invisible as she fell into reverie upon the leaves where he had left her.

In the meantime Alec d'Urberville had pushed on up the slope to clear his genuine doubt as to the quarter of The Chase they were in. He had, in fact, ridden quite at random for over an hour, taking any turning that came to hand in order to prolong companionship with her, and giving far more attention to Tess's moonlit person than to any wayside object. A little rest for the jaded animal being desirable, he did not hasten his search for landmarks. A clamber over the hill into the adjoining vale brought him to the fence of a highway whose contours he recognized, which settled the question of their whereabouts. D'Urberville thereupon turned back; but by this time the moon had quite gone down, and partly on account of the fog The Chase was wrapped in thick darkness, although morning was not far off. He was obliged to advance with outstretched hands to avoid contact with the boughs, and discovered that to hit the exact spot from which he had started was at first entirely beyond him. Roaming up and down, round and round, he at length heard a slight movement of the horse close at hand; and the sleeve of his overcoat unexpectedly caught his foot.

'Tess!' said d'Urberville.

There was no answer. The obscurity was now so great that he could see absolutely nothing but a pale nebulousness at his feet, which represented the white muslin figure he had left upon the dead leaves. Everything else was blackness alike. D'Urberville stooped; and heard a gentle regular breathing. He knelt and bent lower, till her breath warmed his face, and in a moment his cheek was in contact with hers. She was sleeping soundly, and upon her eyelashes there lingered tears.

Darkness and silence ruled everywhere around. Above them rose the primeval yews and oaks of The Chase, in which were poised gentle roosting birds in their last nap; and about them stole the hopping rabbits and hares. But, might some say, where was Tess's guardian angel? where was the providence of her simple faith? Perhaps, like that other god of whom the ironical Tishbite spoke, he was talking, or he was pursuing, or he was in a journey, or he was sleeping and not to be awaked.

Why it was that upon this beautiful feminine tissue, sensitive as gossamer, and practically blank as snow as yet, there should have been traced such a coarse pattern as it was doomed to receive; why so often the coarse appropriates the finer thus, the wrong man the woman, the wrong woman the man, many thousand years of analytical philosophy have failed to explain to our sense of order. One may, indeed, admit the possibility of a retribution lurking in the present catastrophe. Doubtless some of Tess d'Urberville's mailed ancestors rollicking home from a fray had dealt the same measure even more ruthlessly towards peasant girls of their time. But though to visit the sins of the fathers upon the children may be a morality good enough for divinities, it is scorned by average human nature; and it therefore does not mend the matter.

As Tess's own people down in those retreats are never tired of saying among each other in their fatalistic way: 'It was to be.' There lay the pity of it. An immeasurable social chasm was to divide our heroine's personality thereafter from that previous self of hers who stepped from her mother's door to try her fortune at Trantridge poultry-farm.

Thomas Hardy
1840–1928

The Ruined Maid

'Oh 'MELIA, my dear, this does everything crown!
Who could have supposed I should meet you in Town?
And whence such fair garments, such prosperi-ty?' —
'O didn't you know I'd been ruined?' said she.

— 'You left us in tatters, without shoes or socks,
Tired of digging potatoes, and spudding up docks;
And now you've gay bracelets and bright feathers three!' —
'Yes: that's how we dress when we're ruined,' said she.

— 'At home in the barton you said "thee" and 'thou,"
And "thik oon," and "theäs oon," and "t'other"; but now
Your talking quite fits 'ee for high compa-ny!' —
'Some polish is gained with one's ruin,' said she.

— 'Your hands were like paws then, your face blue and bleak
But now I'm bewitched by your delicate cheek,
And your little gloves fit as on any la-dy!' —
'We never do work when we're ruined,' said she.

— 'You used to call home-life a hag-ridden dream,
And you'd sigh, and you'd sock; but at present you seem
To know not of megrims or melancho-ly!' —
'True. One's pretty lively when ruined,' said she.

— 'I wish I had feathers, a fine sweeping gown,
And a delicate face, and could strut about Town!' —
'My dear — a raw country girl, such as you be,
Cannot quite expect that. You ain't ruined,' said she.

Travesties

✿

Ian McEwan
1948–

from Homemade

The narrator of this story is a fourteen-year-old boy.

All the way home I thought about cunt. I saw it in the smile of the conductress, I heard it in the roar of the traffic, I smelt it in the fumes from the shoe-polish factory, conjectured it beneath the skirts of passing housewives, felt it at my finger tips, sensed it in the air, drew it in my mind and at supper, which was toad-in-the-hole, I devoured, as in an unspeakable rite, genitalia of batter and sausage. And for all this I still did not know just exactly what a cunt was. I eyed my sister across the table. I exaggerated a little just now when I said she was an ugly bat – I was beginning to think that perhaps she was not so bad-looking after all. Her teeth protruded, that could not be denied, and if her cheeks were a little too sunken it was not so you would notice in the dark, and when her hair had been washed, as it was now, you could almost pass her off as plain. So it was not surprising that I came to be thinking over my toad-in-the-hole that with some cajoling and perhaps a little honest deceit Connie could be persuaded to think of herself, if only for a few minutes, as something more than a sister, as, let us say, a beautiful young lady, a film star and maybe, Connie, we could slip into bed here and try out this rather moving scene, now you get out of these clumsy pyjamas while I see to the light . . . And armed with this comfortably gained knowledge I could face the awesome Lulu with zeal and abandon, the whole terrifying ordeal would pale into insignificance, and who knows, perhaps I could lay her out there and then, halfway through the peepshow.

I never enjoyed looking after Connie. She was petulant, demanding, spoiled and wanted to play games all the while instead of watching the television. I usually managed to get her to bed an hour early by winding the clock forward. Tonight I wound it back. As soon as my mother and father had left for the dog track I asked Connie which games she would like to play, she could choose anything she liked.

'I don't want to play games with you.'

'Why not?'

'Because you were staring at me all the time through supper.'

'Well, of course I was, Connie. I was trying to think of the games you liked to play best and I was just looking at you, that was all.' Finally she agreed to play hide and seek, which I had suggested with special insistence because our house was of such a size that there were only two rooms you could hide in, and they were both bedrooms. Connie was to hide first. I covered my eyes and counted to thirty, listening all the while to her footsteps in my parents' bedroom directly above, hearing with satisfaction the creak of the bed – she was hiding under the eiderdown, her second favourite place. I shouted 'Coming' and began to mount the stairs. At the bottom of the stairs I do not think I had decided clearly what I was about to do; perhaps just look around, see where things were, draw a mental plan for future reference – after all it would not do to go scaring my little sister who would not think twice about telling my father everything, and that would mean a scene of some sort, laborious lies to invent, shouting and crying and that sort of thing, just at a time when I needed all my energy for the obsession in hand. By the time I reached the top of the stairs, however, the blood having drained from brain to groin, literally, one might say, from sense to sensibility, by the time I was catching my breath on the top stair and closing my moist hand round the bedroom door-handle, I had decided to rape my sister. Gently I pushed the door open and called in a sing-song voice,

'Connieee, where aaare you?' That usually made her giggle, but this time there was no sound. Holding my breath I tip-toed over to the bedside and sang,

'I knooow where youuu are,' and bending down by the tell-tale lump under the eiderdown, I whispered,

'I'm coming to get you,' and began to peel the bulky cover away, softly, almost tenderly, peeking into the dark warmth underneath. Dizzy with expectation I drew it right back, and there, helplessly and innocently stretched out before me were my parents' pyjamas, and even as I was leaping back in surprise I received a blow in the small of my back of such unthinking vigour as can only be inflicted by a sister on her brother. And there was Connie dancing with mirth, the wardrobe door swinging open behind her.

'I saw you, I saw you and you didn't see me!' To relieve my feelings I kicked her shins and sat on the bed to consider what next, while Connie, predictably histrionic, sat on the floor and boo-hooed. I found the noise depressing after a while so I went downstairs and read the paper, certain that soon Connie would follow me down. She did, and she was sulking.

'What game do you want to play now?' I asked her. She sat on the edge of the sofa pouting and sniffing and hating me. I was even considering forgetting the whole plan and giving myself up to an evening's television when I had an idea, an idea of such simplicity, elegance, clarity and formal beauty, an idea which wore the assurance of its own success like a tailor-made suit. There is a game which all home-loving, unimaginative little girls like Connie find irresistible, a game which, ever since she had learned to speak the necessary words, Connie had plagued me to play with her, so that my boyhood years were haunted by her pleadings and exorcised by my inevitable refusals; it was a game, in short, which I would rather be burned at the stake for than have my friends see me play it. And now at last we were going to play Mummies and Daddies.

'*I* know a game you'd like to play, Connie,' I said. Of course she would not reply, but I let my words hang there in the air like bait. 'I know a game *you'd* like to play.' She lifted her head.

'What is it?'

'It's a game you're always wanting to play.'

She brightened. 'Mummies and Daddies?' She was transformed, she was ecstatic. She fetched prams, dolls, stoves, fridges, cots, tea-cups, a washing machine and a kennel from her room and set them up around me in a flutter of organizational zeal.

'Now you go here, no there, and this can be the kitchen and this is the door where you come in and don't tread on there because there's a wall and I come in and see you and I say to you and then you say to me you go out and I make lunch.' I was plunged into the microcosm of the dreary, everyday, ponderous banalities, the horrifying, niggling details of the life of our parents and their friends, the life that Connie so dearly wanted to ape. I went to work and came back, I went to the pub and came back, I posted a letter and came back, I went to the shops and came back, I read a paper, I pinched the Bakelite cheeks of my progeny, I read another paper, pinched some more cheeks, went to work and came back. And Connie? She just cooked on the stove, washed up in the sink unit, washed, fed, put to sleep and roused her sixteen dolls and then poured some more tea – and she was happy. She was the inter-galactic-earth-goddess-housewife, she owned and controlled all around her, she saw all, she knew all, she told me when to go out, when to come in, which room I was in, what to say, how and when to say it. She was happy. She was complete, I have never seen another human so complete, she smiled, wide open, joyous and innocent smiles which I have never seen since – she tasted paradise on earth. And one point she was so blocked with the wonder, the ecstasy of it all, that mid-sentence her words choked up and she sat back on her heels, her eyes glistening, and breathed one long musical sigh of rare and wonderful happiness. It was almost a shame I had it in mind to rape her. Returning from work the twentieth time that half hour I said,

'Connie, we're leaving out one of the most important things that Mummies and Daddies do together.' She could hardly believe we had left anything out and she was curious to know.

'They fuck together, Connie, surely you know about that.'

'Fuck?' On her lips the word sounded strangely meaningless, which in a way I suppose it was, as far as I was concerned. The whole idea was to give it some meaning.

'Fuck? What does that mean?'

'Well, it's what they do at night, when they go to bed at night, just before they go to sleep.'

'Show me.' I explained that we would have to go upstairs and get into bed.

'No, we don't. We can pretend and this can be the bed,' she said, pointing at a square made by the design of the carpet.

'I cannot pretend and show it to you at the same time.' So once again I was climbing the stairs, once again my blood pounding and my manhood proudly stirring. Connie was quite excited too, still delirious with the happiness of the game and pleased at the novel turn it was taking.

'The first thing they do,' I said, as I led her to the bed, 'is to take off all their clothes.' I pushed her on to the bed and, with fingers almost useless with agitation, unbuttoned her pyjamas till she sat naked before me, still sweet-smelling from her bath and giggling with the fun of it all. Then I got undressed too, leaving my pants on so as not to alarm her, and sat by her side. As children we had seen enough of each other's bodies to take our nakedness for granted, though that was some time ago now and I sensed her unease.

'Are you sure this is what they do?'

My own uncertainty was obscured now by lust. 'Yes,' I said, 'it's quite simple. You have a hole there and I put my weenie in it.' She clasped her hand over her mouth, giggling incredulously.

'That's silly. Why do they want to do that?' I had to admit it to myself, there was something unreal about it.

'They do it because it's their way of saying they like each other.' Connie was beginning to think that I was making the whole thing up, which again, in a way I suppose I was. She stared at me, wide-eyed.

'But that's daft, why don't they just tell each other?' I was on the defensive, a mad scientist explaining his new crack-pot invention – coitus – before an audience of sceptical rationalists.

'Look,' I said to my sister, 'it's not only that. It's also a very nice feeling. They do it to get that feeling.'

'To get the feeling?' She still did not quite believe me. 'Get the feeling? What do you mean, get the feeling?'

I said, 'I'll show you.' And at the same time I pushed Connie on to the bed and lay on top of her in the manner I had inferred from the films Raymond and I had seen together. I was still wearing my underpants. Connie stared blankly up at me, not even afraid – in fact, she might have been closer to boredom. I writhed from side to side, trying to push my pants off without getting up.

'I still don't get it,' she complained from underneath me. 'I'm not getting any feeling. Are you getting any feeling?'

'Wait,' I grunted, as I hooked the underpants round the end of my toes with the very tips of my fingers, 'if you just wait a minute I'll show you.' I was beginning to lose my temper with Connie, with myself, with the universe, but mostly with my underpants which snaked determinedly round my ankles. At last I was free. My prick was hard and sticky on Connie's belly and now I began to manoeuvre it between her legs with one hand while I supported the weight of my body with the other. I searched her tiny crevice without the least notion of what I was looking for, but half expecting all the same to be transformed at any moment into a human whirlwind of sensation. I think perhaps I had in mind a warm fleshy chamber, but as I prodded and foraged, jabbed and wheedled, I found nothing other than tight, resisting skin. Meanwhile Connie just lay on her back, occasionally making little comments.

'Ooh, that's where I go wee-wee. I'm sure *our* mummy and daddy don't do this.' My supporting arm was being seared by pins and needles, I was feeling raw and yet still I poked and pushed, in a mood of growing despair. Each time Connie said, 'I still don't get any feeling,' I felt another ounce of my manhood slip away. Finally I had to rest. I sat on the edge of the bed to consider my hopeless failure, while behind me Connie propped herself up on her elbows. After a moment or two I felt the bed begin to shake with silent spasms and, turning, I saw Connie with tears spilling down her screwed-up face, inarticulate and writhing with choked laughter.

'What is it?' I asked, but she could only point vaguely in my direction and groan, and then she lay back on the bed, heaving and helpless with mirth. I sat by her side, not knowing what to think but deciding, as Connie quaked behind me, that another attempt was now out of the question. At last she was able to get out some words. She sat up and pointed at my still erect prick and gasped.

'It looks so . . . it looks so . . .' sank back in another fit, and then managed in one squeal, '*So silly, it looks so silly,*' after which she collapsed again into a high-pitched, squeezed-out titter. I sat there in lonely detumescent blankness, numbed by this final humiliation into the realization that this was no real girl beside me, this was no true representative of that sex; this was no boy, certainly, nor was it finally a girl – it was my sister, after all. I stared down at my limp prick, wondering at its hang-dog look, and just as I was thinking of getting my clothes together, Connie, silent now, touched me on the elbow.

'I know where it goes,' she said, and lay back on the bed, her legs wide apart, something it had not occurred to me to ask her to do. She settled herself among the pillows. 'I know where the hole is.'

I forgot my sister and my prick rose inquisitively, hopefully, to the invitation which Connie was whispering. It was all right with her now, she was at Mummies and Daddies and controlling the game again. With her hand she guided me into her tight, dry little-girl's cunt and we lay perfectly still for a while. I wished Raymond could have seen me, and I was glad he had brought my virginity to my notice, I wished Dinky Lulu could have seen me, in fact if my wishes had been granted I would have had all my friends, all the people I knew, file through the bedroom to catch me in my splendorous pose. For more than sensation, more than any explosion behind my ears, spears through my stomach, searings in my groin or rackings of my soul – more than any of these things, none of which I felt anyway, more then than even the thought of these things, I felt proud, proud to be fucking, even if it were only Connie, my ten-year-old sister, even if it had been a crippled mountain goat I would have been proud to be lying there in that manly position, proud in advance of being able to say 'I have fucked', of belonging intimately and irrevocably to that superior half of humanity who had known coitus, and fertilized the world with it. Connie lay quite still too, her eyes half-closed, breathing deeply – she was asleep. It was way past her bedtime and our strange game had exhausted her. For the first time I moved gently backwards and forwards, just a few times, and came in a miserable, played-out, barely pleasurable way. I woke Connie into indignation.

'You've wet inside me,' and she began to cry. Hardly noticing, I got up and started to get dressed. This may have been one of the most desolate couplings known to copulating mankind, involving lies, deceit, humiliation, incest, my partner falling asleep, my gnat's orgasm and the sobbing which now filled the bedroom, but I was pleased with it, myself, Connie, pleased to let things rest a while, to let the matter drop. I led Connie to the bathroom and began to fill the sink – my parents would be back soon and Connie should be asleep in her bed. I had made it into the adult world finally, I was pleased about that, but right then I did not want to see a naked girl, or any naked thing for a while yet. Tomorrow I would tell Raymond to forget the appointment with Lulu, unless he wanted to go it alone. And I knew for a fact that he would not want that at all.

John Wilmot, Earl of Rochester
1648–80

Song (Fair Chloris)

Fair Chloris in a pigsty lay;
   Her tender herd lay by her.
She slept; in murmuring gruntlings they,
Complaining of the scorching day,
   Her slumbers thus inspire.

She dreamt whilst she with careful pains
   Her snowy arms employed
In ivory pails to fill out grains,
One of her love-convicted swains
   Thus hasting to her cried:

'Fly, nymph! Oh, fly ere 'tis too late
   A dear, loved life to save;
Rescue your bosom pig from fate
Who now expires, hung in the gate
   That leads to Flora's cave.

'Myself had tried to set him free
   Rather than brought the news,
But I am so abhorred by thee
That ev'n thy darling's life from me
   I know thou wouldst refuse.'

Struck with the news, as quick she flies
   As blushes to her face;
Not the bright lightning from the skies,
Nor love, shot from her brighter eyes,
   Move half so swift a pace.

This plot, it seems, the lustful slave
    Had laid against her honor,
Which not one god took care to save,
For he pursues her to the cave
    And throws himself upon her.

Now piercèd is her virgin zone;
    She feels the foe within it.
She hears a broken amorous groan,
The panting lover's fainting moan,
    Just in the happy minute.

Frighted she wakes, and waking frigs.
    Nature thus kindly eased
In dreams raised by her murmuring pigs
And her own thumb between her legs,
    She's innocent and pleased.

Samuel Richardson
1689–1761

from Pamela

Pamela is a virtuous servant in the household of Squire B——, where Mrs Jervis is housekeeper, Mr Jonathan is butler, John is footman and Rachel another servant. Pamela is an epistolary novel, and this is one of the heroine's letters home.

MY DEAR PARENTS – Oh let me take up my complaint, and say, Never was poor creature so unhappy, and so barbarously used, as poor Pamela! Indeed, my dear father and mother, my heart's just broke! I can neither write as I should do, nor let it alone, for to whom but you can I vent my griefs, and keep my poor heart from bursting! Wicked, wicked man! – I have no patience when I think of him! – But yet, don't be frightened – for – I hope – I hope, I am honest! – But if my head and my hand will let me, you shall hear all. – Is there no constable nor headborough, though, to take me out of his house? for I am sure I can safely swear the peace against him: But, alas! he is greater than any constable: he is a justice himself: Such a justice deliver me from! – But God Almighty, I hope, in time, will right me – For He knows the innocence of my heart!

John went your way in the morning; but I have been too much distracted to send by him; and have seen nobody but Mrs Jervis or Rachel, and one I hate to see or be seen by: and indeed I hate now to see anybody. Strange things I have to tell you, that happened since last night, that good Mr Jonathan's letter, and my master's harshness, put me into such a fluster; but I will not keep you in suspense.

I went to Mrs Jervis's chamber; and, oh dreadful! my wicked master had hid himself, base gentleman as he is, in her closet, where she has a few books, and chest of drawers, and such like. I little suspected it; though I used, till this sad night, always to look into that closet and another in the room, and under the bed, ever since the summer-house trick; but never found anything; and so I did not do it then, being fully resolved to be angry with Mrs Jervis for what had happened in the day, and so thought of nothing else.

I sat down on one side of the bed, and she on the other, and we began to undress ourselves; but she on that side next the wicked closet, that held the worst heart in the world [. . .] Hush! said I, Mrs Jervis, did you not hear something stir in the closet? No, silly girl, said she, your fears are always awake. – But indeed, said I, I think I heard something rustle. – May be, says she, the cat may be got there: but I hear nothing.

I was hush; but she said, Pr'ythee, my good girl, make haste to bed. See if the door be fast. So I did, and was thinking to look into the closet; but, hearing no more noise, thought it needless, and so went again and sat myself down on the bed-side, and went on undressing myself. And Mrs Jervis, being by this time undressed, stepped into bed, and bid me hasten, for she was sleepy.

I don't know what was the matter, but my heart sadly misgave me: Indeed, Mr Jonathan's note was enough to make it do so, with what Mrs Jervis had said. I pulled off my stays, and my stockings, and all my clothes to an under-petticoat; and then hearing a rustling again in the closet, I said, Heaven protect us! but before I say my prayers, I must look into this closet. And so was going to it slip-shod, when, oh dreadful! out rushed my master in a rich silk and silver morning gown.

I screamed, and ran to the bed, and Mrs Jervis screamed too; and he said, I'll do you no harm, if you forbear this noise; but othewise take what follows.

Instantly he came to the bed (for I had crept into it, to Mrs Jervis, with my coat on, and my shoes); and taking me in his arms, said, Mrs Jervis, rise, and just step up stairs, to keep the maids from coming down at this noise: I'll do no harm to this rebel.

Oh, for Heaven's sake! for pity's sake! Mrs Jervis, said I, if I am not betrayed, don't leave me; and, I beseech you, raise all the house. No, said Mrs Jervis, I will not stir, my dear lamb; I will not leave you. I wonder at you, sir, said she; and kindly threw herself upon my coat, clasping me round the waist: You shall not hurt this innocent, said she: for I will lose my life in her defence. Are there not, said she, enough wicked ones in the world, for your base purpose, but you must attempt such a lamb as this?

He was desperate angry, and threatened to throw her out of the window; and to turn her out of the house the next morning. You need not, sir, said she; for I will not stay in it. God defend my poor Pamela till tomorrow, and we will both go together. – Says he, let me but expostulate a word or two with you, Pamela. Pray, Pamela, said Mrs Jervis, don't hear a word, except he leaves the bed, and goes to the other end of the room. Ay, out of the room, said I; expostulate tomorrow, if you must expostulate!

I found his hand in my bosom; and when my fright let me know it, I was ready to die; and I sighed and screamed, and fainted away. And still he had his arms about my neck; and Mrs Jervis was about my feet, and upon my coat. And all in a cold dewy sweat was I. Pamela! Pamela! said Mrs Jervis, as she tells me since, O—h, and gave another shriek, my poor Pamela is dead for certain! And so, to be sure, I was for a time; for I knew nothing more of the matter, one fit following another, till about three hours after, as it proved to be, I found myself in bed, and Mrs Jervis sitting upon one side, with her wrapper about her, and Rachel on the other; and no master, for the wicked wretch was gone. But I was so overjoyed, that I hardly could believe myself; and I said, which were my first words, Mrs Jervis, Mrs Rachel, can I be *sure* it is you? Tell me! can I? – Where have I been? Hush, my dear, said Mrs Jervis; you have been in fit after fit. I never saw anybody so frightful in my life!

By this I judged Rachel knew nothing of the matter; and it seems my wicked master had, upon Mrs Jervis's second noise on my fainting away, slipt out, and, as if he had come from his own chamber, disturbed by the screaming, went up to the maids' room (who, hearing the noise, lay trembling, and afraid to stir), and bid them go down, and see what was the matter with Mrs Jervis and me. And he charged Mrs Jervis, and promised to forgive her for what she had said and done, if she would conceal the matter. So the maids came down, and all went up again, when I came to myself a little, except Rachel, who stayed to sit up with me, and bear Mrs Jervis company. I believe they all guess the matter to be bad enough; though they dare not say anything.

When I think of my danger, and the freedoms he actually took, though I believe Mrs Jervis saved me from worse, and she said she did (though what can I think, who was in a fit, and knew nothing of the matter?) I am almost distracted.

At first I was afraid of Mrs Jervis; but I am fully satisfied she is very good, and I should have been lost but for her; and she takes on grievously about it. What would have become of me, had she gone out of the room, to still the maids, as he bid her! He'd certainly have shut her out, and then, mercy on me! what would have become of your poor Pamela?

I must leave off a little; for my eyes and my head are sadly bad. – This was a dreadful trial! This was the worst of all! Oh, that I was out of the power of this dreadfully wicked man! Pray for

Your distressed DAUGHTER.

attributed to Henry Fielding
1707–54

from Shamela

This is an extract from a famous parody of the last-quoted novel.

A letter from Shamela Andrews to Henrietta Maria Honora Andrews

O Madam, I have strange Things to tell you! As I was reading in that charming Book about the Dealings, in comes my Master – to be sure he is a precious One. *Pamela*, says he, what Book is that, I warrant you *Rochester*'s Poems. – No, forsooth, says I, as pertly as I could; why how now Saucy Chops, Boldface, says he – Mighty pretty Words, says I, pert again. – Yes (says he) you are a d—d, impudent, stinking, cursed, confounded Jade, and I have a great Mind to kick your A—. You, kiss — says I. A-gad, says he, and so I will; with that he caught me in his Arms, and kissed me till he made my Face all over Fire. Now this served purely you know, to put upon the Fool for Anger. O! What precious Fools Men are! And so I flung from him in a mighty Rage, and pretended as how I would go out at the Door; but when I came to the End of the Room, I stood still, and my Master cryed out, Hussy, Slut, Saucebox, Boldface, come hither — Yes to be sure, says I; why don't you come, says he; what should I come for, says I; if you don't come to me, I'll come to you, says he; I shan't come to you I assure you, says I. Upon which he run up, caught me in his Arms, and flung me upon a Chair, and began to offer to touch my Under-Petticoat. Sir, says I, you had better not offer to be rude; well, says he, no more I won't then; and away he went out of the Room. I was so mad to be sure I could have cry'd.

Oh what a prodigious Vexation it is to a Woman to be made a Fool of.

Mrs *Jervis*, who had been without, harkening, now came to me. She burst into a violent Laugh the Moment she came in. Well, says she, as soon as she could speak, I have reason to bless myself that I am an Old Woman. Ah Child! if you had known the Jolly Blades of my Age, you would not have been left in the Lurch in this manner. Dear Mrs *Jervis*, says I, don't laugh at one; and to be sure I was a little angry with her. – Come, says she, my dear Honey-suckle, I have one Game to play for you; he shall see you in Bed; he shall, my little Rose-bud, he shall see those pretty, litcle, white, round, panting — and offer'd to pull off my Handkerchief. – Fie, Mrs *Jervis*, says I, you make me blush, and upon my Fackins, I believe she did: She went on thus. I know the Squire likes you, and notwithstanding the Aukwardness of his Proceeding, I am convinced hath some hot Blood in his Veins, which will not let him rest, 'till he hath communicated some of his Warmth to thee my little Angel; I heard him last Night at our Door, trying if it was open, now tonight I will take care it shall be so; I warrant that he makes the second Trial; which if he doth, he shall find us ready to receive him. I will at first counterfeit Sleep, and after a Swoon; so that he will have you naked in his Possession: and then if you are disappointed, a Plague of all young Squires, say I. – And so, Mrs *Jervis*, says I, you would have me yield my self to him, would you; you would have me be a second Time a Fool for nothing. Thank you for that, Mrs *Jervis*. For nothing! marry forbid, says she, you know he hath large Sums of Money, besides abundance of fine Things; and do you think, when you have inflamed him, by giving his Hand a Liberty, with that charming Person; and that you know he may easily think he obtains against your Will, he will not give any thing to come at all —. This will not do, Mrs *Jervis*, answered I. I have heard my Mamma say, (and so you know, Madam, I have) that in her Youth, Fellows have often taken away in the Morning, what they gave over Night. No, Mrs *Jervis*, nothing under a regular taking into Keeping, a settled Settlement, for me, and all my Heirs, all my whole Life-time, shall do the Business — or else cross-legged, is the Word, faith, with *Sham*; and then I snapt my Fingers.

Thursday Night, Twelve o'Clock

Mrs *Jervis* and I are just in Bed, and the Door unlocked; if my Master should come – Odsbobs! I hear him just coming in at the Door. You see I write in the present Tense, as Parson *Williams* says. Well, he is in Bed between us, we both shamming a Sleep, he steals his Hand into my Bosom, which I, as if in my Sleep, press close to me with mine, and then pretend to awake. – I no sooner see him, but I scream out to Mrs *Jervis*, she feigns likewise but just to come to herself; we both begin, she to becall, and I to bescratch very liberally. After having made a pretty free Use of my Fingers, without any great Regard to the Parts I attack'd, I counterfeit a Swoon. Mrs *Jervis* then cries out, O, Sir, what have you done, you have murthered poor *Pamela*: she is gone, she is gone. –

O what a Difficulty it is to keep one's Countenance, when a violent Laugh desires to burst forth.

The poor Booby frighted out of his Wits, jumped out of Bed, and, in his Shirt, sat down by my Bed-Side, pale and trembling, for the Moon shone, and I kept my Eyes wide open, and pretended to fix them in my Head. Mrs *Jervis* apply'd Lavender Water, and Hartshorn, and this, for a full half Hour; when thinking I had carried it on long enough, and being likewise unable to continue the Sport any longer, I began by Degrees to come to my self.

The Squire who had sat all this while speechless, and was almost really in that Condition, which I feigned, the Moment he saw me give Symptoms of recovering my Senses, fell down on his Knees; and O *Pamela*, cryed he, can you forgive me, my injured Maid? by Heaven, I know not whether you are a Man or a Woman, unless by your swelling Breasts. Will you promise to forgive me: I forgive you! D—n you (says I) and d—n you, says he, if you come to that. I wish I had never seen your bold Face, saucy Sow, and so went out of the Room.

O what a silly Fellow is a bashful young Lover!

He was no sooner out of hearing, as we thought, than we both burst into a violent Laugh. Well, says Mrs *Jervis*, I never saw any thing better acted than your Part: But I wish you may not have discouraged him from any future Attempt; especially since his Passions are so cool, that you could prevent his Hands going further than your Bosom. Hang him, answer'd I, he is not quite so cold as that I assure you; our Hands, on neither Side, were idle in the Scuffle, nor have left us any Doubt of each other as to that matter [. . .]

Your Dutiful Daughter,

SHAMELA.

William Shakespeare
1564–1616

from Venus and Adonis

Even as the sun with purple-colour'd face
Had ta'en his last leave of the weeping morn,
Rose-cheek'd Adonis hied him to the chase;
Hunting he lov'd, but love he laugh'd to scorn;
   Sick-thoughted Venus makes amain unto him,
   And like a bold-fac'd suitor 'gins to woo him.

'Thrice fairer than myself,' thus she began,
'The field's chief flower, sweet above compare,
Stain to all nymphs, more lovely than a man,
More white and red than doves or roses are;
   Nature that made thee, with herself at strife,
   Saith that the world hath ending with thy life.

'Vouchsafe, thou wonder, to alight thy steed,
And rein his proud head to the saddle-bow;
If thou wilt deign this favour, for thy meed
A thousand honey secrets shalt thou know:
   Here come and sit, where never serpent hisses;
   And being set, I'll smother thee with kisses:

'And yet not cloy thy lips with loath'd satiety,
But rather famish them amid their plenty,
Making them red and pale with fresh variety;
Ten kisses short as one, one long as twenty:
   A summer's day will seem an hour but short,
   Being wasted in such time-beguiling sport.'

With this she seizeth on his sweating palm,
The precedent of pith and livelihood,
And, trembling in her passion, calls it balm,
Earth's sovereign salve to do a goddess good:
    Being so enrag'd, desire doth lend her force
    Courageously to pluck him from his horse.

Over one arm the lusty courser's rein,
Under her other was the tender boy,
Who blush'd and pouted in a dull disdain,
With leaden appetite, unapt to toy;
    She red and hot as coals of glowing fire,
    He red for shame, but frosty in desire.

The studded bridle on a ragged bough
Nimbly she fastens; O! how quick is love: –
The steed is stalled up, and even now
To tie the rider she begins to prove:
    Backward she push'd him, as she would be thrust,
    And govern'd him in strength, though not in lust.

So soon was she along, as he was down,
Each leaning on their elbows and their hips:
Now doth she stroke his cheek, now doth he frown,
And 'gins to chide, but soon she stops his lips;
    And kissing speaks, with lustful language broken,
    'If thou wilt chide, thy lips shall never open.'

He burns with bashful shame; she with her tears
Doth quench the maiden burning of his cheeks;
Then with her windy sighs and golden hairs
To fan and blow them dry again she seeks:
    He saith she is immodest, blames her miss;
    What follows more she murders with a kiss.

Even as an empty eagle, sharp by fast,
Tires with her beak on feathers, flesh and bone,
Shaking her wings, devouring all in haste,
Till either gorge be stuff'd or prey be gone;
    Even so she kiss'd his brow, his cheek, his chin,
    And where she ends she doth anew begin.

Forc'd to content, but never to obey,
Panting he lies, and breatheth in her face;
She feedeth on the steam, as on a prey,
And calls it heavenly moisture, air of grace;
    Wishing her cheeks were gardens full of flowers,
    So they were dew'd with such distilling showers.

Look! how a bird lies tangled in a net,
So fasten'd in her arms Adonis lies;
Pure shame and aw'd resistance made him fret,
Which bred more beauty in his angry eyes:
    Rain added to a river that is rank
    Perforce will force it overflow the bank.

Still she entreats, and prettily entreats,
For to a pretty ear she tunes her tale;
Still is he sullen, still he lours and frets,
'Twixt crimson shame and anger ashy-pale;
    Being red, she loves him best; and being white,
    Her best is better'd with a more delight.

Look how he can, she cannot choose but love;
And by her fair immortal hand she swears,
From his soft bosom never to remove,
Till he take truce with her contending tears,
    Which long have rain'd, making her cheeks all wet;
    And one sweet kiss shall pay this countless debt.

Upon this promise did he raise his chin
Like a dive-dapper peering through a wave,
Who, being look'd on, ducks as quickly in;
So offers he to give what she did crave;
    But when her lips were ready for his pay,
    He winks, and turns his lips another way.

Never did passenger in summer's heat
More thirst for drink than she for this good turn.
Her help she sees, but help she cannot get;
She bathes in water, yet her fire must burn:
    'O! pity,' 'gan she cry, 'flint-hearted boy:
    'Tis but a kiss I beg; why art thou coy?

'I have been woo'd, as I entreat thee now,
Even by the stern and direful god of war,
Whose sinewy neck in battle ne'er did bow,
Who conquers where he comes in every jar;
    Yet hath he been my captive and my slave,
    And begg'd for that which thou unask'd shalt have.

'Over my altars hath he hung his lance,
His batter'd shield, his uncontrolled crest,
And for my sake hath learn'd to sport and dance,
To toy, to wanton, dally, smile, and jest;
    Scorning his churlish drum and ensign red,
    Making my arms his field, his tent my bed.

'Thus he that overrul'd I oversway'd,
Leading him prisoner in a red-rose chain:
Strong-temper'd steel his stronger strength obey'd,
Yet was he servile to my coy disdain.
    O! be not proud, nor brag not of thy might,
    For mastering her that foil'd the god of fight.

Touch but my lips with those fair lips of thine, –
Though mine be not so fair, yet are they red, –
The kiss shall be thine own as well as mine:
What seest thou in the ground? hold up thy head:
   Look in mine eyeballs, there thy beauty lies;
   Then why not lips on lips, since eyes in eyes?

'Art thou asham'd to kiss? then wink again,
And I will wink; so shall the day seem night;
Love keeps his revels where there are but twain;
Be bold to play, our sport is not in sight:
   These blue-vein'd violets whereon we lean
   Never can blab, nor know not what we mean.

'The tender spring upon thy tempting lip
Shows thee unripe, yet mayst thou well be tasted:
Make use of time, let not advantage slip;
Beauty within itself should not be wasted:
   Fair flowers that are not gather'd in their prime
   Rot and consume themselves in little time.'

William Golding
1911–

from Free Fall

I sent a message in by the porter. Mr Mountjoy wishes to speak to Miss Ifor.

'Sammy!'

It was a quarter to eight in the morning.

'I had to come and look at you. To make sure you were real.'

'But how did you get here at this time?'

'I wanted to see you.'

'But how – '

'I wanted – oh that? I've been walking all night, keeping ahead of it.'

'But – '

'You are my sanity, Beatrice. I had to come and see you. Now everything is all right.'

'You'll be late, Sammy, you must go. Are you all right?'

Compunction in compulsion, almost weeping. What is madness after all? Can a man who pretends to be mad claim to be sane?

Compulsion, weeping.

'I have to do it. I don't know why. I have to.'

'Oh look, Sammy – here I'm not supposed to – I'll see you to the bus stop. Come on. You know the number? You're to go straight to bed.'

'You won't leave me?'

'Look – dear!'

'As soon as you can then – the very first moment – '

'I promise.'

The bus top was among branches part of the way. I was shaking and shuddering by myself with no need to act. I was muttering like a drunk man.

'I don't understand. I don't know anything. I'm on rails. I have to. Have to. There is too much life. I could kick myself or kill

[252]

myself. Is my living to be nothing but moving like an insect? Scuttering, crawling? I could go away. Could I? Could I go away? Across the sea where the painted walls wait for me, I might. I am tied by this must.'

The muscles of the chest get tautened, the sinews stand out in the wrists, the heart beats faster till the air is eaten up with red shapes expanding; and then you understand that you ought to breathe again; for even if compulsion is a pitiless thing a man does not have to let it take charge of his physical reflexes, no, he can suffer emotionally without starving himself of air – there, I thought, I have breathed the load off my back.

She came to me malleable, and at the same time authoritative, for she was very firm about eating regularly and so on. She was very sweet. She only put up a token fight. She was my sanity. I would take any consequences that ensued would I not, who was so breathlessly assuring her that there would be no consequences. And then Beatrice of four years' fever lay back obediently, closed her eyes and placed one clenched fist bravely on her forehead as though she were about to be injected for T.A.B.

And what of Sammy?

There could be no consequences because there was no cause.

What precisely was he after? Why should it be that at this most triumphant or at least enjoyable moment of his career, the sight of the victim displayed humble, acquiescent and frightened should not only be less stimulating than the least of his sexual inventions but should even be damping and impossible? No, said his body, no not this at all. That was not the thing I meant, thing I wanted. How far was I right to think myself obsessed with sex when that potency which is assumed in all literature was not mine to use at the drop of a knicker? It seemed then that some co-operation was essential. If she were to make of herself a victim I could not be her executioner. If she were to be frightened, then I was ashamed in my very flesh that she should be frightened of me. This did not seem to me to tally with the accepted version of a man who was either wholly incapable or heroically ready, aye ready. There were gradations. But neither I nor Beatrice were prepared to admit them. On the other hand my feelings about her were without doubt obsessive if not pathological. Should they not then make my achievement of her easy? But she, out of my suggested madness and her own religious taboos, was incapable of thinking about this moment, this pre-marital deed, without a sense that was at once one of sin, one of fear, one of love and consequently one of drama. Unconsciously we were both setting ourselves to music. The gesture with which she opened her knees was, so to speak, operatic, heroic, dramatic and daunting. I could not accompany her. My instrument was flat.

William Shakespeare
1564–1616

from Richard III

The Duke of Gloucester, later Richard III, woos Anne at the funeral of her father-in-law, whom he has murdered, having already stabbed to death her husband, Edward, Prince of Wales.

Enter the corpse of KING HENRY *the sixth, Gentlemen with halberds to guard it;* LADY ANNE *being the mourner.*

ANNE: Set down, set down your honourable load –
    If honour may be shrouded in a hearse –
    Whilst I awhile obsequiously lament
    The untimely fall of virtuous Lancaster.
    Poor key-cold figure of a holy king!
    Pale ashes of the house of Lancaster!
    Thou bloodless remnant of that royal blood!
    Be it lawful that I invocate thy ghost,
    To hear the lamentations of poor Anne,
    Wife to thy Edward, to thy slaughtered son,
    Stabb'd by the selfsame hand that made these wounds!
    Lo, in these windows that let forth thy life
    I pour the helpless balm of my poor eyes.
    Cursed be the hand that made these fatal holes!
    Cursed be the heart that had the heart to do it!
    Cursed the blood that let this blood from hence!
    More direful hap betide that hated wretch,
    That makes us wretched by the death of thee,
    Than I can wish to adders, spiders, toads,
    Or any creeping venom'd thing that lives!
    If ever he have child, abortive be it,
    Prodigious, and untimely brought to light,
    Whose ugly and unnatural aspect

May fright the hopeful mother at the view;
And that be heir to his unhappiness!
If ever he have wife, let her be made
As miserable by the death of him,
As I am made by my poor lord and thee!
Come, now towards Chertsey with your holy load,
Taken from Paul's to be interred there;
And still, as you are weary of the weight,
Rest you, whiles I lament King Henry's corse.
(*Enter* GLOUCESTER.)

GLOU: Stay, you that bear the corse, and set it down.

ANNE: What black magician conjures up this fiend,
To stop devoted charitable deeds?

GLOU: Villians, set down the corse; or, by Saint Paul,
I'll make a corse of him that disobeys.

GENT: My lord, stand back, and let the coffin pass.

GLOU: Unmanner'd dog! stand thou, when I command:
Advance thy halberd higher than my breast,
Or, by Saint Paul, I'll strike thee to my foot,
And spurn upon thee, beggar, for thy boldness.

ANNE: What, do you tremble? are you all afraid?
Alas, I blame you not; for you are mortal,
And mortal eyes cannot endure the devil.
Avaunt, thou dreadful minister of hell!
Thou hadst but power over his mortal body,
His soul thou canst not have; therefore, be gone.

GLOU: Sweet saint, for charity, be not so curst.

ANNE: Foul devil, for God's sake, hence, and trouble us not;
For thou hast made the happy earth thy hell,
Fill'd it with cursing cries and deep exclaims.
If thou delight to view thy heinous deeds,
Behold this pattern of thy butcheries.
O, gentlemen, see, see! dead Henry's wounds
Open their congeal'd mouths and bleed afresh.
Blush, blush, thou lump of foul deformity;
For 'tis thy presence that exhales this blood
From cold and empty veins, where no blood dwells;
Thy deed, inhuman and unnatural,
Provokes this deluge most unnatural.

O God, which this blood madest, revenge his death!
O earth, which this blood drink'st, revenge his death!
Either heaven with lightning strike the murderer dead,
Or earth, gape open wide and eat him quick,
As thou dost swallow up this good king's blood,
Which his hell-govern'd arm hath butchered!

GLOU: Lady, you know no rules of charity,
Which renders good for bad, blessings for curses.

ANNE: Villain, thou know'st no law of God nor man:
No beast so fierce but knows some touch of pity.

GLOU: But I know none, and therefore am no beast.

ANNE: O wonderful, when devils tell the truth!

GLOU: More wonderful, when angels are so angry.
Vouchsafe, divine perfection of a woman,
Of these supposed evils, to give me leave,
By circumstance, but to acquit myself.

ANNE: Vouchsafe, defused infection of a man,
For these known evils, but to give me leave,
By circumstance, to curse thy cursed self.

GLOU: Fairer than tongue can name thee, let me have
Some patient leisure to excuse myself.

ANNE: Fouler than heart can think thee, thou canst make
No excuse current, but to hang thyself.

GLOU: By such despair, I should accuse myself.

ANNE: And, by despairing, shouldst thou stand excused
For doing worthy vengeance on thyself,
Which didst unworthy slaughter upon others.

GLOU: Say that I slew them not?

ANNE: Why, then they are not dead:
But dead they are, and, devilish slave, by thee.

GLOU: I did not kill your husband.

ANNE: Why, then he is alive.

GLOU: Nay, he is dead; and slain by Edward's hand.

ANNE: In thy foul throat thou liest: Queen Margaret saw
Thy murderous falchion smoking in his blood;
The which thou once didst bend against her breast,
But that thy brothers beat aside the point.

GLOU: I was provoked by her slanderous tongue,
Which laid their guilt upon my guiltless shoulders.

ANNE: Thou wast provoked by thy bloody mind,
　　Which never dreamt on aught but butcheries:
　　Didst thou not kill this king?
GLOU:　　　　　　　　　　I grant ye.
ANNE: Dost grant me, hedgehog? then, God grant me too
　　Thou mayst be damned for that wicked deed!
　　O, he was gentle, mild, and virtuous!
GLOU: The fitter for the King of heaven, that hath him.
ANNE: He is in heaven, where thou shalt never come.
GLOU: Let him thank me, that holp to send him thither;
　　For he was fitter for that place than earth.
ANNE: And thou unfit for any place but hell.
GLOU: Yes, one place else, if you will hear me name it.
ANNE: Some dungeon.
GLOU:　　　　　　　Your bed-chamber.
ANNE: Ill rest betide the chamber where thou liest!
GLOU: So will it, madam, till I lie with you.
ANNE: I hope so.
GLOU:　　　　　I know so. But, gentle Lady Anne,
　　To leave this keen encounter of our wits,
　　And fall somewhat into a slower method,
　　Is not the causer of the timeless deaths
　　Of these Plantagenets, Henry and Edward,
　　As blameful as the executioner?
ANNE: Thou art the cause, and most accursed effect.
GLOU: Your beauty was the cause of that effect;
　　Your beauty, which did haunt me in my sleep
　　To undertake the death of all the world,
　　So I might live one hour in your sweet bosom.
ANNE: If I thought that, I tell thee, homicide,
　　These nails should rend that beauty from my cheeks.
GLOU: These eyes could never endure sweet beauty's wreck;
　　You should not blemish it, if I stood by:
　　As all the world is cheered by the sun,
　　So I by that; it is my day, my life.
ANNE: Black night o'ershade thy day, the death thy life!
GLOU: Curse not thyself, fair creature; thou art both.
ANNE: I would I were, to be revenged on thee.
GLOU: It is a quarrel most unnatural,

To be revenged on him that loveth you.

ANNE: It is a quarrel just and reasonable,

To be revenged on him that slew my husband.

GLOU: He that bereft thee, lady, of thy husband,

Did it to help thee to a better husband.

ANNE: His better doth not breathe upon the earth.

GLOU: He lives that loves you better than he could.

ANNE: Name him.

GLOU: Plantagenet.

ANNE: Why, that was he.

GLOU: The selfsame name, but one of better nature.

ANNE: Where is he?

GLOU: Here. (*She spitteth at him.*) Why dost thou
spit at me?

ANNE: Would it were mortal poison, for thy sake!

GLOU: Never came poison from so sweet a place.

ANNE: Never hung poison on a fouler toad.

Out of my sight! thou dost infect my eyes.

GLOU: Thine eyes, sweet lady, have infected mine.

ANNE: Would they were basilisks, to strike thee dead!

GLOU: I would they were, that I might die at once;

For now they kill me with a living death.

Those eyes of thine from mine have drawn salt tears,

Shamed their aspect with store of childish drops:

These eyes, which never shed remorseful tear,

No, when my father York and Edward wept,

To hear the piteous moan that Rutland made

When black-faced Clifford shook his sword at him;

Nor when thy warlike father, like a child,

Told the sad story of my father's death,

And twenty times made pause to sob and weep,

That all the standers-by had wet their cheeks,

Like trees bedash'd with rain: in that sad time

My manly eyes did scorn an humble tear;

And what these sorrows could not thence exhale,

Thy beauty hath, and made them blind with weeping.

I never sued to friend nor enemy;

My tongue could never learn sweet smoothing words;

But, now thy beauty is proposed my fee,

My proud heart sues, and prompts my tongue to speak.
(*She looks scornfully at him.*)
Teach not thy lips such scorn, for they were made
For kissing, lady, not for such contempt.
If thy revengeful heart cannot forgive,
Lo, here I lend thee this sharp-pointed sword;
Which if thou please to hide in this true bosom,
And let the soul forth that adoreth thee,
I lay it naked to the deadly stroke,
And humbly beg the death upon my knee.
(*He lays his breast open: she offers at it with his sword.*)
Nay, do not pause; for I did kill King Henry,
But 'twas thy beauty that provoked me.
Nay, now dispatch; 'twas I that stabb'd young Edward,
But 'twas thy heavenly face that set me on.
(*Here she lets fall the sword.*)
Take up the sword again, or take up me.
ANNE: Arise, dissembler: though I wish thy death,
    I will not be the executioner.
GLOU: Then bid me kill myself, and I will do it.
ANNE: I have already.
GLOU: Tush, that was in thy rage:
    Speak it again, and, even with the word,
    That hand, which, for thy love, did kill thy love,
    Shall, for thy love, kill a far truer love;
    To both their deaths shalt thou be accessary.
ANNE: I would I knew thy heart.
GLOU: 'Tis figured in my tongue.
ANNE: I fear me both are false.
GLOU: Then never man was true.
ANNE: Well, well, put up your sword.
GLOU: Say, then, my peace is made.
ANNE: That shall you know hereafter.
GLOU: But shall I live in hope?
ANNE: All men, I hope, live so.
GLOU: Vouchsafe to wear this ring.
ANNE: To take is not to give.
GLOU: Look, how this ring encompasseth thy finger,
    Even so thy breast encloseth my poor heart;

Wear both of them, for both of them are thine.
And if thy poor devoted suppliant may
But beg one favour at thy gracious hand,
Thou dost confirm his happiness for ever.

ANNE: What is it?

GLOU: That it would please thee leave these sad designs
To him that hath more cause to be a mourner,
And presently repair to Crosby Place;
Where, after I have solemnly interr'd
At Chertsey monastery this noble king,
And wet his grave with my repentant tears,
I will with all expedient duty see you:
For divers unknown reasons, I beseech you,
Grant me this boon.

ANNE: With all my heart; and much it joys me too,
To see you are become so penitent.
Tressel and Berkeley, go along with me.

GLOU: Bid me farewell,

ANNE: 'Tis more than you deserve;
But since you teach me how to flatter you,
Imagine I have said farewell already.

(*Exeunt* LADY ANNE, TRESSEL *and* BERKELEY.)

GLOU: Sirs, take up the corse.

GENT: Towards Chertsey, noble lord?

GLOU: No, to White-Friars; there attend my coming.

(*Exeunt all but* GLOUCESTER.)
Was ever woman in this humour woo'd?
Was ever women in this humour won?
I'll have her; but I will not keep her long.
What! I, that kill'd her husband and his father,
To take her in her heart's extremest hate,
With curses in her mouth, tears in her eyes,
The bleeding witness of her hatred by;
Having God, her conscience, and these bars against me,
And I nothing to back my suit at all,
But the plain devil and dissembling looks,
And yet to win her, all the world to nothing!
Ha!
Hath she forgot already that brave prince,

Edward, her lord, whom I, some three months since,
Stabb'd in my angry mood at Tewksbury?
A sweeter and a lovelier gentleman,
Framed in the prodigality of nature,
Young, valiant, wise, and, no doubt, right royal,
The spacious world cannot again afford:
And will she yet debase her eyes on me,
That cropp'd the golden prime of this sweet prince,
And made her widow to a woful bed?
On me, whose all not equals Edward's moiety?
On me, that halt and am unshapen thus?
My dukedom to a beggarly denier,
I do mistake my person all this while:
Upon my life, she finds, although I cannot,
Myself to be a marvellous proper man.
I'll be at charges for a looking-glass,
And entertain some score or two of tailors,
To study fashions to adorn my body:
Since I am crept in favour with myself,
I will maintain it with some little cost.
But first I'll turn yon fellow in his grave;
And then return lamenting to my love.
Shine out, fair sun, till I have bought a glass,
That I may see my shadow as I pass.
(*Exit.*)

John Milton
1608-74

from Paradise Lost, Book v

Now Morn her rosie steps in th' Eastern Clime
Advancing, sow'd the earth with Orient Pearle,
When *Adam* wak't, so customd, for his sleep
Was Aerie light from pure digestion bred,
And temperat vapors bland, which th' only sound
Of leaves and fuming rills, *Aurora's* fan,
Lightly dispers'd, and the shrill Matin Song
Of Birds on every bough; so much the more
His wonder was to find unwak'nd *Eve*
With Tresses discompos'd, and glowing Cheek,
As through unquiet rest: he on his side
Leaning half-rais'd, with look of cordial Love
Hung over her enamour'd, and beheld
Beautie, which whether waking or asleep,
Shot forth peculiar Graces; then with voice
Milde, as when *Zephyrus* on *Flora* breathes,
Her hand soft touching, whisperd thus. Awake
My fairest, my espous'd, my latest found,
Heav'ns last best gift, my ever new delight,
Awake, the morning shines, and the fresh field
Calls us, we lose the prime, to mark how spring
Our tended Plants, how blows the Citron Grove,
What drops the Myrrhe, and what the balmie Reed,
How Nature paints her colours, how the Bee
Sits on the Bloom extracting liquid sweet.
    Such whispering wak'd her, but with startl'd eye
On *Adam*, whom imbracing, thus she spake.
    O Sole in whom my thoughts find all repose,
My Glorie, my Perfection, glad I see
Thy face, and Morn return'd, for I this Night,
Such night till this I never pass'd, have dream'd,

If dream'd, not as I oft am wont, of thee,
Works of day pass't, or morrows next designe,
But of offence and trouble, which my mind
Knew never till this irksom night; methought
Close at mine ear one call'd me forth to walk
With gentle voice, I thought it thine; it said,
Why sleepst thou *Eve*? now is the pleasant time,
The cool, the silent, save where silence yields
To the night-warbling Bird, that now awake
Tunes sweetest his love-labor'd song; now reignes
Full Orb'd the Moon, and with more pleasing light
Shadowie sets off the face of things; in vain,
If none regard; Heav'n wakes with all his eyes,
Whom to behold but thee, Natures desire,
In whose sight all things joy, with ravishment
Attracted by thy beauty still to gaze.
I rose as at thy call, but found thee not;
To find thee I directed then my walk;
And on, methought, alone I pass'd through ways
That brought me on a sudden to the Tree
Of interdicted Knowledge: fair it seem'd,
Much fairer to my Fancie then by day:
And as I wondring lookt, beside it stood
One shap'd and wing'd like one of those from Heav'n
By us oft seen; his dewie locks distill'd
Ambrosia; on that Tree he also gaz'd;
And O fair Plant, said he, with fruit surcharg'd,
Deigns none to ease thy load and taste thy sweet,
Nor God, nor Man; is Knowledge so despis'd?
Or envie, or what reserve forbids to taste?
Forbid who will, none shall from me withhold
Longer thy offerd good, why else set here?
This said he paus'd not, but with ventrous Arme
He pluckt, he tasted; mee damp horror chil'd
At such bold words voucht with a deed so bold:
But he thus overjoy'd, O Fruit Divine,
Sweet of thy self, but much more sweet thus cropt,
Forbidd'n here, it seems, as onely fit
For God's, yet able to make Gods of Men:

And why not Gods of Men, since good, the more
Communicated, more abundant growes,
The Author not impair'd, but honourd more?
Here, happie Creature, fair Angelic *Eve*,
Partake thou also; happie though thou art,
Happier thou mayst be, worthier canst not be:
Taste this, and be henceforth among the Gods
Thy self a Goddess, not to Earth confind,
But somtimes in the Air, as wee, somtimes
Ascend to Heav'n, by merit thine, and see
What life the Gods live there, and such live thou.
So saying, he drew nigh, and to me held,
Even to my mouth of that same fruit held part
Which he had pluckt; the pleasant savourie smell
So quick'nd appetite, that I, methought,
Could not but taste. Forthwith up to the Clouds
With him I flew, and underneath beheld
The Earth outstretcht immense, a prospect wide
And various: wondring at my flight and change
To this high exaltation; suddenly
My Guide was gon, and I, me thought, sunk down,
And fell asleep; but O how glad I wak'd
To find this but a dream!

John Keats
1795–1821

from Lamia

*In return for a favour, Lamia has asked the god Hermes to allow her
metamorphosis from a snake back into a woman, because she has fallen in love
with Lycius, a young man from Corinth. Hermes has agreed before leaving
her alone.*

   Left to herself, the serpent now began
To change; her elfin blood in madness ran,
Her mouth foam'd, and the grass, therewith besprent,
Wither'd at dew so sweet and virulent;
Her eyes in torture fix'd, and anguish drear,
Hot, glaz'd, and wide, with lid-lashes all sear,
Flash'd phosphor and sharp sparks, without one cooling
    tear.
The colours all inflam'd throughout her train,
She writh'd about, convuls'd with scarlet pain:
A deep volcanian yellow took the place
Of all her milder-mooned body's grace;
And, as the lava ravishes the mead,
Spoilt all her silver mail, and golden brede;
Made gloom of all her frecklings, streaks and bars,
Eclips'd her crescents, and lick'd up her stars:
So that, in moments few, she was undrest
Of all her sapphires, greens, and amethyst,
And rubious-argent: of all these bereft,
Nothing but pain and ugliness were left.
Still shone her crown; that vanish'd, also she
Melted and disappear'd as suddenly;
And in the air, her new voice luting soft,
Cried, 'Lycius! gentle Lycius!' – Borne aloft

With the bright mists about the mountains hoar
These words dissolv'd: Crete's forests heard no more.

Whither fled Lamia, now a lady bright,
A full-born beauty new and exquisite?
She fled into that valley they pass o'er
Who go to Corinth from Cenchreas' shore;
And rested at the foot of those wild hills,
The rugged founts of the Peræan rills,
And of that other ridge whose barren back
Stretches, with all its mist and cloudy rack,
South-westward to Cleone. There she stood
About a young bird's flutter from a wood,
Fair, on a sloping green of mossy tread,
By a clear pool, wherein she passioned
To see herself escap'd from so sore ills,
While her robes flaunted with the daffodils.

Ah, happy Lycius! – for she was a maid
More beautiful than ever twisted braid,
Or sigh'd, or blush'd, or on spring-flowered lea
Spread a green kirtle to the minstrelsy:
A virgin purest lipp'd, yet in the lore
Of love deep learned to the red heart's core:
Not one hour old, yet of sciential brain
To unperplex bliss from its neighbour pain;
Define their pettish limits, and estrange
Their points of contact, and swift counterchange;
Intrigue with the specious chaos, and dispart
Its most ambiguous atoms with sure art;
As though in Cupid's college she had spent
Sweet days a lovely graduate, still unshent,
And kept his rosy terms in idle languishment.

Why this fair creature chose so fairily
By the wayside to linger, we shall see;
But first 'tis fit to tell how she could muse
And dream, when in the serpent prison-house,
Of all she list, strange or magnificent:

How, ever, where she will'd, her spirit went;
Whether to faint Elysium, or where
Down through tress-lifting waves the Nereids fair
Wind into Thetis' bower by many a pearly stair;
Or where God Bacchus drains his cups divine,
Stretch'd out, at ease, beneath a glutinous pine;
Or where in Pluto's gardens palatine
Mulciber's columns gleam in far piazzian line.
And sometimes into cities she would send
Her dream, with feast and rioting to blend;
And once, while among mortals dreaming thus,
She saw the young Corinthian Lycius
Charioting foremost in the envious race,
Like a young Jove with calm uneager face,
And fell into a swooning love of him.
Now on the moth-time of that evening dim
He would return that way, as well she knew,
To Corinth from the shore; for freshly blew
The eastern soft wind, and his galley now
Grated the quaystones with her brazen prow
In port Cenchreas, from Egina isle
Fresh anchor'd; whither he had been awhile
To sacrifice to Jove, whose temple there
Waits with high marble doors for blood and incense rare.
Jove heard his vows, and better'd his desire;
For by some freakful chance he made retire
From his companions, and set forth to walk,
Perhaps grown wearied of their Corinth talk:
Over the solitary hills he fared,
Thoughtless at first, but ere eve's star appeared
His phantasy was lost, where reason fades,
In the calm'd twilight of Platonic shades.
Lamia beheld him coming, near, more near –
Close to her passing, in indifference drear,
His silent sandals swept the mossy green;
So neighbour'd to him, and yet so unseen
She stood: he pass'd, shut up in mysteries,
His mind wrapp'd like his mantle, while her eyes
Follow'd his steps, and her neck regal white

Turn'd – syllabling thus, 'Ah, Lycius bright,
And will you leave me on the hills alone?
Lycius, look back! and be some pity shown.'
He did; not with cold wonder fearingly,
But Orpheus-like at an Eurydice;
For so delicious were the words she sung,
It seem'd he had lov'd them a whole summer long:
And soon his eyes had drunk her beauty up,
Leaving no drop in the bewildering cup,
And still the cup was full, – while he, afraid
Lest she should vanish ere his lip had paid
Due adoration, thus began to adore;
Her soft look growing coy, she saw his chain so sure:
'Leave thee alone! Look back! Ah, Goddess, see
Whether my eyes can ever turn from thee!
For pity do not this sad heart belie –
Even as thou vanishest so I shall die.
Stay! though a Naiad of the rivers, stay!
To thy far wishes will thy streams obey:
Stay! though the greenest woods be thy domain,
Alone they can drink up the morning rain:
Though a descended Pleiad, will not one
Of thine harmonious sisters keep in tune
Thy spheres, and as thy silver proxy shine?
So sweetly to these ravish'd ears of mine
Came thy sweet greeting, that if thou shouldst fade
Thy memory will waste me to a shade: –
For pity do not melt!' – 'If I should stay,'
Said Lamia, 'here, upon this floor of clay,
And pain my steps upon these flowers too rough,
What canst thou say or do of charm enough
To dull the nice remembrance of my home?
Thou canst not ask me with thee here to roam
Over these hills and vales, where no joy is, –
Empty of immortality and bliss!
Thou art a scholar, Lycius, and must know
That finer spirits cannot breathe below
In human climes, and live: Alas! poor youth,
What taste of purer air hast thou to soothe

My essence? What serener palaces,
Where I may all my many senses please,
And by mysterious sleights a hundred thirsts appease?
It cannot be – Adieu!' So said, she rose
Tiptoe with white arms spread. He, sick to lose
The amorous promise of her lone complain,
Swoon'd, murmuring of love, and pale with pain.
The cruel lady, without any show
Of sorrow for her tender favourite woe,
But rather, if her eyes could brighter be,
With brighter eyes and slow amenity,
Put her new lips to his, and gave afresh
The life she had so tangled in her mesh:
And as he from one trance was wakening
Into another, she began to sing,
Happy in beauty, life, and love, and every thing,
A song of love, too sweet for earthly lyres,
While, like held breath, the stars drew in their panting fires.
And then she whisper'd in such trembling tone,
As those who, safe together met alone
For the first time through many anguish'd days,
Use other speech than looks; bidding him raise
His drooping head, and clear his soul of doubt,
For that she was a woman, and without
Any more subtle fluid in her veins
Than throbbing blood, and that the self-same pains
Inhabited her frail-strung heart as his.
And next she wonder'd how his eyes could miss
Her face so long in Corinth, where, she said,
She dwelt but half retir'd, and there had led
Days happy as the gold coin could invent
Without the aid of love; yet in content
Till she saw him, as once she pass'd him by,
Where 'gainst a column he leant thoughtfully
At Venus' temple porch, 'mid baskets heap'd
Of amorous herbs and flowers, newly reap'd
Late on that eve, as 'twas the night before
The Adonian feast; whereof she saw no more,
But wept alone those days, for why should she adore?

Lycius from death awoke into amaze,
To see her still, and singing so sweet lays;
Then from amaze into delight he fell
To hear her whisper woman's lore so well;
And every word she spake entic'd him on
To unperplex'd delight and pleasure known.
Let the mad poets say whate'er they please
Of the sweets of Fairies, Peris, Goddesses,
There is not such a treat among them all,
Haunters of cavern, lake, and waterfall,
As a real woman, lineal indeed
From Pyrrha's pebbles or old Adam's seed.
Thus gentle Lamia judg'd, and judg'd aright,
That Lycius could not love in half a fright,
So threw the goddess off, and won his heart
More pleasantly by playing woman's part,
With no more awe than what her beauty gave,
That, while it smote, still guaranteed to save.
Lycius to all made eloquent reply,
Marrying to every word a twinborn sigh;
And last, pointing to Corinth, ask'd her sweet,
If 'twas too far that night for her soft feet.
The way was short, for Lamia's eagerness
Made, by a spell, the triple league decrease
To a few paces; not at all surmised
By blinded Lycius, so in her comprized.
They pass'd the city gates, he knew not how,
So noiseless, and he never thought to know.

Christina Rossetti
1830–94

Goblin Market

Morning and evening
Maids heard the goblins cry:
'Come buy our orchard fruits,
Come buy, come buy:
Apples and quinces,
Lemons and oranges,
Plump unpecked cherries,
Melons and raspberries,
Bloom-down-cheeked peaches,
Swart-headed mulberries,
Wild free-born cranberries,
Crab-apples, dewberries,
Pine-apples, blackberries,
Apricots, strawberries; –
All ripe together
In summer weather, –
Morns that pass by,
Fair eves that fly;
Come buy, come buy:
Our grapes fresh from the vine,
Pomegranates full and fine,
Dates and sharp bullaces,
Rare pears and greengages,
Damsons and bilberries,
Taste them and try:
Currants and gooseberries,
Bright-fire-like barberries,
Figs to fill your mouth,
Citrons from the South,
Sweet to tongue and sound to eye;

Come buy, come buy.'
Evening by evening
Among the brookside rushes,
Laura bowed her head to hear,
Lizzie veiled her blushes:
Crouching close together
In the cooling weather,
With clasping arms and cautioning lips,
With tingling cheeks and finger tips.
'Lie close,' Laura said,
Pricking up her golden head:
'We must not look at goblin men,
We must not buy their fruits:
Who knows upon what soil they fed
Their hungry thirsty roots?'
'Come buy,' call the goblins
Hobbling down the glen.
'Oh,' cried Lizzie, 'Laura, Laura,
You should not peep at goblin men.'
Lizzie covered up her eyes,
Covered close lest they should look;
Laura reared her glossy head,
And whispered like the restless brook:
'Look, Lizzie, look, Lizzie,
Down the glen tramp little men.
One hauls a basket,
One bears a plate,
One lugs a golden dish
Of many pounds' weight.
How fair the vine must grow
Whose grapes are so luscious;
How warm the wind must blow
Through those fruit bushes.'
'No,' said Lizzie: 'No, no, no;
Their offers should not charm us,
Their evil gifts would harm us.'
She thrust a dimpled finger
In each ear, shut eyes and ran:
Curious Laura chose to linger

Wondering at each merchant man.
One had a cat's face,
One whisked a tail,
One tramped at a rat's pace,
One crawled like a snail,
One like a wombat prowled obtuse and furry,
One like a ratel tumbled hurry skurry.
She heard a voice like voice of doves
Cooing all together:
They sounded kind and full of loves
In the pleasant weather.

Laura stretched her gleaming neck
Like a rush-imbedded swan,
Like a lily from the beck,
Like a moonlit poplar branch,
Like a vessel at the launch
When its last restraint is gone.

Backwards up the mossy glen
Turned and trooped the goblin men,
With their shrill repeated cry,
'Come buy, come buy.'
When they reached where Laura was
They stood stock still upon the moss,
Leering at each other,
Brother with queer brother;
Signalling each other,
Brother with sly brother.
One set his basket down,
One reared his plate;
One began to weave a crown
Of tendrils, leaves, and rough nuts brown
(Men sell not such in any town);
One heaved the golden weight
Of dish and fruit to offer her:
'Come buy, come buy,' was still their cry.
Laura stared, but did not stir,
Longed but had no money.

The whisk-tailed merchant bade her taste
In tones as smooth as honey,
The cat-faced purr'd,
The rat-paced spoke a word
Of welcome, and the snail-paced even was heard;
One parrot-voiced and jolly
Cried 'Pretty Goblin' still for 'Pretty Polly';
One whistled like a bird.

But sweet-tooth Laura spoke in haste:
'Good Folk, I have no coin;
To take were to purloin:
I have no copper in my purse,
I have no silver either,
And all my gold is on the furze
That shakes in windy weather
Above the rusty heather.'
'You have much gold upon your head,'
They answered all together:
'Buy from us with a golden curl.'
She clipped a precious golden lock,
She dropped a tear more rare than pearl,
Then sucked their fruit globes fair or red.
Sweeter than honey from the rock,
Stronger than man-rejoicing wine,
Clearer than water flowed that juice;
She never tasted such before,
How should it cloy with length of use?
She sucked and sucked and sucked the more
Fruits which that unknown orchard bore:
She sucked until her lips were sore;
Then flung the emptied rinds away
But gathered up one kernel stone,
And knew not was it night or day
As she turned home alone.

Lizzie met her at the gate
Full of wise upbraidings:

'Dear, you should not stay so late,
Twilight is not good for maidens;
Should not loiter in the glen
In the haunts of goblin men.
Do you not remember Jeanie,
How she met them in the moonlight,
Took their gifts both choice and many,
Ate their fruits and wore their flowers
Plucked from bowers
Where summer ripens at all hours?
But ever in the noonlight
She pined and pined away;
Sought them by night and day,
Found them no more, but dwindled and grew grey;
Then fell with the first snow,
While to this day no grass will grow
Where she lies low:
I planted daisies there a year ago
That never blow.
You should not loiter so.'
'Nay, hush,' said Laura:
'Nay, hush, my sister:
I ate and ate my fill,
Yet my mouth waters still:
To-morrow night I will
Buy more;' and kissed her.
'Have done with sorrow;
I'll bring you plums to-morrow
Fresh on their mother twigs,
Cherries worth getting;
You cannot think what figs
My teeth have met in,
What melons icy-cold
Piled on a dish of gold
Too huge for me to hold,
What peaches with a velvet nap,
Pellucid grapes without one seed:
Odorous indeed must be the mead
Whereon they grow, and pure the wave they drink

With lilies at the brink,
And sugar-sweet their sap.'

Golden head by golden head,
Like two pigeons in one nest
Folded in each other's wings,
They lay down in their curtained bed:
Like two blossoms on one stem,
Like two flakes of new-fall'n snow,
Like two wands of ivory
Tipped with gold for awful kings.
Moon and stars gazed in at them,
Wind sang to them lullaby,
Lumbering owls forebore to fly,
Not a bat flapped to and fro
Round their nest:
Cheek to cheek and breast to breast
Locked together in one nest.

Early in the morning
When the first cock crowed his warning,
Neat like bees, as sweet and busy,
Laura rose with Lizzie:
Fetched in honey, milked the cows,
Aired and set to rights the house,
Kneaded cakes of whitest wheat,
Cakes for dainty mouths to eat,
Next churned butter, whipped up cream,
Fed their poultry, sat and sewed;
Talked as modest maidens should:
Lizzie with an open heart,
Laura in an absent dream,
One content, one sick in part;
One warbling for the mere bright day's delight,
One longing for the night.

At length slow evening came:
They went with pitchers to the reedy brook;

Lizzie most placid in her look,
Laura most like a leaping flame.
They drew the gurgling water from its deep.
Lizzie plucked purple and rich golden flags,
Then turning homeward said: 'The sunset flushes
Those furthest loftiest crags;
Come, Laura, not another maiden lags.
No wilful squirrel wags,
The beasts and birds are fast asleep.'
But Laura loitered still among the rushes,
And said the bank was steep.

And said the hour was early still,
The dew not fall'n, the wind not chill;
Listening ever, but not catching
The customary cry,
'Come buy, come buy,'
With its iterated jingle
Of sugar-baited words:
Not for all her watching
Once discerning even one goblin
Racing, whisking, tumbling, hobbling –
Let alone the herds
That used to tramp along the glen,
In groups or single,
Of brisk fruit-merchant men.

Till Lizzie urged, 'O Laura, come;
I hear the fruit-call, but I dare not look:
You should not loiter longer at this brook:
Come with me home.
The stars rise, the moon bends her arc,
Each glow-worm winks her spark,
Let us get home before the night grows dark:
For clouds may gather
Though this is summer weather,
Put out the lights and drench us through;
Then if we lost our way what should we do?'

Laura turned cold as stone
To find her sister heard that cry alone,
That goblin cry,
'Come buy our fruits, come buy.'
Must she then buy no more such dainty fruit?
Must she no more such succous pasture find,
Gone deaf and blind?
Her tree of life drooped from the root:
She said not one word in her heart's sore ache:
But peering thro' the dimness, nought discerning,
Trudged home, her pitcher dripping all the way;
So crept to bed, and lay
Silent till Lizzie slept;
Then sat up in a passionate yearning,
And gnashed her teeth for baulked desire, and wept
As if her heart would break.

Day after day, night after night,
Laura kept watch in vain
In sullen silence of exceeding pain.
She never caught again the goblin cry,
'Come buy, come buy;' –
She never spied the goblin men
Hawking their fruits along the glen:
But when the noon waxed bright
Her hair grew thin and grey;
She dwindled, as the fair full moon doth turn
To swift decay and burn
Her fire away.

One day remembering her kernel-stone
She set it by a wall that faced the south;
Dewed it with tears, hoped for a root,
Watched for a waxing shoot,
But there came none.
It never saw the sun,
It never felt the trickling moisture run:
While with sunk eyes and faded mouth
She dreamed of melons, as a traveller sees

False waves in desert drouth
With shade of leaf-crowned trees,
And burns the thirstier in the sandful breeze.

She no more swept the house,
Tended the fowls or cows,
Fetched honey, kneaded cakes of wheat,
Brought water from the brook:
But sat down listless in the chimney-nook
And would not eat.

Tender Lizzie could not bear
To watch her sister's cankerous care,
Yet not to share.
She night and morning
Caught the goblins' cry:
'Come buy our orchard fruits,
Come buy, come buy:' —
Beside the brook, along the glen,
She heard the tramp of goblin men,
The voice and stir
Poor Laura could not hear;
Longed to buy fruit to comfort her,
But feared to pay too dear.
She thought of Jeanie in her grave,
Who should have been a bride;
But who for joys brides hopes to have
Fell sick and died
In her gay prime,
In earliest winter time,
With the first glazing rime,
With the first snow-fall of crisp winter time.

Till Laura dwindling
Seemed knocking at Death's door.
Then Lizzie weighed no more
Better and worse;
But put a silver penny in her purse,

Kissed Laura, crossed the heath with clumps of furze
At twilight, halted by the brook:
And for the first time in her life
Began to listen and look.

Laughed every goblin
When they spied her peeping:
Came towards her hobbling,
Flying, running, leaping,
Puffling and blowing,
Chuckling, clapping, crowing,
Clucking and gobbling,
Mopping and mowing,
Full of airs and graces,
Pulling wry faces,
Demure grimaces,
Cat-like and rat-like,
Ratel- and wombat-like,
Snail-paced in a hurry,
Parrot-voiced and whistler,
Helter skelter, hurry skurry,
Chattering like magpies,
Fluttering like pigeons,
Gliding like fishes, –
Hugged her and kissed her:
Squeezed and caressed her:
Stretched up their dishes,
Panniers, and plates:
'Look at our apples
Russet and dun,
Bob at our cherries,
Bite at our peaches,
Citrons and dates,
Grapes for the asking,
Pears red with basking
Out in the sun,
Plums on their twigs;
Pluck them and suck them, –
Pomegranates, figs.'

'Good folk,' said Lizzie,
Mindful of Jeanie:
'Give me much and many:'
Held out her apron,
Tossed them her penny.
'Nay, take a seat with us,
Honour and eat with us,'
They answered grinning:
'Our feast is but beginning.
Night yet is early,
Warm and dew-pearly,
Wakeful and starry:
Such fruits as these
No man can carry;
Half their bloom would fly,
Half their dew would dry,
Half their flavour would pass by.
Sit down and feast with us,
Be welcome guest with us,
Cheer you and rest with us.' –
'Thank you,' said Lizzie: 'But one waits
At home alone for me:
So without further parleying,
If you will not sell me any
Of your fruits though much and many,
Give me back my silver penny
I tossed you for a fee.' –
They began to scratch their pates,
No longer wagging, purring,
But visibly demurring,
Grunting and snarling.
One called her proud,
Cross-grained, uncivil;
Their tones waxed loud,
Their looks were evil.
Lashing their tails
They trod and hustled her,
Elbowed and jostled her,
Clawed with their nails,

Barking, mewing, hissing, mocking
Tore her gown and soiled her stocking,
Twitched her hair out by the roots,
Stamped upon her tender feet,
Held her hands and squeezed their fruits
Against her mouth to make her eat.

White and golden Lizzie stood,
Like a lily in a flood, –
Like a rock of blue-veined stone
Lashed by tides obstreperously, –
Like a beacon left alone
In a hoary roaring sea,
Sending up a golden fire, –
Like a fruit-crowned orange-tree
White with blossoms honey-sweet
Sore beset by wasp and bee, –
Like a royal virgin town
Topped with gilded dome and spire
Close beleaguered by a fleet
Mad to tug her standard down.

One may lead a horse to water,
Twenty cannot make him drink.
Though the goblins cuffed and caught her,
Coaxed and fought her,
Bullied and besought her,
Scratched her, pinched her black as ink,
Kicked and knocked her,
Mauled and mocked her,
Lizzie uttered not a word;
Would not open lip from lip
Lest they should cram a mouthful in:
But laughed in heart to feel the drip
Of juice that syruped all her face,
And lodged in dimples of her chin,
And streaked her neck which quaked like curd.
At last the evil people,
Worn out by her resistance,

Flung back her penny, kicked their fruit
Along whichever road they took,
Not leaving root or stone or shoot;
Some writhed into the ground,
Some dived into the brook
With ring and ripple,
Some scudded on the gale without a sound,
Some vanished in the distance.

In a smart, ache, tingle,
Lizzie went her way;
Knew not was it night or day;
Sprang up the bank, tore thro' the furze,
Threaded copse and dingle,
And heard her penny jingle
Bouncing in her purse, –
Its bounce was music to her ear.
She ran and ran
As if she feared some goblin man
Dogged her with gibe or curse
Or something worse:
But not one goblin skurried after,
Nor was she pricked by fear;
The kind heart made her windy-paced
That urged her home quite out of breath with haste
And inward laughter.

She cried, 'Laura,' up the garden,
'Did you miss me?
Come and kiss me.
Never mind my bruises,
Hug me, kiss me, suck my juices
Squeezed from goblin fruits for you,
Goblin pulp and goblin dew.
Eat me, drink me, love me;
Laura, make much of me;
For your sake I have braved the glen
And had to do with goblin merchant men.'

Laura started from her chair,
Flung her arms up in the air,
Clutched her hair:
'Lizzie, Lizzie, have you tasted
For my sake the fruit forbidden?
Must your light like mine be hidden,
Your young life like mine be wasted,
Undone in mine undoing,
And ruined in my ruin,
Thirsty, cankered, goblin-ridden?' –
She clung about her sister,
Kissed and kissed and kissed her:
Tears once again
Refreshed her shrunken eyes,
Dropping like rain
After long sultry drouth;
Shaking with aguish fear, and pain,
She kissed, and kissed her with a hungry mouth.

Her lips began to scorch,
That juice was wormwood to her tongue,
She loathed the feast:
Writhing as one possessed she leaped and sung,
Rent all her robe, and wrung
Her hands in lamentable haste,
And beat her breast.
Her locks streamed like the torch
Borne by a racer at full speed,
Or like the mane of horses in their flight,
Or like an eagle when she stems the light
Straight toward the sun,
Or like a caged thing freed,
Or like a flying flag when armies run.
Swift fire spread through her veins, knocked at her heart,
Met the fire smouldering there
And overbore its lesser flame;
She gorged on bitterness without a name:
Ah fool, to choose such part

Of soul-consuming care!
Sense failed in the mortal strife:
Like the watch-tower of a town
Which an earthquake shatters down,
Like a lightning-stricken mast,
Like a wind-uprooted tree
Spun about,
Like a foam-topped waterspout
Cast down headlong in the sea,
She fell at last;
Pleasure past and anguish past,
Is it death or is it life?

Life out of death.
That night long Lizzie watched by her,
Counted her pulse's flagging stir,
Felt for her breath,
Held water to her lips, and cooled her face
With tears and fanning leaves.
But when the first birds chirped about their eaves,
And early reapers plodded to the place
Of golden sheaves,
And dew-wet grass
Bowed in the morning winds so brisk to pass,
And new buds with new day
Opened of cup-like lilies on the stream,
Laura awoke as from a dream,
Laughed in the innocent old way,
Hugged Lizzie but not twice or thrice;
Her gleaming locks showed not one thread of grey,
Her breath was sweet as May,
And light danced in her eyes.

Days, weeks, months, years
Afterwards, when both were wives
With children of their own;
Their mother-hearts beset with fears,
Their lives bound up in tender lives;
Laura would call the little ones

And tell them of her early prime,
Those pleasant days long gone
Of not-returning time:
Would talk about the haunted glen,
The wicked quaint fruit-merchant men,
Their fruits like honey to the throat
But poison in the blood
(Men sell not such in any town):
Would tell them how her sister stood
In deadly peril to do her good,
And win the fiery antidote:
Then joining hands to little hands
Would bid them cling together, —
'For there is no friend like a sister
In calm or stormy weather;
To cheer one on the tedious way,
To fetch one if one goes astray,
To lift one if one totters down,
To strengthen whilst one stands.'

Oliver Goldsmith
1730–74

---

from The Vicar of Wakefield

Song

When lovely woman stoops to folly,
   And finds too late that men betray,
What charm can sooth her melancholy,
   What art can wash her guilt away?

The only art her guilt to cover,
   To hide her shame from every eye,
To give repentance to her lover,
   And wring his bosom, is – to die.

Cyril Tourneur
1575?–1626

from The Revenger's Tragedy

*The Duchess wishes to seduce her stepson, the bastard, Spurio, to revenge
herself on her husband for failing to acquit one of her own sons, who is in
prison for rape. Spurio, in turn, wishes to revenge himself on his father and
the world in general because he is a bastard.*

SPURIO: Madam, your grace so private?
    My duty on your hand.
DUCHESS: Upon my hand, sir! troth, I think you'd fear
    To kiss my hand too, if my lip stood there.
SPURIO: Witness I would not, madam. (*Kisses her.*)
DUCHESS: 'Tis a wonder,
    For ceremony has made many fools!
    It is as easy way unto a duchess,
    As to a hatted dame, if her love answer:
    But that by timorous honours, pale respects,
    Idle degrees of fear, men make their ways
    Hard of themselves. What, have you thought of me?
SPURIO: Madam, I ever think of you in duty,
    Regard, and –
DUCHESS: Pooh! upon my love, I mean.
SPURIO: I would 'twere love; but 'tis a fouler name
    Than lust: you are my father's wife – your grace may guess
      now
    What I could call it.
DUCHESS: Why, th'art his son but falsely;
    'Tis a hard question whether he begot thee.
SPURIO: I' faith, 'tis true: I'm an uncertain man
    Of more uncertain woman. Maybe, his groom
    O' the stable begot me; you know I know not!
    He could ride a horse well, a shrewd suspicion, marry! –

He was wondrous tall: he had his length, i' faith.
For peeping over half-shut holyday windows,
Men would desire him light. When he was afoot
He made a goodly show under a pent-house;
And when he rid, his hat would check the signs,
And clatter barbers' basons.

DUCHESS: Nay, set you a-horseback once,
You'll ne'er light off.

SPURIO: Indeed, I am a beggar.

DUCHESS: That's the more sign thou'rt great. –
But to our love:
Let it stand firm both in thy thought and mind,
That the duke was thy father, as no doubt then
He bid fair for't – thy injury is the more;
For had he cut thee a right diamond,
Thou had'st been next set in the dukedom's ring,
When his worn self, like age's easy slave,
Had dropped out of the collet into th' grave.
What wrong can equal this? canst thou be tame,
And think upon't?

SPURIO: No, mad, and think upon't.

DUCHESS: Who would not be revenged of such a father,
E'en in the worst way? I would thank that sin,
That could most injure him, and be in league with it.
O, what a grief 'tis that a man should live
But once i' the world, and then to live a bastard –
The curse o' the womb, the thief of nature,
Begot against the seventh commandment,
Half-damned in the conception by the justice
Of that unbribèd everlasting law.

SPURIO: O, I'd a hot-backed devil to my father.

DUCHESS: Would not this mad e'en patience, make blood
rough?
Who but an eunuch would not sin? his bed,
By one false minute disinherited.

SPURIO: Ay, there's the vengeance that my birth was wrapped
in!
I'll be revenged for all: now, hate, begin;
I'll call foul incest but a venial sin.

DUCHESS: Cold still! in vain then must a duchess woo?
SPURIO: Madam, I blush to say what I will do.
DUCHESS: Thence flew sweet comfort. Earnest, and farewell.
    (*Kisses him.*)
SPURIO: O, one incestuous kiss picks open hell.
DUCHESS: Faith, now, old duke, my vengeance shall reach high,
    I'll arm thy brow with woman's heraldry. (*Exit.*)
SPURIO: Duke, thou didst do me wrong; and, by thy act
    Adultery is my nature.
    Faith, if the truth were known, I was begot
    After some gluttonous dinner; some stirring dish
    Was my first father, when deep healths went round,
    And ladies' cheeks were painted red with wine,
    Their tongues, as short and nimble as their heels,
    Uttering words sweet and thick; and when they rose,
    Were merrily disposed to fall again.
    In such a whispering and withdrawing hour,
    When base male-bawds kept sentinel at stair-head,
    Was I stol'n softly. O damnation meet!
    The sin of feasts, drunken adultery!
    I feel it swell me; my revenge is just!
    I was begot in impudent wine and lust.

Aldous Huxley
1894–1963

from Point Counter Point

Denis Burlap is forty, and the editor of his periodical, the Literary World. *Thirty-five-year-old Beatrice Gilray works for him, and is also his landlady. Mark Rampion is an acquaintance of both, a character allegedly based on D. H. Lawrence.*

Burlap came home to find Beatrice, as usual, waiting up for him. Sitting – for such was the engagingly child-like habit he had formed during the last few weeks – on the floor at her feet, his head, with the little pink tonsure in the middle of the dark curls, against her knee, he sipped his hot milk and talked of Rampion. An extraordinary man, a great man, even. Great? queried Beatrice, disapprovingly. She didn't like to hear greatness attributed to any living man (the dead were a different matter; they were dead), unless it was to Denis himself. Hardly *great*, she insisted jealously. Well, perhaps not quite. But very nearly. If he hadn't that strange insensitiveness to spiritual values, that prejudice, that blind spot. The attitude was comprehensible. Rampion was reacting against something which had gone too far in one direction; but in the process of reacting he had gone too far in the other. His incapacity to understand St Francis, for example. The grotesque and really hideous things he could say about the saint. That was extraordinary and deplorable.

'What does he say?' asked Beatrice severely. Since knowing Burlap, she had taken St Francis under her protection.

Burlap gave her an account, a little expurgated, of what Rampion had said. Beatrice was indignant. How could he say such things? How did he dare? It was an outrage. Yes, it was a defect in him, Burlap admitted, a real defect. But so few people, he added in charitable palliation, were born with a real feeling for spiritual beauty. Rampion was an extraordinary man in many ways, but it was as though he lacked that extra sense-organ which enables men like St Francis to see the beauty that is beyond earthly beauty. In a rudimentary form he himself, he thought, had the power. How rarely he met anyone who seemed to be like him! Almost everybody was in this respect a stranger. It was like seeing normally in a country where most people were colour blind. Didn't Beatrice feel that too? For of course she was one of the rare clear-seeing ones. He had felt it at once, the first time he met her. Beatrice nodded gravely. Yes, she too felt like that. Burlap smiled up at her; he knew it. She felt proud and important. Rampion's idea of love, for example; Burlap shook his head. So extraordinarily gross and animal and corporeal.

'Dreadful,' said Beatrice feelingly. Denis, she was thinking, was so different. Tenderly she looked down at the head that reposed, so trustingly, against her knee. She adored the way his hair curled, and his very small, beautiful ears, and even the pink bare spot on the top of his crown. That little pink tonsure was somehow rather engagingly pathetic. There was a long silence.

Burlap at last profoundly sighed. 'How tired I am!' he said.

'You ought to go to bed.'

'Too tired even to move.' He pressed his cheek more heavily against her knee and shut his eyes.

Beatrice raised her hand, hesitated a moment, dropped it again, then raised it once more and began to run her fingers soothingly through his dark curls. There was another long silence.

'Ah, don't stop,' he said, when at last she withdrew her hand. 'It's so comforting. Such a virtue seems to go out from you. You'd almost cured my headache.'

'You've got a headache?' asked Beatrice, her solicitude running as usual to a kind of anger. 'Then you simply must go to bed,' she commanded.

'But I'm so happy here.'

'No, I insist.' Her protective motherliness was thoroughly aroused. It was a bullying tenderness.

'How cruel you are!' Burlap complained, rising reluctantly to his feet. Beatrice was touched with compunction. 'I'll stroke your head when you're in bed,' she promised. She too now regretted that soft warm silence, that speechless intimacy, which her outburst of domineering solicitude had too abruptly shattered.

She justified herself by an explanation. The headache would return if he didn't go to sleep the moment it was cured. And so on.

Burlap had been in bed nearly ten minutes when she came to keep her promise. She was dressed in a green dressing-gown and her yellow hair was plaited into a long thick pigtail that swung heavily as she moved, like the heavy plaited tail of a cart-horse at a show.

'You look about twelve with that pigtail hanging down your back,' said Burlap, enchanted.

Beatrice laughed, rather nervously, and sat down on the edge of the bed. He raised his hand and took hold of the thick plait. 'Too charming,' he said. 'It simply invites pulling.' He gave a little tug at it, playfully.

'Look out,' she warned. 'I'll pull back, in spite of your headache.' She took hold of one of his dark curls.

'Pax, pax!' he begged, reverting to the vocabulary of the preparatory school. 'I'll let go. The real reason,' he added, 'why little boys don't like fighting with little girls is simply that little girls are so much more ruthless and ferocious.'

Beatrice laughed again. There was a silence. She felt a little breathless and fluttering, as one feels when one is anxiously expecting something to happen. 'Head bad?' she asked.

'Rather bad.'

She stretched out a hand and touched his forehead.

'Your hand's magical,' he said. With a quick unexpected movement he wriggled round sideways under the sheets and laid his head on her lap. 'There,' he whispered and, with a sigh of contentment, closed his eyes.

For a moment Beatrice was taken aback, almost frightened. That dark head lying hard and heavy on her thighs – it seemed strange, terrifying. She had to suppress a little shudder before she could feel glad at the confiding childishness of his movement. She began stroking his forehead, stroking his scalp through the thick dark curls. Time passed. The soft warm silence enveloped them once more, the dumb intimacy of contact was re-established. She was no longer domineering in her protective solicitude, only tender. The armour of her hardness was as though melted away from her, melted away in this warm intimacy along with the terrors which made it necessary.

Burlap sighed again. He was in a kind of blissful doze of sensual passivity.

'Better?' she asked in a soft whisper.

'Still rather bad on the side,' he whispered back. 'Just over the ear.' And he rolled his head over so that she could more easily reach the painful spot, rolled it over so that his face was pressed against her belly, her soft belly that stirred so livingly with her breathing, that was so warm and yielding against his face.

At the touch of his face against her body Beatrice felt a sudden renewal of those spasmodic creepings of apprehension. Her flesh was terrified by the nearness of that physical intimacy. But as Burlap did not stir, as he made no dangerous gesture, no movement towards a closer contact, the terrors died gradually down and their flutterings served only to enhance and intensify that wonderful warm emotion of tenderness which succeeded them. She ran her fingers through his hair, again and again. The warmth of his breathing was against her belly. She shivered a little; her happiness fluttered with apprehensions and anticipations. Her flesh trembled, but was somehow joyful; was afraid and yet curious; shrank, but took warmth at the contact and even, through its terrors, timidly desired.

'Better?' she whispered again.

He made a little movement with his head and pressed his face closer to her soft flesh.

'Shall I stop now?' she went on, 'shall I go away?'

Burlap raised his head and looked at her. 'No, no,' he implored. 'Don't go. Not yet. Don't break the magic. Stay here for a moment longer. Lie down here for a moment under the quilt. For a moment.'

Without speaking she stretched herself out beside him and he drew the quilt over her, he turned out the light.

The fingers that caressed her arm under its wide sleeve touched delicately, touched spiritually and as it were disembodiedly, like the fingers of those inflated rubber gloves that brush so thrillingly against one's face in the darkness of séances, bringing comfort from the Great Beyond and a message of affection from the loved ones who have passed over. To caress and yet be a spiritualized rubber glove at a séance, to make love but as though from the Great Beyond – that was Burlap's talent. Softly, patiently, with an infinite disembodied gentleness he went on caressing. Beatrice's armour was melted quite away. It was the soft young-girlish, tremulous core of her that Burlap caressed with that delicate touch of spirit fingers from the Great Beyond. Her armour was gone; but she felt so wonderfully safe with Denis. She felt no fears, or at least only such faint breathless flutterings of her still almost childish flesh as served to quicken her happiness. She felt so wonderfully safe even when – after what had seemed a delicious eternity of patiently repeated caresses from wrist to shoulder and back again – the spirit hand reached out of the Beyond and touched her breast. Delicately, almost disembodiedly it touched, like a skin of rubber stuffed with air; spiritually it slid over the rounded flesh, and its angelic fingers lingered along the skin. At the first touch the round breast shuddered; it had its private terrors within Beatrice's general happiness and sense of security. But patiently, gently, unalarmingly, the spirit hand repeated its caress again, again, till the reassured and at last eager breast longed for its return and her whole body was alive with the tingling ramifications of the breast's desires. In the darkness the eternities prolonged themselves.

Leda and the Swan

A sudden blow: the great wings beating still
Above the staggering girl, her thighs caressed
By the dark webs, her nape caught in his bill,
He holds her helpless breast upon his breast.

How can those terrified vague fingers push
The feathered glory from her loosening thighs?
And how can body, laid in that white rush,
But feel the strange heart beating where it lies?

A shudder in the loins engenders there
The broken wall, the burning roof and tower
And Agamemnon dead.
                  Being so caught up,
So mastered by the brute blood of the air,
Did she put on his knowledge with his power
Before the indifferent beak could let her drop?

Lilian Bowes-Lyon
1895–1949

Leda

Remember still the first, impetuous form
His person took, when like a pool your mind
Contained the sun, though furious the storm
That struck your reed-bed of a body blind.

Revive your wonder that his thrashing breath
Was every violet's, yet an outlaw wind's.
So strong the river rolls; not even death
Can stop it rippling over rush-lit hands.

Love, you were more than rover, robber, ranger;
More than a serpent throat, or silvered thighs.
Alas! We lose the fiery fellow-stranger.
Light on the water hurts our human eyes.

Bram Stoker
1847–1912

from Dracula

*Lucy, formerly engaged to Arthur, has died and become a vampire after being
bitten by Dracula. This extract from the diary of Dr Seward, head of a
lunatic asylum and himself a former suitor of Lucy, describes how he and
Arthur and Quincey Morris, yet another erstwhile suitor, track down Lucy
and free her from the ranks of the undead, under the leadership of the
vampirologist, Professor Van Helsing. The scene is Highgate Cemetery.*

There was a long spell of silence, a big, aching void, and then from
the Professor a keen 'S-s-s-s!' He pointed; and far down the avenue
of yews we saw a white figure advance – a dim white figure, which
held something dark at its breast. The figure stopped, and at the
moment a ray of moonlight fell between the masses of driving
clouds and showed in startling prominence a dark-haired woman,
dressed in the cerements of the grave. We could not see the face,
for it was bent down over what we saw to be a fair-haired child.
There was a pause and a sharp little cry, such as a child gives in
sleep, or a dog as it lies before the fire and dreams. We were
starting forward, but the Professor's warning hand, seen by us as
he stood behind a yew-tree, kept us back; and then as we looked
the white figure moved forward again. It was now near enough for
us to see clearly, and the moonlight still held. My own heart grew
cold as ice, and I could hear the gasp of Arthur, as we recognized
the features of Lucy Westenra. Lucy Westenra, but yet how
changed. The sweetness was turned to adamantine, heartless
cruelty, and the purity to voluptuous wantonness. Van Helsing
stepped out, and, obedient to his gesture, we all advanced too; the
four of us ranged in a line before the door of the tomb. Van Helsing
raised his lantern and drew the slide; by the concentrated light
that fell on Lucy's face we could see that the lips were crimson with

fresh blood, and that the stream had trickled over her chin and stained the purity of her lawn death-robe.

We shuddered with horror. I could see by the tremulous light that even Van Helsing's iron nerve had failed. Arthur was next to me, and if I had not seized his arm and held him up, he would have fallen.

When Lucy – I call the thing that was before us Lucy because it bore her shape – saw us she drew back with an angry snarl, such as a cat gives when taken unawares; then her eyes ranged over us. Lucy's eyes in form and colour; but Lucy's eyes unclean and full of hell-fire, instead of the pure, gentle orbs we knew. At that moment the remnant of my love passed into hate and loathing; had she then to be killed, I could have done it with savage delight. As she looked, her eyes blazed with unholy light, and the face became wreathed with a voluptuous smile. Oh, God, how it made me shudder to see it! With a careless motion, she flung to the ground, callous as a devil, the child that up to now she had clutched strenuously to her breast, growling over it as a dog growls over a bone. The child gave a sharp cry, and lay there moaning. There was a cold-bloodedness in the act which wrung a groan from Arthur; when she advanced to him with outstretched arms and a wanton smile, he fell back and hid his face in his hands.

She still advanced, however, and with a languorous, voluptuous grace, said: –

'Come to me, Arthur. Leave these others and come to me. My arms are hungry for you. Come, and we can rest together. Come, my husband, come!'

There was something diabolically sweet in her tones – something of the tingling of glass when struck – which rang through the brains even of us who heard the words addressed to another. As for Arthur, he seemed under a spell; moving his hands from his face, he opened wide his arms. She was leaping for them, when Van Helsing sprang forward and held between them his little golden crucifix. She recoiled from it, and, with a suddenly distorted face, full of rage, dashed past him as if to enter the tomb.

When within a foot or two of the door, however, she stopped as if arrested by some irresistible force. Then she turned, and her face was shown in the clear burst of moonlight and by the lamp, which had now no quiver from Van Helsing's iron nerves. Never did I see such baffled malice on a face; and never, I trust, shall such ever be seen again by mortal eyes. The beautiful colour became livid, the eyes seemed to throw out sparks of hell-fire, the brows were wrinkled as though the folds of the flesh were the coils of Medusa's snakes, and the lovely, blood-stained mouth grew to an open square, as in the passion masks of the Greeks and Japanese. If ever a face meant death – if looks could kill – we saw it at that moment.

And so for full half a minute, which seemed an eternity, she remained between the lifted crucifix and the sacred closing of her means of entry. Van Helsing broke the silence by asking Arthur: –

'Answer me, oh my friend! Am I to proceed in my work?'

Arthur threw himself on his knees, and hid his face in his hands, as he answered: –

'Do as you will, friend; do as you will. There can be no horror like this ever any more!' and he groaned in spirit. Quincey and I simultaneously moved towards him, and took his arms. We could hear the click of the closing lantern as Van Helsing held it down; coming close to the tomb, he began to remove from the chinks some of the sacred emblem which he had placed there. We all looked on in horrified amazement as we saw, when he stood back, the woman, with a corporeal body as real at the moment as our own, pass in through the interstice where scarce a knife-blade could have gone. We all felt a glad sense of relief when we saw the Professor calmly restoring the strings of putty to the edges of the door.

When this was done, he lifted the child and said: –

'Come now, my friends; we can do no more till tomorrow. There is a funeral at noon, so here we shall all come before long after that. The friends of the dead will all be gone by two, and when the sexton lock the gate we shall remain. Then there is more to do; but not like this of tonight. As for this little one, he is not much harmed, and by tomorrow night he shall be well. We shall leave him where the police will find him, as on the other night and then to home.' Coming close to Arthur, he said: –

'My friend Arthur, you have had sore trial; but after, when you will look back, you will see how it was necessary. You are now in the bitter waters, my child. By this time tomorrow, you will, please God, have passed them, and have drunk of the sweet waters; so do not mourn overmuch. Till then I shall not ask you to forgive me.'

Arthur and Quincey came home with me, and we tried to cheer each other on the way. We had left the child in safety, and were tired; so we all slept with more or less reality of sleep.

29 *September, night*. – A little before twelve o'clock we three – Arthur, Quincey Morris, and myself – called for the Professor. It was odd to notice that by common consent we had all put on black clothes. Of course, Arthur wore black, for he was in deep mourning, but the rest of us wore it by instinct. We got to the churchyard by half-past one, and strolled about, keeping out of official observation, so that when the gravediggers had completed their task, and the sexton, under the belief that every one had gone, had locked the gate, we had the place all to ourselves. Van Helsing, instead of his little black bag, had with him a long leather one, something like a cricketing bag; it was manifestly of fair weight.

When we were alone and had heard the last of the footsteps die out up the road, we silently, and as if by ordered intention, followed the Professor to the tomb. He unlocked the door, and we entered, closing it behind us. Then he took from his bag the lantern, which he lit, and also two wax candles, which, when lighted, he stuck, by melting their own ends, on other coffins, so that they might give light sufficient to work by. When he again lifted the lid off Lucy's coffin we all looked – Arthur trembling like an aspen – and saw that the body lay there in all its death-beauty. But there was no love in my own heart, nothing but loathing for the foul Thing which had taken Lucy's shape without her soul. I could see even Arthur's face grow hard as he looked. Presently he said to Van Helsing: –

'Is this really Lucy's body, or only a demon in her shape?'

'It is her body, and yet not it. But wait a while, and you shall see her as she was, and is.'

She seemed like a nightmare of Lucy as she lay there; the pointed teeth, the bloodstained, voluptuous mouth – which it made one shudder to see – the whole carnal and unspiritual appearance, seeming like a devilish mockery of Lucy's sweet purity. Van Helsing, in his methodical manner, began taking the various contents from his bag and placing them ready for use. First he took out a soldering iron and some plumbing solder, and then a small oil-lamp, which gave out, when lit in a corner of the tomb, gas which burned at fierce heat with a blue flame; then his operating knives, which he placed to hand; and last a round wooden stake, some two and a half or three inches thick and about three feet long. One end of it was hardened by charring in the fire, and was sharpened to a fine point. With this stake came a heavy hammer, such as in households is used in a coal-cellar for breaking the lumps. To me, a doctor's preparations for work of any kind are stimulating and bracing, but the effect of these things on both Arthur and Quincey was to cause them a sort of consternation. They both, however, kept their courage, and remained silent and quiet.

When all was ready, Van Helsing said: —

'Before we do anything, let me tell you this; it is out of the lore and experience of the ancients and of all those who have studied the powers of the Un-Dead. When they become such, there comes with the change the curse of immortality; they cannot die, but must go on age after age adding new victims and multiplying the evils of the world; for all that die from the preying of the Un-Dead become themselves Un-Dead, and prey on their kind. And so the circle goes on ever widening, like as the ripples from a stone thrown in the water. Friend Arthur, if you had met that kiss which you know of before poor Lucy die; or again, last night when you open your arms to her, you would in time, when you had died, have become *nosferatu*, as they call it in Eastern Europe, and would all time make more of those Un-Deads that so have fill us with horror. The career of this so unhappy dear lady is but just begun. Those children whose blood she suck are not as yet so much the worse; but if she live on, Un-Dead, more and more they lose their blood, and by her power over them they come to her; and so she draw their blood with that so wicked mouth. But if she die in truth, then all cease; the tiny wounds of the throats disappear, and they go back to their plays unknowing ever of what has been. But of the most blessed of all, when this now Un-Dead be made to rest as true dead, then the soul of the poor lady whom we love shall again be free. Instead of working wickedness by night and growing more debased in the assimilation of it by day, she shall take her place with the other Angels. So that, my friend, it will be a blessed hand for her that shall strike the blow that sets her free. To this I am willing; but is there none amongst us who has a better right? Will it be no joy to think of hereafter in the silence of the night when sleep is not: "It was my hand that sent her to the stars; it was the hand of him that loved her best; the hand that of all she would herself have chosen, had it been to her to choose"? Tell me if there be such a one amongst us?'

. We all looked at Arthur. He saw, too, what we all did, the infinite kindness which suggested that his should be the hand which would restore Lucy to us as a holy, and not an unholy, memory; he stepped forward and said bravely, though his hand trembled, and his face was as pale as snow: –

'My true friend, from the bottom of my broken heart I thank you. Tell me what I am to do, and I shall not falter!' Van Helsing laid a hand on his shoulder, and said: –

'Brave lad! A moment's courage, and it is done. This stake must be driven through her. It will be a fearful ordeal – be not deceived in that – but it will be only a short time, and you will then rejoice more than your pain was great; from this grim tomb you will emerge as though you tread on air. But you must not falter when once you have begun. Only think that we, your true friends, are round you, and that we pray for you all the time.'

'Go on,' said Arthur hoarsely. 'Tell me what I am to do.'

'Take this stake in your left hand, ready to place the point over the heart, and the hammer in your right. Then when we begin our prayer for the dead – I shall read him. I have here the book, and the others shall follow – strike in God's name, that so all may be well with the dead that we love, and that the Un-Dead pass away.'

Arthur took the stake and the hammer, and when once his mind was set on action his hands never trembled nor even quivered. Van Helsing opened his missal and began to read, and Quincey and I followed as well as we could. Arthur placed the point over the heart, and as I looked I could see its dint in the white flesh. Then he struck with all his might.

The Thing in the coffin writhed; and a hideous, blood-curdling screech came from the opened red lips. The body shook and quivered and twisted in wild contortions; the sharp white teeth champed together till the lips were cut, and the mouth was smeared with a crimson foam. But Arthur never faltered. He looked like a figure of Thor as his untrembling arm rose and fell, driving deeper and deeper the mercy-bearing stake, whilst the blood from the pierced heart welled and spurted up around it. His face was set, and high duty seemed to shine through it; the sight of it gave us courage, so that our voices seemed to ring through the little vault.

And then the writhing and quivering of the body became less, and the teeth ceased to champ, and the face to quiver. Finally it lay still. The terrible task was over.

The hammer fell from Arthur's hand. He reeled and would have fallen had we not caught him. The great drops of sweat sprang out on his forehead, and his breath came in broken gasps. It had indeed been an awful strain on him; and had he not been forced to his task by more than human considerations he could never have gone through with it. For a few minutes we were so taken up with him that we did not look towards the coffin. When we did, however, a murmur of startled surprise ran from one to the other of us. We gazed so eagerly that Arthur rose, for he had been seated on the ground, and came and looked too; and then a glad, strange light broke over his face and dispelled altogether the gloom of horror that lay upon it.

There in the coffin lay no longer the foul Thing that we had so dreaded and grown to hate that the work of her destruction was yielded as a privilege to the one best entitled to it, but Lucy as we had seen her in her life, with her face of unequalled sweetness and purity. True that there were there, as we had seen them in life, the traces of care and pain and waste; but these were all dear to us, for they marked her truth to what we knew. One and all we felt that the holy calm that lay like sunshine over the wasted face and form was only an earthly token and symbol of the calm that was to reign for ever.

Van Helsing came and laid his hand on Arthur's shoulder, and said to him: –

'And now, Arthur, my friend, dear lad, am I not forgiven?'

The reaction of the terrible strain came as he took the old man's hand in his, and raising it to his lips, pressed it, and said: –

'Forgiven! God bless you that you have given my dear one her soul again, and me peace.' He put his hands on the Professor's shoulder, and laying his head on his breast, cried for a while silently, whilst we stood unmoving. When he raised his head Van Helsing said to him: –

'And now, my child, you may kiss her. Kiss her dead lips if you will, as she would have you to, if for her to choose. For she is not a grinning devil now – not any more a foul Thing for all eternity. No longer she is the devil's Un-Dead. She is God's true dead, whose soul is with Him!'

Arthur bent and kissed her, and then we sent him and Quincey out of the tomb; the Professor and I sawed the top off the stake, leaving the point of it in the body. Then we cut off the head and filled the mouth with garlic. We soldered up the leaden coffin, screwed on the coffin-lid, and gathering up our belongings, came away. When the Professor locked the door he gave the key to Arthur.

Siren Song

Anon

from The Book of Genesis

Now the serpent was more subtil than any beast of the field which the LORD God had made. And he said unto the woman, Yea, hath God said, Ye shall not eat of every tree of the garden?

And the woman said unto the serpent, We may eat of the fruit of the trees of the garden:

But of the fruit of the tree which *is* in the midst of the garden, God hath said, Ye shall not eat of it, neither shall ye touch it, lest ye die.

And the serpent said unto the woman, Ye shall not surely die:

For God doth know that in the day ye eat thereof, then your eyes shall be opened, and ye shall be as gods, knowing good and evil.

And when the woman saw that the tree *was* good for food, and that it *was* pleasant to the eyes, and a tree to be desired to make *one* wise, she took of the fruit thereof, and did eat, and gave also unto her husband with her; and he did eat.

And the eyes of them both were opened, and they knew that they *were* naked; and they sewed fig leaves together, and made themselves aprons.

And they heard the voice of the LORD God walking in the garden in the cool of the day: and Adam and his wife hid themselves from the presence of the LORD God amongst the trees of the garden.

And the LORD God called unto Adam, and said unto him, Where *art* thou?

And he said, I heard thy voice in the garden, and I was afraid, because I *was* naked; and I hid myself.

And he said, Who told thee that thou *wast* naked? Hast thou eaten of the tree, whereof I commanded thee that thou shouldest not eat?

And the man said, The woman whom thou gavest *to be* with me, she gave me of the tree, and I did eat.

And the LORD God said unto the woman, What *is* this *that* thou hast done? And the woman said, The serpent beguiled me, and I did eat.

And the LORD God said unto the serpent, Because thou hast done this, thou *art* cursed above all cattle, and above every beast of the field; upon thy belly shalt thou go, and dust shalt thou eat all the days of thy life:

And I will put enmity between thee and the woman, and between thy seed and her seed; it shall bruise thy head, and thou shalt bruise his heel.

Unto the woman he said, I will greatly multiply thy sorrow and thy conception; in sorrow thou shalt bring forth children; and thy desire *shall be* to thy husband, and he shall rule over thee.

And unto Adam he said, Because thou hast hearkened unto the voice of thy wife, and hast eaten of the tree, of which I commanded thee, saying, Thou shalt not eat of it: cursed *is* the ground for thy sake; in sorrow shalt thou eat *of* it all the days of thy life;

Thorns also and thistles shall it bring forth to thee; and thou shalt eat the herb of the field;

In the sweat of thy face shalt thou eat bread, till thou return unto the ground; for out of it wast thou taken: for dust thou *art*, and unto dust shalt thou return.

And Adam called his wife's name Eve; because she was the mother of all living.

Unto Adam also and to his wife did the LORD God make coats of skins, and clothed them.

And the LORD God said, Behold, the man is become as one of us, to know good and evil: and now, lest he put forth his hand, and take also of the tree of life, and eat, and live for ever:

Therefore the LORD God sent him forth from the garden of Eden, to till the ground from whence he was taken.

So he drove out the man; and he placed at the east of the garden of Eden Cherubims, and a flaming sword which turned every way, to keep the way of the tree of life.

🔖

John Milton
1608–74

---

from Paradise Lost, Book IX

Eve tempts Adam

Hast thou not wondered, *Adam*, at my stay?
Thee I have misst, and thought it long, depriv'd
Thy presence, agonie of love till now
Not felt, nor shall be twice, for never more
Mean I to trie, what rash untri'd I sought,
The pain of absence from thy sight. But strange
Hath bin the cause, and wonderful to heare:
This Tree is not as we are told, a Tree
Of danger tasted, nor to evil unknown
Op'ning the way, but of Divine effect
To open Eyes, and make them Gods who taste;
And hath bin tasted such: the Serpent wise,
Or not restraind as wee, or not obeying,
Hath eat'n of the fruit, and is become,
Not dead, as we are threatn'd, but thenceforth
Endu'd with human voice and human sense,
Reasoning to admiration, and with mee
Perswasively hath so prevaild, that I
Have also tasted, and have also found
Th' effects to correspond, opener mine Eyes,
Dimm erst, dilated Spirits, ampler Heart,
And growing up to Godhead; which for thee
Chiefly I sought, without thee can despise.
For bliss, as thou hast part, to me is bliss,
Tedious, unshar'd with thee, and odious soon.
Thou therefore also taste, that equal Lot
May joyne us, equal Joy, as equal Love;
Least thou not tasting, different degree

Disjoyne us, and I then too late renounce
Deitie for thee, when Fate will not permit.

   Thus *Eve* with Countnance blithe her storie told;
But in her Cheek distemper flushing glowd.
On th' other side, *Adam*, soon as he heard
The fatal Trespass don by *Eve*, amaz'd,
Astonied stood and Blank, while horror chill
Ran through his veins, and all his joynts relax'd;
From his slack hand the Garland wreath'd for *Eve*
Down drop'd, and all the faded Roses shed:
Speechless he stood and pale, till thus at length
First to himself he inward silence broke.

   O fairest of Creation, last and best
Of all Gods works, Creature in whom excell'd
Whatever can to sight or thought be formd,
Holy, divine, good, amiable, or sweet!
How art thou lost, how on a sudden lost,
Defac't, deflourd, and now to Death devote?
Rather how hast thou yeelded to transgress
The strict forbiddance, how to violate
The sacred Fruit forbidd'n! som cursed fraud
Of Enemie hath beguil'd thee, yet unknown,
And mee with thee hath ruind, for with thee
Certain my resolution is to Die;
How can I live without thee, how forgoe
Thy sweet Converse and Love so dearly joyn'd,
To live again in these wilde Woods forlorn?
Should God create another *Eve*, and I
Another Rib afford, yet loss of thee
Would never from my heart; no no, I feel
The Link of Nature draw me: Flesh of Flesh,
Bone of my Bone thou art, and from thy State
Mine never shall be parted, bliss or woe.

   So having said, as one from sad dismay
Recomforted, and after thoughts disturbd
Submitting to what seemd remediless,
Thus in calm mood his Words to *Eve* he turnd.

   Bold deed thou hast presum'd, adventurous *Eve*,
And peril great provok't, who thus hath dar'd

Had it been onely coveting to Eye
That sacred Fruit, sacred to abstinence,
Much more to taste it under banne to touch.
But past who can recall, or don undoe?
Not God Omnipotent, nor Fate, yet so
Perhaps thou shalt not Die, perhaps the Fact
Is not so hainous now, foretasted Fruit,
Profan'd first by the Serpent, by him first
Made common and unhallowd ere our taste;
Nor yet on him found deadly, he yet lives,
Lives, as thou saidst, and gaines to live as Man
Higher degree of Life, inducement strong
To us, as likely tasting to attaine
Proportional ascent, which cannot be
But to be Gods, or Angels Demi-gods.
Nor can I think that God, Creator wise,
Though threatning, will in earnest so destroy
Us his prime Creatures, dignifi'd so high,
Set over all his Works, which in our Fall,
For us created, needs with us must faile,
Dependent made; so God shall uncreate,
Be frustrate, do, undo, and labour loose,
Not well conceav'd of God, who though his Power
Creation could repeate, yet would be loath
Us to abolish, least the Adversary
Triumph and say; Fickle their State whom God
Most Favors, who can please him long; Mee first
He ruind, now Mankind; whom will he next?
Matter of scorne, not to be given the Foe,
However I with thee have fixt my Lot,
Certain to undergoe like doom, if Death
Consort with thee, Death is to mee as Life;
So forcible within my heart I feel
The Bond of Nature draw me to my owne,
My own in thee, for what thou art is mine;
Our State cannot be severd, we are one,
One Flesh; to loose thee were to loose my self.
    So *Adam*, and thus *Eve* to him repli'd.
O glorious trial of exceeding Love,

Illustrious evidence, example high!
Ingaging me to emulate, but short
Of thy perfection, how shall I attaine,
Adam, from whose deare side I boast me sprung,
And gladly of our Union heare thee speak,
One Heart, one Soul in both; whereof good prooff
This day affords, declaring thee resolvd,
Rather then Death or aught then Death more dread
Shall separate us, linkt in Love so deare,
To undergoe with mee one Guilt, one Crime,
If any be, of tasting this fair Fruit,
Whose vertue, for of good still good proceeds,
Direct, or by occasion hath presented
This happie trial of thy Love, which else
So eminently never had bin known.
Were it I thought Death menac't would ensue
This my attempt, I would sustain alone
The worst, and not perswade thee, rather die
Deserted, then oblige thee with a fact
Pernicious to thy Peace, chiefly assur'd
Remarkably so late of thy so true,
So faithful Love unequald; but I feel
Farr otherwise th' event, not Death, but Life
Augmented, op'nd Eyes, new Hopes, new Joyes,
Taste so Divine, that what of sweet before
Hath toucht my sense, flat seems to this, and harsh.
On my experience, *Adam*, freely taste,
And fear of Death deliver to the Windes.
    So saying, she embrac'd him, and for joy
Tenderly wept, much won that he his Love
Had so enobl'd, as of choice to incurr
Divine displeasure for her sake, or Death.
In recompence (for such compliance bad
Such recompence best merits) from the bough
She gave him of that fair enticing Fruit
With liberal hand: he scrupl'd not to eat
Against his better knowledge, not deceav'd,
But fondly overcome with Femal charm.
Earth trembl'd from her entrails, as again

In pangs, and Nature gave a second groan,
Skie lowr'd and muttering Thunder, som sad drops
Wept at compleating of the mortal Sin
Original; while *Adam* took no thought,
Eating his fill, nor *Eve* to iterate
Her former trespass fear'd, the more to soothe
Him with her lov'd societie, that now
As with new Wine intoxicated both
They swim in mirth, and fansie that they feel
Divinitie within them breeding wings
Wherewith to scorne the Earth: but that false Fruit
Farr other operation first displaid,
Carnal desire enflaming, hee on *Eve*
Began to cast lascivious Eyes, she him
As wantonly repaid; in Lust they burne:
Till *Adam* thus 'gan *Eve* to dalliance move,

    Eve, now I see thou art exact of taste,
And elegant, of Sapience no small part,
Since to each meaning savour we apply,
And Palate call judicious; I the praise
Yeild thee, so well this day thou hast purvey'd.
Much pleasure we have lost, while we abstain'd
From this delightful Fruit, nor known till now
True relish, tasting; if such pleasure be
In things to us forbidden, it might be wish'd,
For this one Tree had bin forbidden ten.
But come, so well refresh't, now let us play,
As meet is, after such delicious Fare;
For never did thy Beautie since the day
I saw thee first and wedded thee, adorn'd
With all perfections, so enflame my sense
With ardor to enjoy thee, fairer now
Then ever, bountie of this vertuous Tree.

    So said he, and forbore not glance or toy
Of amorous intent, well understood
Of *Eve*, whose Eye darted contagious Fire.
Her hand he seis'd, and to a shadie bank,
Thick overhead with verdant roof imbowr'd
He led her nothing loath; Flours were the Couch,

Pansies, and Violets, and Asphodel,
And Hyacinth, Earths freshest softest lap.
There they thir fill of Love and Loves disport
Took largely, of thir mutual guilt the Seale,
The solace of thir sin, till dewie sleep
Oppress'd them, wearied with thir amorous play.

🔥

Christopher Marlowe
1564–93

from Doctor Faustus

*Faustus has made a pact with Mephistophilis to surrender his soul to the
Devil in return for twenty-four years of life with Mephistophilis giving him
whatever he demands. Faustus is now nearing the end of his time on earth.*

(*Enter an* OLD MAN *to* FAUSTUS *and* MEPHISTOPHILIS.)
OLD MAN: Ah, Doctor Faustus, that I might prevail
    To guide thy steps unto the way of life,
    By which sweet path thou mayst attain the goal
    That shall conduct thee to celestial rest!
    Break heart, drop blood, and mingle it with tears,
    Tears falling from repentant heaviness
    Of thy most vile and loathsome filthiness,
    The stench whereof corrupts the inward soul
    With such flagitious crimes of heinous sin
    As no commiseration may expel,
    But mercy, Faustus, of thy Saviour sweet,
    Whose blood alone must wash away thy guilt.
FAUST: Where art thou, Faustus? wretch, what hast thou done?
    Damn'd art thou, Faustus, damn'd; despair and die!
    Hell calls for right, and with a roaring voice
    Says, 'Faustus, come; thine hour is come;'
    And Faustus will come to do thee right.
    (MEPHISTOPHILIS *gives him a dagger.*)
OLD MAN: Ah, stay, good Faustus, stay thy desperate steps!
    I see an angel hovers o'er thy head,
    And, with a vial full of precious grace,
    Offers to pour the same into thy soul:
    Then call for mercy, and avoid despair.
FAUST: Ah, my sweet friend, I feel
    Thy words to comfort my distressed soul!

Leave me a while to ponder on my sins.

OLD MAN: I go, sweet Faustus; but with heavy cheer,
Fearing the ruin of thy hopeless soul. (*Exit.*)

FAUST: Accursed Faustus, where is mercy now?
I do repent; and yet I do despair:
Hell strives with grace for conquest in my breast:
What shall I do to shun the snares of death?

MEPH: Thou traitor, Faustus, I arrest thy soul
For disobedience to my sovereign lord:
Revolt, or I'll in piece-meal tear thy flesh.

FAUST: Sweet Mephistophilis, entreat thy lord
To pardon my unjust presumption,
And with my blood again I will confirm
My former vow I made to Lucifer.

MEPH: Do it, then, quickly, with unfeigned heart,
Lest greater danger do attend thy drift.

FAUST: Torment, sweet friend, that base and crooked age,
That durst dissuade me from thy Lucifer,
With greatest torments that our hell affords.

MEPH: His faith is great; I cannot touch his soul;
But what I may afflict his body with
I will attempt, which is but little worth.

FAUST: One thing, good servant, let me crave of thee,
To glut the longing of my heart's desire, –
That I might have unto my paramour
That heavenly Helen which I saw of late,
Whose sweet embracings may extinguish clean
Those thoughts that do dissuade me from my vow,
And keep mine oath I made to Lucifer.

MEPH: Faustus, this, or what else thou shalt desire,
Shall be perform'd in twinkling of an eye.
(*Enter* HELEN.)

FAUST: Was this the face that launch'd a thousand ships?
And burnt the topless towers of Ilium? –
Sweet Helen, make me immortal with a kiss. – (*Kisses her.*)
Her lips suck forth my soul: see, where it flies –
Come, Helen, come, give me my soul again.
Here will I dwell, for heaven is in these lips,
And all is dross that is not Helena.

I will be Paris, and for love of thee,
Instead of Troy, shall Wertenberg be sack'd;
And I will combat with weak Menelaus,
And wear thy colours on my plumed crest;
Yes, I will wound Achilles in the heel,
And then return to Helen for a kiss.
O, thou art fairer than the evening air
Clad in the beauty of a thousand stars;
Brighter art thou than flaming Jupiter
When he appear'd to hapless Semele;
More lovely than the monarch of the sky
In wanton Arethusa's azur'd arms;
And none but thou shalt be my paramour! (*Exeunt.*)
(*Enter the* OLD MAN.)

OLD MAN: Accursed Faustus, miserable man,
That from thy soul exclud'st the grace of heaven,
And fly'st the throne of his tribunal-seat!
(*Enter* DEVILS.)
Satan begins to sift me with his pride:
As in this furnace God shall try my faith,
My faith vile hell, shall triumph over thee,
Ambitious fiends, see how the heavens smile
At your repulse, and laugh your state to scorn!
Hence, hell! for hence I fly unto my God.
(*Exeunt – on one side,* DEVILS, *on the other,* OLD MAN.)

Laurie Lee
1914–

from Cider with Rosie

The day Rosie Burdock decided to take me in hand was a motionless day of summer, creamy, hazy, and amber-coloured, with the beech trees standing in heavy sunlight as though clogged with wild wet honey. It was the time of hay-making, so when we came out of school Jack and I went to the farm to help.

The whirr of the mower met us across the stubble, rabbits jumped like firecrackers about the fields, and the hay smelt crisp and sweet. The farmer's men were all hard at work, raking, turning, and loading. Tall, whiskered fellows forked the grass, their chests like bramble patches. The air swung with their forks and the swathes took wing and rose like eagles to the tops of the wagons. The farmer gave us a short fork each and we both pitched in with the rest . . .

I stumbled on Rosie behind a haycock, and she grinned up at me with the sly, glittering eyes of her mother. She wore her tartan frock and cheap brass necklace, and her bare legs were brown with hay-dust.

'Get out a there,' I said. 'Go on.'

Rosie had grown and was hefty now, and I was terrified of her. In her cat-like eyes and curling mouth I saw unnatural wisdoms more threatening than anything I could imagine. The last time we'd met I'd hit her with a cabbage stump. She bore me no grudge, just grinned.

'I got summat to show ya.'

'You push off,' I said.

I felt dry and dripping, icy hot. Her eyes glinted, and I stood rooted. Her face was wrapped in a pulsating haze and her body seemed to flicker with lightning.

'You thirsty?' she said.

'I ain't, so there.'

'You be,' she said. 'C'mon.'

So I struck the fork into the ringing ground and followed her, like doom.

We went a long way, to the bottom of the field, where a wagon stood half-loaded. Festoons of untrimmed grass hung down like curtains all around it. We crawled underneath, between the wheels, into a herb-scented cave of darkness. Rosie scratched about, turned over a sack, and revealed a stone jar of cider.

'It's cider,' she said. 'You ain't to drink it though. Not much of it, any rate.'

Huge and squat, the jar lay on the grass like an unexploded bomb. We lifted it up, unscrewed the stopper, and smelt the whiff of fermented apples. I held the jar to my mouth and rolled my eyes sideways, like a beast at a waterhole. 'Go on,' said Rosie. I took a deep breath . . .

Never to be forgotten, that first long secret drink of golden fire, juice of those valleys and of that time, wine of wild orchards, of russet summer, of plump red apples, and Rosie's burning cheeks. Never to be forgotten, or ever tasted again . . .

I put down the jar with a gulp and a gasp. Then I turned to look at Rosie. She was yellow and dusty with buttercups and seemed to be purring in the gloom; her hair was rich as a wild bee's nest and her eyes were full of stings. I did not know what to do about her, nor did I know what not to do. She looked smooth and precious, a thing of unplumbable mysteries, and perilous as quicksand.

'Rosie . . .' I said, on my knees, and shaking.

She crawled with a rustle of grass towards me, quick and superbly assured. Her hand in mine was like a small wet flame which I could neither hold nor throw away. Then Rosie, with a remorseless, reedy strength, pulled me down from my tottering perch, pulled me down, down into her wide green smile and into the deep subaqueous grass.

Then I remember little, and that little, vaguely. Skin drums beat in my head. Rosie was close-up, salty, an invisible touch, too near to be seen or measured. And it seemed that the wagon under which we lay went floating away like a barge, out over the valley where we rocked unseen, swinging on motionless tides.

Then she took off her boots and stuffed them with flowers. She did the same with mine. Her parched voice crackled like flames in my ears. More fires were started. I drank more cider. Rosie told me outrageous fantasies. She liked me, she said, better than Walt, or Ken, Boney Harris, or even the curate. And I admitted to her, in a loud, rough voice, that she was even prettier than Betty Gleed. For a long time we sat with our mouths very close, breathing the same hot air. We kissed, once only, so dry and shy, it was like two leaves colliding in air.

At last the cuckoos stopped singing and slid into the woods. The mowers went home and left us. I heard Jack calling as he went down the lane, calling my name till I heard him no more. And still we lay in our wagon of grass tugging at each other's hands, while her husky, perilous whisper drugged me and the cider beat gongs in my head . . .

Night came at last, and we crawled out from the wagon and stumbled together towards home. Bright dew and glow-worms shone over the grass, and the heat of the day grew softer. I felt like a giant; I swung from the trees and plunged my arms into nettles just to show her. Whatever I did seemed valiant and easy. Rosie carried her boots, and smiled.

There was something about that evening which dilates the memory, even now. The long hills slavered like Chinese dragons, crimson in the setting sun. The shifting lane lassoed my feet and tried to trip me up. And the lake, as we passed it, rose hissing with waves and tried to drown us among its cannibal fish.

Perhaps I fell in – though I don't remember. But here I lost Rosie for good. I found myself wandering home alone, wet through, and possessed by miracles. I discovered extraordinary tricks of sight. I could make trees move and leap-frog each other, and turn bushes into roaring trains. I could lick up the stars like acid drops and fall flat on my face without pain. I felt magnificent, fateful, and for the first time in my life, invulnerable to the perils of night.

When at last I reached home, still dripping wet, I was bursting with power and pleasure. I sat on the chopping-block and sang 'Fierce Raged the Tempest' and several other hymns of that nature. I went on singing till long after supper-time, bawling alone in the dark. Then Harold and Jack came and frog-marched me to bed. I was never the same again . . .

❧

Edmund Spenser
1552?–99

from The Faerie Queene Book II, Canto xii

The knight Guyon visits the Bower of Bliss of the enchantress, Acrasia.

There the most daintie Paradise on ground,
　It selfe doth offer to his sober eye,
　In which all pleasures plenteously abound,
　And none does others happinesse enuye:
　The painted flowres, the trees vpshooting hye,
　The dales for shade, the hilles for breathing space,
　The trembling groues, the Christall running by;
　And that, which all faire workes doth most aggrace,
The art, which all that wrought, appeared in no place.

One would haue thought, (so cunningly, the rude,
　And scorned parts were mingled with the fine,)
　That nature had for wantonesse ensude
　Art, and that Art at nature did repine;
　So striuing each th'other to vndermine,
　Each did the others worke more beautifie;
　So diff'ring both in willes, agreed in fine:
　So all agreed through sweete diuersitie,
This Gardin to adorne with all varietie.

And in the midst of all, a fountaine stood,
　Of richest substaunce, that on earth might bee,
　So pure and shiny, that the siluer flood
　Through euery channell running one might see;
　Most goodly it with curious imageree
　Was ouer-wrought, and shapes of naked boyes,
　Of which some seemd with liuely iollitee,
　To fly about, playing their wanton toyes,
Whilest others did them selues embay in liquid ioyes.

And ouer all, of purest gold was spred,
    A trayle of yuie in his natiue hew:
    For the rich mettall was so coloured,
    That wight, who did not well auis'd it vew,
    Would surely deeme it to be yuie trew:
    Low his lasciuious armes adown did creepe,
    That themselues dipping in the siluer dew,
    Their fleecy flowres they tenderly did steepe,
Which drops of Christall seemd for wantones to weepe.

Infinit streames continually did well
    Out of this fountaine, sweet and faire to see,
    The which into an ample lauer fell,
    And shortly grew to so great quantitie,
    That like a little lake it seemd to bee;
    Whose depth exceeded not three cubits hight,
    That through the waues one might the bottom see,
    All pau'd beneath with Iaspar shining bright,
That seemd the fountaine in that sea did sayle vpright.

And all the margent round about was set,
    With shady Laurell trees, thence to defend
    The sunny beames, which on the billowes bet,
    And those which therein bathed, mote offend.
    As *Guyon* hapned by the same to wend,
    Two naked Damzelles he therein espyde,
    Which therein bathing, seemed to contend,
    And wrestle wantonly, ne car'd to hyde,
Their dainty parts from vew of any, which them eyde.

Sometimes the one would lift the other quight
    Aboue the waters, and then downe againe
    Her plong, as ouer maistered by might,
    Where both awhile would couered remaine,
    And each the other from to rise restraine;
    The whiles their snowy limbes, as through a vele,
    So through the Christall waues appeared plaine:
    Then suddeinly both would themselues vnhele,
And th'amarous sweet spoiles to greedy eyes reuele.

As that faire Starre, the messenger of morne,
  His deawy face out of the sea doth reare:
  Or as the *Cyprian* goddesse, newly borne
  Of th'Oceans fruitfull froth, did first appeare:
  Such seemed they, and so their yellow heare
  Christalline humour dropped downe apace.
  Whom such when *Guyon* saw, he drew him neare,
  And somewhat gan relent his earnest pace,
His stubborne brest gan secret pleasaunce to embrace.

The wanton Maidens him espying, stood
  Gazing a while at his vnwonted guise;
  Then th'one her selfe low ducked in the flood,
  Abasht, that her a straunger did a vise:
  But th'other rather higher did arise,
  And her two lilly paps aloft displayd,
  And all, that might his melting hart entise
  To her delights, she vnto him bewrayd:
The rest hid vnderneath, him more desirous made.

With that, the other likewise vp arose,
  And her faire lockes, which formerly were bownd
  Vp in one knot, she low adowne did lose:
  Which flowing long and thick, her cloth'd arownd,
  And th'yuorie in golden mantle gownd:
  So that faire spectacle from him was reft,
  Yet that, which reft it, no lesse faire was fownd:
  So hid in lockes and waues from lookers theft,
Nought but her louely face she for his looking left.

Withall she laughed, and she blusht withall,
  That blushing to her laughter gaue more grace,
  And laughter to her blushing, as did fall:
  Now when they spide the knight to slacke his pace,
  Them to behold, and in his sparkling face
  The secret signes of kindled lust appeare,
  Their wanton meriments they did encreace,
  And to him beckned, to approch more neare,
And shewd him many sights, that courage cold could reare.

On which when gazing him the Palmer saw,
   He much rebukt those wandring eyes of his,
   And counseld well, him forward thence did draw.
   Now are they come nigh to the *Bowre of blis*
   Of her fond fauorites so nam'd amis:
   When thus the Palmer; Now Sir, well auise;
   For here the end of all our trauell is:
   Here wonnes *Acrasia*, whom we must surprise,
Else she will slip away, and all our drift despise.

Eftsoones they heard a most melodious sound,
   Of all that mote delight a daintie eare,
   Such as attonce might not on liuing ground,
   Saue in this Paradise, be heard elswhere:
   Right hard it was, for wight, which did it heare,
   To read, what manner musicke that mote bee:
   For all that pleasing is to liuing eare,
   Was there consorted in one harmonee,
Birdes, voyces, instruments, windes, waters, all agree.

The ioyous birdes shrouded in chearefull shade,
   Their notes vnto the voyce attempred sweet;
   Th'Angelicall soft trembling voyces made
   To th'instruments diuine respondence meet:
   The siluer sounding instruments did meet
   With the base murmure of the waters fall:
   The waters fall with difference discreet,
   Now soft, now loud, vnto the wind did call:
The gentle warbling wind low answered to all.

There, whence that Musick seemed heard to bee,
   Was the faire Witch her selfe now solacing,
   With a new Louer, whom through sorceree
   And witchcraft, she from farre did thither bring:
   There she had him now layd a slombering,
   In secret shade, after long wanton ioyes:
   Whilst round about them pleasauntly did sing
   Many faire Ladies, and lasciuious boyes,
That euer mixt their song with light licentious toyes.

And all that while, right ouer him she hong,
   With her false eyes fast fixed in his sight,
   As seeking medicine, whence she was stong,
   Or greedily depasturing delight:
   And oft inclining downe with kisses light,
   For feare of waking him, his lips bedewd,
   And through his humid eyes did sucke his spright,
   Quite molten into lust and pleasure lewd;
Wherewith she sighed soft, as if his case she rewd.

The whiles some one did chaunt this louely lay;
   Ah see, who so faire thing doest faine to see,
   In springing flowre the image of thy day;
   Ah see the Virgin Rose, how sweetly shee
   Doth first peepe forth with bashfull modestee,
   That fairer seemes, the lesse ye see her may;
   Lo see soone after, how more bold and free
   Her bared bosome she doth broad display;
Loe see soone after, how she fades, and falles away.

So passeth, in the passing of a day,
   Of mortall life the leafe, the bud, the flowre,
   Ne more doth flourish after first decay,
   That earst was sought to decke both bed and bowre,
   Of many a Ladie, and many a Paramowre:
   Gather therefore the Rose, whilest yet is prime,
   For soone comes age, that will her pride deflowre:
   Gather the Rose of loue, whilest yet is time,
Whilest louing thou mayst loued be with equall crime.

He ceast and then gan all the quire of birdes
   Their diuerse notes t'attune vnto his lay,
   As in approuance of his pleasing words.
   The constant paire heard all, that he did say,
   Yet swarued not, but kept their forward way,
   Through many couert groues, and thickets close,
   In which they creeping did at last display
   That wanton Ladie, with her louer lose,
Whose sleepie head she in her lap did soft dispose.

Vpon a bed of Roses she was layd,
    As faint through heat, or dight to pleasant sin,
    And was arayd, or rather disarayd,
    All in a vele of silke and siluer thin,
    That hid no whit her alablaster skin,
    But rather shewd more white, if more might bee:
    More subtile web *Arachne* cannot spin,
    Nor the fine nets, which oft we wouen see
Of scorched deaw, do not in th'aire more lightly flee.

Her snowy brest was bare to readie spoyle
    Of hungry eies, which n'ote therewith be fild,
    And yet through languour of her late sweet toyle,
    Few drops, more cleare then Nectar, forth distild,
    That like pure Orient perles adowne it trild,
    And her faire eyes sweet smyling in delight,
    Moystened their fierie beames, with which she thrild
    Fraile harts, yet quenched not; like starry light
Which sparckling on the silent waues, does seeme more bright.

The young man sleeping by her, seemd to bee
    Some goodly swayne of honorable place,
    That certes it great pittie was to see
    Him his nobilitie so foule deface;
    A sweet regard, and amiable grace,
    Mixed with manly sternnesse did appeare
    Yet sleeping, in his well proportiond face,
    And on his tender lips the downy heare
Did now but freshly spring, and silken blossomes beare.

His warlike armes, the idle instruments
    Of sleeping praise, were hong vpon a tree,
    And his braue shield, full of old moniments,
    Was fowly ra'st, that none the signes might see;
    Ne for them, ne for honour cared hee,
    Ne ought, that did to his aduauncement tend,
    But in lewd loues, and wastfull luxuree,
    His dayes, his goods, his bodie he did spend:
O horrible enchantment, that him so did blend.

🔥

Thomas Malory
d. 1471

from Le Morte d'Arthur

Elaine seduces Launcelot through Dame Brisen's magic.

King Arthur had been in France, and had made war upon the
mighty King Claudas, and had won much of his lands. And when
the king was come again he let cry a great feast, that all lords and
ladies of all England should be there, but if it were such as were
rebellious against him.

And when Dame Elaine, the daughter of King Pelles, heard of
this feast she went to her father and required him that he would
give her leave to ride to that feast. The king answered: I will well
ye go thither, but in any wise as ye love me and will have my
blessing, that ye be well beseen in the richest wise; and look that ye
spare not for no cost; ask and ye shall have all that you needeth.
Then by the advice of Dame Brisen, her maiden, all thing was
apparelled unto the purpose, that there was never no lady more
richlier beseen. So she rode with twenty knights, and ten ladies,
and gentlewomen, to the number of an hundred horses. And when
she came to Camelot, King Arthur and Queen Guenever said, and
all the knights, that Dame Elaine was the fairest and the best
beseen lady that ever was seen in that court. And anon as King
Arthur wist that she was come he met her and saluted her, and so
did the most part of all the knights of the Round Table, both Sir
Tristram, Sir Bleoberis, and Sir Gawaine, and many more that I
will not rehearse. But when Sir Launcelot saw her he was so
ashamed, and that because he drew his sword on the morn when
he had lain by her, that he would not salute her nor speak to her;
and yet Sir Launcelot thought she was the fairest woman that ever
he saw in his life-days.

But when Dame Elaine saw Sir Launcelot that would not speak
unto her she was so heavy that she weened her heart would have

to-brast; for wit you well, out of measure she loved him. And then Elaine said unto her woman, Dame Brisen: The unkindness of Sir Launcelot slayeth me near. Ah, peace, madam, said Dame Brisen, I will undertake that this night he shall lie with you, an ye would hold you still. That were me liefer, said Dame Elaine, than all the gold that is above the earth. Let me deal, said Dame Brisen. So when Elaine was brought unto Queen Guenever either made other good cheer by countenance, but nothing with hearts. But all men and women spake of the beauty of Dame Elaine, and of her great riches.

Then, at night, the queen commanded that Dame Elaine should sleep in a chamber nigh her chamber, and all under one roof; and so it was done as the queen commanded. Then the queen sent for Sir Launcelot and bade him come to her chamber that night: Or else I am sure, said the queen, that ye will go to your lady's bed, Dame Elaine, by whom ye gat Galahad. Ah, madam, said Sir Launcelot, never say ye so, for that I did was against my will. Then, said the queen, look that ye come to me when I send for you. Madam, said Launcelot, I shall not fail you, but I shall be ready at your commandment. This bargain was soon done and made between them, but Dame Brisen knew it by her crafts, and told it to her lady, Dame Elaine. Alas, said she, now shall I do? Let me deal, said Dame Brisen, for I shall bring him by the hand even to your bed, and he shall ween that I am Queen Guenever's messenger. Now well is me, said Dame Elaine, for all the world I love not so much as I do Sir Launcelot.

So when time came that all folks were abed, Dame Brisen came to Sir Launcelot's bed's side and said: Sir Launcelot du Lake, sleep you? My lady, Queen Guenever, lieth and awaiteth upon you. O my fair lady, said Sir Launcelot, I am ready to go with you where ye will have me. So Sir Launcelot threw upon him a long gown, and his sword in his hand; and then Dame Brisen took him by the finger and led him to her lady's bed, Dame Elaine; and then she departed and left them in bed together. Wit you well the lady was glad, and so was Sir Launcelot, for he weened that he had had another in his arms.

Now leave we them kissing and clipping, as was kindly thing; and now speak we of Queen Guenever that sent one of her women unto Sir Launcelot's bed; and when she came there she found the bed cold, and he was away; so she came to the queen and told her all. Alas, said the queen, where is that false knight become? Then the queen was nigh out of her wit, and then she writhed and weltered as a mad woman, and might not sleep a four or five hours. Then Sir Launcelot had a condition that he used of custom, he would clatter in his sleep, and speak oft of his lady, Queen Guenever. So as Sir Launcelot had waked as long as it had pleased him, then by course of kind he slept, and Dame Elaine both. And in his sleep he talked and clattered as a jay, of the love that had been betwixt Queen Guenever and him. And so as he talked so loud the queen heard him thereas she lay in her chamber; and when she heard him so clatter she was nigh wood and out of her mind, and for anger and pain wist not what to do. And then she coughed so loud that Sir Launcelot awaked, and he knew her hemming. And then he knew well that he lay not by the queen; and therewith he leapt out of his bed as he had been a wood man, in his shirt, and the queen met him in the floor; and thus she said: False traitor knight that thou art, look thou never abide in my court, and avoid my chamber, and not so hardy, thou false traitor knight that thou art, that ever thou come in my sight. Alas, said Sir Launcelot; and therewith he took such an heartly sorrow at her words that he fell down to the floor in a swoon. And therewithal Queen Guenever departed. And when Sir Launcelot awoke of his swoon, he leapt out at a bay window into a garden, and there with thorns he was all to-scratched in his visage and his body; and so he ran forth he wist not whither, and was wild wood as ever was man; and so he ran two year, and never man might have grace to know him.

🜊

John Keats
1795–1821

La Belle Dame sans Merci

1

O what can ail thee Knight at arms
  Alone and palely loitering?
The sedge has withered from the Lake
  And no birds sing!

2

O what can ail thee Knight at arms
  So haggard, and so woe begone?
The Squirrel's granary is full
  And the harvest's done.

3

I see a lilly on thy brow
  With anguish moist and fever dew,
And on thy cheeks a fading rose
  Fast withereth too –

4

I met a Lady in the Meads
  Full beautiful, a faery's child
Her hair was long, her foot was light
  And her eyes were wild –

5

I made a Garland for her head,
  And bracelets too, and fragrant Zone
She look'd at me as she did love
  And made sweet moan –

6

I set her on my pacing steed
  And nothing else saw all day long
For sidelong would she bend and sing
  A faery's song –

7

She found me roots of relish sweet
  And honey wild and manna dew
And sure in language strange she said
  I love thee true –

8

She took me to her elfin grot
  And there she wept and sigh'd full sore,
And there I shut her wild wild eyes
  With kisses four.

9

And there she lulled me asleep
  And there I dream'd Ah Woe betide!
The latest dream I ever dreamt
  On the cold hill side

10

I saw pale Kings, and Princes too
  Pale warriors death pale were they all
They cried La belle dame sans merci
  Thee hath in thrall.

11

I saw their starv'd lips in the gloam
  With horrid warning gaped wide,
And I awoke, and found me here
  On the cold hill's side

And this is why I sojourn here
   Alone and palely loitering;
Though the sedge is withered from the Lake
   And no birds sing – . . .

🕯

William Shakespeare
1564–1616

---

from Antony and Cleopatra

*Mæcenas and Agrippa are welcoming Enobarbus to Rome, on his arrival
from Egypt with Antony.*

MÆC: Welcome from Egypt, sir.

ENO: Half the heart of Cæsar, worthy Mæcenas! My
honourable friend, Agrippa!

AGR: Good Enobarbus!

MÆC: We have cause to be glad that matters are so well
digested. You stayed well by't in Egypt.

ENO: Ay, sir; we did sleep day out of countenance, and made
the night light with drinking.

MÆC: Eight wild-boars roasted whole at a breakfast, and but
twelve persons there; is this true?

ENO: This was but as a fly by an eagle: we had much more
monstrous matter of feast, which worthily deserved noting.

MÆC: She's a most triumphant lady, if report be square to her.

ENO: When she first met Mark Antony, she pursed up his
heart, upon the river of Cydnus.

AGR: There she appeared indeed, or my reporter devised well
for her.

ENO: I will tell you.
The barge she sat in, like a burnish'd throne,
Burn'd on the water: the poop was beaten gold;
Purple the sails, and so perfumed that
The winds were love-sick with them; the oars were silver,
Which to the tune of flutes kept stroke and made
The water which they beat to follow faster,
As amorous of their strokes. For her own person,
It beggar'd all description: she did lie
In her pavilion, cloth-of-gold of tissue,

O'er-picturing that Venus where we see
The fancy outwork nature: on each side her
Stood pretty dimpled boys, like smiling Cupids,
With divers-colour'd fans, whose wind did seem
To glow the delicate cheeks which they did cool,
And what they undid did.

AGR: O, rare for Antony!

ENO: Her gentlewomen, like the Nereides,
So many mermaids, tended her i' the eyes,
And made their bends adornings: at the helm
A seeming mermaid steers: the silken tackle
Swell with the touches of those flower-soft hands,
That yarely frame the office. From the barge
A strange invisible perfume hits the sense
Of the adjacent wharfs. The city cast
Her people out upon her; and Antony,
Enthroned i' the market-place, did sit alone,
Whistling to the air; which, but for vacancy,
Had gone to gaze on Cleopatra too,
And made a gap in nature.

AGR: Rare Egyptian!

ENO: Upon her landing, Antony sent to her,
Invited her to supper: she replied,
It should be better he became her guest,
Which she entreated: our courteous Antony,
Whom ne'er the word of 'No' woman heard speak,
Being barber'd ten times o'er, goes to the feast,
And, for his ordinary, pays his heart
For what his eyes eat only.

‍

Oscar Wilde
1854–1900

from Salomé

Jokanaan is John the Baptist, prisoner of Salomé's stepfather, Herod.

JOKANAAN: Who is this woman who is looking at me? I will not
have her look at me. Wherefore doth she look at me with
her golden eyes, under her gilded eyelids? I know not who
she is. I do not wish to know who she is. Bid her begone. It
is not to her that I would speak.

SALOMÉ: I am Salomé, daughter of Herodias, Princess of
Judaea.

JOKANAAN: Back! daughter of Babylon! Come not near the
chosen of the Lord. Thy mother hath filled the earth with
the wine of her iniquities, and the cry of her sins hath come
up to the ears of God.

SALOMÉ: Speak again, Jokanaan. Thy voice is wine to me.

THE YOUNG SYRIAN: Princess! Princess! Princess!

SALOMÉ: Speak again! Speak again, Jokanaan, and tell me
what I must do.

JOKANAAN: Daughter of Sodom, come not near me! But cover
thy face with a veil, and scatter ashes upon thine head, and
get thee to the desert and seek out the Son of Man.

SALOMÉ: Who is he, the Son of Man? Is he as beautiful as thou
art, Jokanaan?

JOKANAAN: Get thee behind me! I hear in the palace the
beatings of the wings of the angel of death.

THE YOUNG SYRIAN: Princess, I beseech thee to go within.

JOKANAAN: Angel of the Lord God, what dost thou here with
thy sword? Whom seekest thou in this foul palace? The day
of him who shall die in a robe of silver has not yet come.

SALOMÉ: Jokanaan!

JOKANAAN: Who speaketh?

[337]

SALOMÉ: Jokanaan, I am amorous of thy body! Thy body is white like the lilies of a field that the mower hath never mowed. Thy body is white like the snows that lie on the mountains, like the snows that lie on the mountains of Judaea, and come down into the valleys. The roses in the garden of the Queen of Arabia are not so white as thy body. Neither the roses in the garden of the Queen of Arabia, the perfumed garden of spices of the Queen of Arabia, nor the feet of the dawn when they light on the leaves, nor the breast of the moon when she lies on the breast of the sea. . . . There is nothing in the world so white as thy body. Let me touch thy body.

JOKANAAN: Back! daughter of Babylon! By woman came evil into the world. Speak not to me. I will not listen to thee. I listen but to the voice of the Lord God.

SALOMÉ: Thy body is hideous. It is like the body of a leper. It is like a plastered wall where vipers have crawled; like a plastered wall where the scorpions have made their nest. It is like a whitened sepulchre full of loathsome things. It is horrible, thy body is horrible. It is of thy hair that I am enamoured, Jokanaan. Thy hair is like clusters of grapes, like the clusters of black grapes that hang from the vine trees of Edom in the land of the Edomites. Thy hair is like the cedars of Lebanon, like the great cedars of Lebanon that give their shade to the lions and to the robbers who would hide themselves by day. The long black nights, when the moon hides her face, when the stars are afraid, are not so black. The silence that dwells in the forest is not so black. There is nothing in the world so black as thy hair . . . Let me touch thy hair.

JOKANAAN: Back, daughter of Sodom! Touch me not. Profane not the temple of the Lord God.

SALOMÉ: Thy hair is horrible. It is covered with mire and dust. It is like a crown of thorns which they have placed on thy forehead. It is like a knot of black serpents writhing round thy neck. I love not thy hair . . . It is thy mouth that I desire, Jokanaan. Thy mouth is like a band of scarlet on a tower of ivory. It is like a pomegranate cut with a knife of ivory. The pomegranate-flowers that blossom in the gardens of Tyre, and are redder than roses, are not so red. The red blasts of trumpets that herald the approach of kings, and make afraid the enemy, are not so red. Thy mouth is redder than the feet of those who tread the wine in the wine-press. Thy mouth is redder than the feet of the doves who haunt the temples and are fed by the priests. It is redder than the feet of him who cometh from a forest where he hath slain a lion, and seen gilded tigers. Thy mouth is like a branch of coral that fishers have found in the twilight of the sea, the coral that they keep for the kings! . . . It is like the vermilion that the Moabites find in the mines of Moab, the vermilion that the kings take from them. It is like the bow of the King of the Persians, that is painted with vermilion, and is tipped with coral. There is nothing in the world so red as thy mouth. . . . Let me kiss thy mouth.

JOKANAAN: Never! daughter of Babylon! Daughter of Sodom! Never.

SALOMÉ: I will kiss thy mouth, Jokanaan. I will kiss thy mouth.

THE YOUNG SYRIAN: Princess, Princess, thou who art like a garden of myrrh, thou who art the dove of all doves, look not at this man, look not at him! Do not speak such words to him. I cannot suffer them. . . . Princess, Princess, do not speak these things.

SALOMÉ: I will kiss thy mouth, Jokanaan.

THE YOUNG SYRIAN: Ah!

(*He kills himself and falls between* SALOMÉ *and* JOKANAAN.)

THE PAGE OF HERODIAS: The young Syrian has slain himself! The young captain has slain himself! He has slain himself who was my friend! I gave him a little box of perfumes and earrings wrought in silver, and now he has killed himself! Ah, did he not foretell that some misfortune would happen? I, too, foretold it, and it has happened. Well I knew that the moon was seeking a dead thing, but I knew not that it was he whom she sought. Ah! why did I not hide him from the moon? If I had hidden him in a cavern she would not have seen him.

FIRST SOLDIER: Princess, the young captain has just killed himself.

[339]

SALOMÉ: Let me kiss thy mouth, Jokanaan.

JOKANAAN: Art thou not afraid, daughter of Herodias? Did I not tell thee that I had heard in the palace the beatings of the wings of the angel of death, and hath he not come, the angel of death?

SALOMÉ: Let me kiss thy mouth.

JOKANAAN: Daughter of adultery, there is but one who can save thee, it is He of whom I spake. Go seek Him. He is in a boat on the sea of Galilee, and He talketh with His disciples. Kneel down on the shore of the sea, and call unto Him by His name. When He cometh to thee (and to all who call on Him He cometh), bow thyself at His feet and ask of Him the remission of thy sins.

SALOMÉ: Let me kiss thy mouth.

JOKANAAN: Cursed be thou! daughter of an incestuous mother, be thou accursed!

SALOMÉ: I will kiss thy mouth, Jokanaan.

JOKANAAN: I do not wish to look at thee. I will not look at thee, thou art accursed, Salomé, thou art accursed.
(*He goes down into the cistern.*)

SALOMÉ: I will kiss thy mouth, Jokanaan; I will kiss thy mouth.

After Jokanaan has been executed in the cistern which is his prison, Salomé addresses these words to the severed head on its silver shield.

SALOMÉ: Ah! thou wouldst not suffer me to kiss thy mouth, Jokanaan. Well! I will kiss it now. I will bite it with my teeth as one bites a ripe fruit. Yes, I will kiss thy mouth, Jokanaan. I said it; did I not say it? I said it. Ah! I will kiss it now . . . But wherefore dost thou not look at me, Jokanaan? Thine eyes that were so terrible, so full of rage and scorn, are shut now. Wherefore are they shut? Open thine eyes! Lift up thine eyelids, Jokanaan! Wherefore dost thou not look at me? Art thou afraid of me, Jokanaan, that thou wilt not look at me? . . . And thy tongue, that was like a red snake darting poison, it moves no more, it says nothing now, Jokanaan, that scarlet viper that spat its venom upon me. It is strange, is it not? How is it that the red viper stirs no longer? . . . Thou wouldst have none of me, Jokanaan. Thou didst reject me. Thou didst speak evil words against me. Thou didst treat me as a harlot, as a wanton, me, Salomé, daughter of Herodias, Princess of Judaea! Well, Jokanaan, I still live, but thou, thou art dead, and thy head belongs to me. I can do with it what I will. I can throw it to the dogs and to the birds of the air. That which the dogs leave, the birds of the air shall devour. . . . Ah, Jokanaan, Jokanaan, thou wert the only man that I have loved. All other men are hateful to me. But thou, thou wert beautiful! Thy body was a column of ivory set on a silver socket. It was a garden full of doves and of silver lilies. It was a tower of silver decked with shields of ivory. There was nothing in the world so white as thy body. There was nothing in the world so black as thy hair. In the whole world there was nothing so red as thy mouth. Thy voice was a censer that scattered strange perfumes, and when I looked on thee I heard a strange music. Ah! wherefore didst thou not look at me, Jokanaan? Behind thine hands and thy curses thou didst hide thy face. Thou didst put upon thine eyes the covering of him who would see his God. Well, thou hast seen thy God, Jokanaan, but me, me, thou didst never see. If thou hadst seen me thou wouldst have loved me. I, I saw thee, Jokanaan, and I loved thee. Oh, how I loved thee! I love thee yet, Jokanaan, I love thee only . . . I am athirst for thy beauty; I am hungry for thy body; and neither wine nor fruits can appease my desire. What shall I do now, Jokanaan? Neither the floods nor the great waters can quench my passion. I was a princess, and thou didst scorn me. I was a virgin, and thou didst take my virginity from me. I was chaste, and thou didst fill my veins with fire . . . Ah! ah! wherefore didst thou not look at me, Jokanaan? If thou hadst looked at me thou hadst loved me. Well I know that thou wouldst have loved me, and the mystery of love is greater than the mystery of death. Love only should one consider.

❧

Anon
14th century

---

from Sir Gawain and the Green Knight

Sir Gawain, on a quest from King Arthur's court to fight with a giant knight dressed in green, is resting during the Christmas festivities at the castle of Hautdesert. This is the third and final scene where a hunt is linked with an attempt at seduction. It is Bertilak, Gawain's host, who is leading the fox hunt while his wife visits their guest in his bed-chamber. The two men have a pledge to exchange what they have gained during the day.

The sun rises red amid radiant clouds,
Sails into the sky, and sends forth his beams.
They let loose the hounds by a leafy wood;
The rocks all round re-echo to their horns;
Soon some have set off in pursuit of the fox,
Cast about with craft for a clearer scent;
A young dog yaps, and is yelled at in turn;
His fellows fall to sniffing, and follow his lead,
Running in a rabble on the right track,
And he scampers all before; they discover him soon,
And when they see him with sight they pursue him the faster,
Railing at him rudely with a wrathful din.
Often he reverses over rough terrain.
Or loops back to listen in the lee of a hedge;
At last, by a little ditch, he leaps over the brush,
Comes into a clearing at a cautious pace.
Then he thought through his wiles to have thrown off the
    hounds
Till he was ware, as he went, of a waiting station
Where three athwart his path threatened him at once,
                    all gray,
            Quick as a flash he wheels
            And darts off in dismay.

[342]

With hard luck at his heels
He is off to the wood away.

Then it was heaven on earth to hark to the hounds
When they had come on their quarry, coursing together!
Such harsh cries and howls they hurled at his head
As all the cliffs with a crash had come down at once.
Here he was hailed, when huntsmen met him;
Yonder they yelled at him, yapping and snarling;
There they cried 'Thief!' and threatened his life,
And ever the harriers at his heels, that he had no rest.
Often he was menaced when he made for the open,
And often rushed in again, for Reynard was wily;
And so he leads them a merry chase, the lord and his men,
In this manner on the mountains, till midday or near,
While our hero lies at home in wholesome sleep
Within the comely curtains on the cold morning.
But the lady, as love would allow her no rest,
And pursuing ever the purpose that pricked her heart,
Was awake with the dawn, and went to his chamber
In a fair flowing mantle that fell to the earth,
All edged and embellished with ermines fine;
No hood on her head, but heavy with gems
Were her fillet and the fret that confined her tresses;
Her face and her fair throat freely displayed;
Her bosom all but bare, and her back as well.
She comes in at the chamber-door, and closes it with care,
Throws wide a window – then waits no longer,
But hails him thus airily with her artful words.
                              with cheer:
          'Ah, man, how can you sleep?
          The morning is so clear!'
          Though dreams have drowned him deep,
          He cannot choose but hear.

Deep in his dreams he darkly mutters
As a man may that mourns, with many grim thoughts
Of that day when destiny shall deal him his doom
When he greets his grim host at the Green Chapel

[343]

And must bow to his buffet, bating all strife.
But when he sees her at his side he summons his wits.
Breaks from the black dreams, and blithely answers.
That lovely lady comes laughing sweet,
Sinks down at his side, and salutes him with a kiss.
He accords her fair welcome in courtliest style;
He sees her so glorious, so gaily attired.
So faultless her features, so fair and so bright.
His heart swelled swiftly with surging joys.
They melt into mirth with many a fond smile,
And there was bliss beyond telling between those two,
                    at height.
            Good were their words of greeting;
            Each joyed in other's sight;
            Great peril attends that meeting
            Should Mary forget her knight.

For that high-born beauty so hemmed him about,
Made so plain her meaning, the man must needs
Either take her tendered love or distastefully refuse.
His courtesy concerned him, lest crass he appear,
But more his soul's mischief, should he commit sin
And belie his loyal oath to the lord of that house.
'God forbid!' said the bold knight, 'That shall not befall!'
With a little fond laugher he lightly let pass
All the words of special weight that were sped his way:
'I find you much at fault,' the fair one said.
'Who can be cold toward a creature so close by your side,
Of all women in this world most wounded in heart,
Unless you have a sweetheart, one you hold dearer,
And allegiance to that lady so loyally knit
That you will never love another, as now I believe.
And, sir, if it be so, then say it, I beg you:
By all your heart holds dear, hide it no longer
                    with guile.'
            'Lady, by Saint John.'
            He answers with a smile.
            'Lover have I none,
            Nor will have, yet awhile.'

'Those words,' said the woman, 'are the worst of all,
But I have had my answer, and hard do I find it!
Kiss me now kindly; I can but go hence
To lament my life long like a maid lovelorn.'
She inclines her head quickly and kisses the knight,
Then straightens with a sigh, and says as she stands,
'Now, dear, ere I depart, do me this pleasure:
Give me some little gift, your love or the like,
That I may think on you, man, and mourn the less.'
'Now by heaven,' said he, 'I wish I had here
My most precious possession, to put it in your hands,
For your deeds, beyond doubt, have often deserved
A repayment far passing my power to bestow.
But a love-token, lady, were of little avail:
It is not to your honor to have at this time
A glove as a guerdon from Gawain's hand.
And I am here on an errand in unknown realms
And have no bearers with baggage with becoming gifts,
Which distresses me, madame, for your dear sake.
A man must keep within his compass: account it neither grief
                              nor slight.'
                    'Nay, noblest knight alive,'
                    Said that beauty of body white.
                    'Though you be loath to give,
                    Yet you shall take, by right.'

She reached out a rich ring, wrought all of gold,
With a splendid stone displayed on the band
That flashed before his eyes like a fiery sun;
It was worth a king's wealth, you may well believe.
But he waved it away with these ready words:
'Before God, good lady, I forego all gifts;
None have I to offer, nor any will I take.'
And she urged it on him eagerly, and ever he refused,
And vowed in very earnest, prevail she would not.
And she sad to find it so, and said to him then,
'If my ring is refused for its rich cost —
You would not be my debtor for so dear a thing —
I shall give you my girdle; you gain less thereby.'

[345]

She released a knot lightly, and loosened a belt
That was caught about her kirtle, the bright cloak beneath,
Of a gay green silk, with gold overwrought,
And the borders all bound with embroidery fine,
And this she presses upon him, and pleads with a smile,
Unworthy though it were, that it would not be scorned.
But the man still maintains that he means to accept
Neither gold nor any gift, till by God's grace
The fate that lay before him was fully achieved.
'And be not offended, fair lady, I beg,
And give over your offer, for ever I must
                  decline.
        I am grateful for favor shown
        Past all deserts of mine.
        And ever shall be your own
        True servant, rain or shine.'

'Now does my present displease you,' she promptly inquired.
'Because it seems in your sight so simple a thing?
And belike, as it is little, it is less to praise,
But if the virtue that invests it were verily known,
It would be held, I hope, in higher esteem.
For the man that possesses this piece of silk,
If he bore it on his body, belted about,
There is no hand under heaven that could hew him down.
For he could not be killed by any craft on earth.'
Then the man began to muse, and mainly he thought
It was a pearl for his plight, the peril to come
When he gains the Green Chapel to get his reward:
Could he escape unscathed, the scheme were noble!
Then he bore with her words and withstood them no more,
And she repeated her petition and pleaded anew,
And he granted it, and gladly she gave him the belt,
And besought him for her sake to conceal it well,
Lest the noble lord should know — and the knight agrees
That not a soul save themselves shall see it thenceforth
                  with sight.
        He thanked her with fervent heart:
        As often as ever he might:

> Three times, before they part,
> She has kissed the stalwart knight.

Then the lady took her leave, and left him there,
For more mirth with that man she might not have.
When she was gone, Sir Gawain got from his bed,
Arose and arrayed him in his rich attire;
Tucked away the token the temptress had left.
Laid it reliably where he looked for it after.
And then with good cheer to the chapel he goes,
Approached a priest in private, and prayed to be taught
To lead a better life and lift up his mind,
Lest he be among the lost when he must leave this world.
And shamefaced at shrift he showed his misdeeds
From the largest to the least, and asked the Lord's mercy,
And called on his confessor to cleanse his soul,
And he absolved him of his sins as safe and as clean
As if the dread Day of Judgment should dawn on the morrow.
And then he made merry amid the fine ladies
With deft-footed dances and dalliance light,
As never until now, while the afternoon wore
>   away.
> He delighted all around him,
> And all agreed, that day,
> They never before had found him
> So gracious and so gay.

Now peaceful be his pasture, and love play him fair!
The host is on horseback, hunting afield;
He has finished off this fox that he followed so long:
As he leapt a low hedge to look for the villain
Where he heard all the hounds in hot pursuit,
Reynard comes racing out of a rough thicket,
And all the rabble in a rush, right at his heels.
The man beholds the beast, and bides his time,
And bares his bright sword, and brings it down hard,
And he blenches from the blade, and backward he starts;
A hound hurries up and hinders that move,
And before the horse's feet they fell on him at once

And ripped the rascal's throat with a wrathful din.
The lord soon alighted and lifted him free,
Swiftly snatched him up from the snapping jaws,
Holds him over his head, halloos with a will,
And the dogs bayed the dirge, that had done him to death.
Hunters hastened thither with horns at their lips,
Sounding the assembly till they saw him at last.
When that comely company was come in together,
All that bore bugles blew them at once,
And the others all hallooed, that had no horns.
It was the merriest medley that ever a man heard,
The racket that they raised for Sir Reynard's soul
                              that died.
              Their hounds they praised and fed.
              Fondling their heads with pride,
              And they took Reynard the Red
              And stripped away his hide.

And then they headed homeward, for evening had come,
Blowing many a blast on their bugles bright.
The lord at long last alights at his house,
Finds fire on the hearth where the fair knight waits,
Sir Gawain the good, that was glad in heart.
With the ladies, that loved him, he lingered at ease;
He wore a rich robe of blue, that reached to the earth
And a surcoat lined softly with sumptuous furs:
A hood of the same hue hung on his shoulders;
With bands of bright ermine embellished were both.
He comes to meet the man amid all the folk,
And greets him good-humouredly, and gaily he says,
'I shall follow forthwith the form of our pledge
That we framed to good effect amid fresh-filled cups.'
He clasps him accordingly and kisses him thrice,
As amiably and as earnestly as ever he could.
'By heaven,' said the host, 'you have had some luck
Since you took up this trade, if the terms were good.'
'Never trouble about the terms,' he returned at once,
'Since all that I owe here is openly paid.'
'Marry!' said the other man, 'mine is much less,

For I have hunted all day, and nought have I got
But this foul fox pelt, the fiend take the goods!
Which but poorly repays those precious things
That you have cordially conferred, those kisses three
                         so good.'
                  'Enough!' said Sir Gawain;
                  'I thank you, by the rood!'
                  And how the fox was slain
                  He told him, as they stood.

&

Thomas Hardy
1840–1928

from Jude the Obscure

Jude Fawley is a naive young stonemason who aspires to gain admission to the university at Christminster. He is interrupted as he is walking home from work one day, planning his future. This extract is taken from the serial version of Jude the Obscure, *which was entitled* The Simpletons.

'Ha, ha, ha! Hoity-toity!' The sounds were expressed in light voices on the other side of the hedge, but he did not notice them. His thoughts went on:

' – Euripides, Plato, Aristotle, Lucretius, Epictetus, Seneca, Antoninus. Then I must master other things: the Fathers thoroughly; Bede and ecclesiastical history generally; a smattering of Hebrew – I only know the letters as yet – '

'Hoity-toity!'

' – but I can work hard. I have staying power in abundance, thank God! and it is that which tells . . . Yes, Christminster shall be my Alma Mater; and I'll be her beloved son, in whom she shall be well pleased.'

In his deep concentration on these transactions of the future, Jude's walk had slackened, and he was now standing quite still, looking at the ground as though the future were thrown thereon by a magic lantern. On a sudden something smacked him sharply in the ear, and he became aware that a soft cold substance had been flung at him, and had fallen at his feet.

A glance told him what it was – a piece of flesh, portion of a recently killed pig, which the countrymen used for greasing their boots, as it was useless for any other purpose. Pigs were rather plentiful hereabout, being bred and fattened in large numbers in certain parts of North Wessex.

On the other side of the hedge was a stream, whence, as he now for the first time realized, had come the slight sounds of voices and laughter that had mingled with his dreams. He mounted the bank and looked over the fence. On the further side of the stream stood a small homestead, having a garden and pigsties attached; in front of it, beside the brook, three young women were kneeling, with buckets and platters beside them containing heaps of pigs' chitterlings, which they were washing in the running water. One or two pairs of eyes slyly glanced up, and perceiving that his attention had at last been attracted, and that he was watching them, they braced themselves for inspection by putting their mouths demurely into shape and recommencing their rinsing operations with assiduity.

'Thank you!' said Jude, severely.

'I *didn't* throw it, I tell you!' asserted one girl to her neighbor, as if unconscious of the young man's presence.

'Nor I,' the second answered.

'Oh, Anny, how can you!' said the third.

'If I had thrown anything at all, it shouldn't have been such a vulgar thing as that!'

'Pooh! I don't care for him!' And they laughed and continued their work, without looking up, still ostentatiously accusing each other.

Jude grew sarcastic as he wiped the spot where the clammy flesh had struck him.

'*You* didn't do it! Oh no!' he said to the upstream one of the three.

She whom he addressed was a fine dark-eyed girl, not exactly handsome, but capable of passing as such at a little distance, despite some coarseness of skin and fibre. She had a round and prominent bosom, full lips, perfect teeth, and the rich complexion of a Cochin hen's egg. She was a complete and substantial female human – no more, no less; and Jude was almost certain that to her was attributable the enterprise of throwing the lump of offal at him.

'That you'll never be told,' said she, decidedly.

'Whoever did it was wasteful of other people's property.'

'Oh, that's nothing. The pig is my father's.'

'But you want it back, I suppose?'

'Oh yes; if you like to give it me.'

'Shall I throw it across, or will you come to the plank above here for me to hand it to you?'

Perhaps she foresaw an opportunity; for somehow or other the eyes of the brown girl rested in his own when he had said the words, and there was a momentary flash of intelligence, a dumb announcement of affinity *in posse*, between herself and him, which, so far as Jude Fawley was concerned, had no sort of premeditation in it. She saw that he had singled her out from the three, as a woman is singled out in such cases, for no reasoned purpose of further acquaintance, but in commonplace obedience to conjunctive orders from headquarters, unconsciously received by unfortunate men when the last intention of their lives is to be occupied with the feminine.

Springing to her feet, she said: 'Don't throw it! Give it to me.'

Jude was now aware that the intrinsic value of the missile had nothing to do with her request. He set down his basket of tools, raked out with his stick the scrap of flesh from the ditch, and got over the hedge. They walked in parallel lines, one on each bank of the stream, towards the small plank bridge. As the girl drew nearer to it, she gave, without Jude perceiving it, an adroit little suck to the interior of each of her cheeks in succession, by which curious and original manœuvre she brought as by magic upon its smooth and rotund surface a perfect dimple, which she was able to retain there as long as she continued to smile. This production of dimples at will was a not unknown operation, which many attempted, but only a few succeeded in accomplishing.

They met in the middle of the plank, and Jude held out his stick with the fragment of pig dangling therefrom, looking elsewhere the while.

She, too, looked in another direction, and took the piece as though ignorant of what her hand was doing. She hung it temporarily on the rail of the bridge, and then, by a species of mutual curiosity, they both turned.

'You don't think I threw it?'

'Oh no.'

'It belongs to father, and he med have been in a taking if he had wanted it. He makes it into dubbin.'

'What made either of the others throw it, I wonder?' Jude asked, politely accepting her assertion, though he had very large doubts as to its truth.

'Impudence. Don't tell folk it was I, mind!'

'How can I? I don't know your name.'

'Ah, no. Shall I tell it to you?'

'Do!'

'Arabella Donn. I'm living here.'

'I must have known it if I had often come this way. But I mostly go straight along the highroad.'

'My father is a pig-breeder, and these girls are helping me wash the innerds for black-puddings and chitterlings.'

They talked a little more and a little more, as they stood regarding the slip of flesh dangling from the hand-rail of the bridge. The unvoiced call of woman to man, which was uttered very distinctly by Arabella's personality, held Jude to the spot against his intention – almost against his will, and in a way new to his experience. It is scarcely an exaggeration to say that till this moment Jude had never looked at a woman to consider her as such, but had vaguely regarded the sex as beings outside his life and purposes. He gazed from her eyes to her mouth, thence to her shoulders, and to her full round naked arms, wet, mottled with the chill of the water, and firm as marble.

'What a nice-looking girl you are!' he murmured, though the words had not been necessary to express his sense of her magnetism.

'Ah, you should see me Sundays!' she said, piquantly.

'I don't suppose I could?' he answered.

'That's for you to think on. There's nobody after me just now, though there med be in a week or two.' She had spoken this without a smile, and the dimples disappeared.

Jude felt himself drifting strangely, but could not help it. 'Will you let me?'

'I don't mind.'

By this time she had managed to get back one dimple by turning her face aside for a moment and repeating the odd little sucking operation before mentioned, Jude being still unconscious of more than a general impression of her appearance. 'Next Sunday?' he hazarded. 'Tomorrow, that is?'

'Yes.'

'Shall I call?'

'Yes.'

She brightened with a little glow of triumph, swept him almost tenderly with her eyes in turning, and throwing the offal out of the way upon the grass, rejoined her companions.

Stevie Smith
1902–71

The River God

(Of the River Mimram in Hertfordshire)

I may be smelly and I may be old,
Rough in my pebbles, reedy in my pools,
But where my fish float by I bless their swimming
And I like the people to bathe in me, especially women.
But I can drown the fools
Who bathe too close to the weir, contrary to rules.
And they take a long time drowning
As I throw them up now and then in a spirit of clowning.
Hi yih, yippity-yap, merrily I flow,
O I may be an old foul river but I have plenty of go.
Once there was a lady who was too bold
She bathed in me by the tall black cliff where the water
     runs cold,
So I brought her down here
To be my beautiful dear.
Oh will she stay with me will she stay
This beautiful lady, or will she go away?
She lies in my beautiful deep river bed with many a weed
To hold her, and many a waving reed.
Oh who would guess what a beautiful white face lies there
Waiting for me to smoothe and wash away the fear
She looks at me with. Hi yih, do not let her
Go. There is no one on earth who does not forget her
Now. They say I am a foolish old smelly river
But they do not know of my wide original bed
Where the lady waits, with her golden sleepy head.
If she wishes to go I will not forgive her.

Liz Lochhead
1947–

What The Pool Said, On Midsummer's Day

I've led you by my garrulous banks, babbling
on and on till – drunk on air
and sure it's only water talking –
you come at last to my silence.
Listen, I'm dark
and still and deep enough.
Even this hottest gonging sun
on this longest day
can't white me out.
What are you waiting for?
I lie here, inviting, winking you in.

The woman was easy.
Like to like, I called her, she came.
In no time I had her
out of herself, slipping on my water-stockings,
leaning into, being cupped and clasped
in my green glass bra.
But it's you I want, and you know it, man.
I watch you, stripped, knee-deep
in my shallows, telling yourself
that what makes you gasp
and balls your gut
is not my coldness but your own fear.

– Your reasonable fear,
what's true in me admits it.
(Though deeper, oh
older than any reason).
Yes, I could
drown you, you
could foul my depths, it's not
unheard of. What's fish
in me could make flesh of you,
my wet weeds against your thigh, it
could turn nasty.
I could have you
gulping fistfuls fighting yourself
back from me.

I get darker and darker, suck harder.
On-the-brink man, you
wish I'd flash and dazzle again.
You'd make a fetish of zazzing dragonflies?
You want I should zip myself up
with the kingfisher's flightpath, be beautiful?
I say no tricks. I say just trust,
I'll soak through your skin and
slake your thirst.

I watch. You clench,
clench and come into me.

Index of Authors
and Works

ANONYMOUS
from The Book of Genesis   309
from Sir Gawain and the Green
     Knight   342
Jankin, the clerical seducer   46
from The Lustful Turk   206

JANE AUSTEN 1775–1817
from Sanditon   35

APHRA BEHN 1640–89
The Willing Mistriss   152

WILLIAM BLAKE 1757–1827
The Sick Rose   177

LILIAN BOWES-LYON 1895–1949
Leda   298

MALCOLM BRADBURY 1932–
from Rates of Exchange   22

JOHN BRAINE 1922–86
from Room at the Top   42

GEORGE GORDON, LORD BYRON
     1788–1824
from Don Juan   145

ANGELA CARTER 1940–
from Heroes and Villains   153

WILLIAM CONGREVE 1670–1729
from Love for Love   3
from The Way of the World   63

JENNIFER DAWSON 1929–
from The Ha-Ha   218

DANIEL DEFOE 1660?–1731
from Moll Flanders   167

JOHN DONNE 1571/2–1631
Going to Bed   6

HENRY FIELDING 1707–54
from Joseph Andrews   124
from Shamela (attributed)   244
from Tom Jones   19

E. M. FORSTER 1879–1970
from Arthur Snatchfold   113

WILLIAM GOLDING 1911–
from Free Fall   252

OLIVER GOLDSMITH 1730–74
Song (*from* The Vicar of Wakefield)   288

GRAHAM GREENE 1904–
Chagrin in Three Parts   8

RADCLYFFE HALL 1886–1943
from The Well of Loneliness   48

THOMAS HARDY 1840–1928
from Jude the Obscure   350
The Ruined Maid   227
from Tess of the d'Urbervilles   221

ROBERT HERRICK 1591–1674
Delight in Disorder   21

THOMAS HEYWOOD 1574?–1641
Jupiter and Ganimede   59

ALDOUS HUXLEY 1894–1963
from Point Counter Point   292

BEN JONSON 1572–1637
from The Alchemist   78
from Volpone   37

MOLLY KEANE 1904–
from Time after Time   135

JOHN KEATS 1795–1821
La Belle Dame sans Merci   332
from Lamia   266

PHILIP LARKIN 1922–86
Deceptions   166

D. H. LAWRENCE 1885–1930
from Sons and Lovers   149

LAURIE LEE 1914–
from Cider with Rosie   320

JOHN LEHMANN 1907–
from In the Purely Pagan Sense   57

MATTHEW G. LEWIS 1775–1818
from The Monk   194

WYNDHAM LEWIS 1884–1957
from Cantleman's Spring-Mate   103

LIZ LOCHHEAD 1947–
What The Pool Said, On
    Midsummer's Day   356

IAN MCEWAN 1948–
from Homemade   231

SARA MAITLAND 1949–
from Virgin Territory   198

THOMAS MALORY d. 1471
from Le Morte d'Arthur (Launcelot
    is tricked by Dame Brisen)   329
from Le Morte d'Arthur (Sir Pelleas
    and the Lady Ettard)   74

MARY DE LA RIVIERE MANLEY 1663–1724
from The New Atalantis   158

CHRISTOPHER MARLOWE 1564–93
from Doctor Faustus   317
from Hero and Leander   32

ANDREW MARVELL 1621–78
To his Coy Mistress   52

[361]

THOMAS MIDDLETON 1570?–1627
from Women Beware Women 109
with WILLIAM ROWLEY 1585?–1642?
from The Changeling 129

JOHN MILTON 1608–74
from Paradise Lost (Book v) 263
from Paradise Lost (Book ix: Satan
 tempts Eve) 92
from Paradise Lost (Book ix: Eve
 tempts Adam) 311

BRIAN PATTEN 1946–
Party Piece 54

SYLVIA PLATH 1932–1963
from The Bell Jar 139

SAMUEL RICHARDSON 1689–1761
from Clarissa 178
from Pamela 240

CHRISTINA ROSSETTI 1830–94
Goblin Market 272

WILLIAM SHAKESPEARE 1564–1616
from Antony and Cleopatra 335
from Measure for Measure 188
from Richard iii 255
from Venus and Adonis 247

STEVIE SMITH 1902–71
The River God 355

EDMUND SPENSER 1552?–99
from The Faerie Queene (Book ii) 323

BRAM STOKER 1847–1912
from Dracula 299

CYRIL TOURNEUR 1575?–1626
from The Revenger's Tragedy 289

BARRY UNSWORTH 1930–
from Mooncranker's Gift 84

JOHN WEBSTER 1580?–1625?
from The White Devil 15

[362]

OSCAR WILDE 1854–1900
from Salomé   337

JOHN WILMOT, EARL OF
   ROCHESTER 1648–80
from Sodom (attributed)   156
Song (Fair Chloris)   238

WILLIAM WORDSWORTH 1770–1850
The Thorn   210

WILLIAM WYCHERLEY 1640?–1716
from The Country Wife   118

W. B. YEATS 1865–1939
Leda and the Swan   297

Acknowledgements

For permission to reprint copyright material, the publishers gratefully acknowledge the following:

Jonathan Cape Limited, the Executors of the Lilian Bowes-Lyon Estate and E. P. Dutton for 'Leda' from *Collected Poems* by Lilian Bowes-Lyon, copyright © 1948 by Lilian Bowes-Lyon; Martin Secker & Warburg Limited and Alfred A. Knopf, Inc., for extract from *Rates of Exchange* by Malcolm Bradbury, copyright © 1983 by Malcolm Bradbury; David Higham Associates for extract from *Room at the Top* by John Braine (Penguin, 1959); Elaine Markson and Deborah Rogers for extract from *Heroes and Villains* by Angela Carter, copyright © by Angela Carter 1969 (Penguin 1981); David Higham Associates for extract from *The Ha-Ha* by Jennifer Dawson (Virago, 1985); Edward Arnold and the Trustees of the Late E. M. Forster Estate for 'Arthur Snatchfold' from *The Life to Come and Other Stories* (Edward Arnold, 1972); Harcourt Brace Jovanovich, Inc. and Faber and Faber Limited for extract from *Free Fall* by William Golding, copyright © 1959 by William Golding; Laurence Pollinger, William Heinemann Limited, The Bodley Head Limited and Viking Penguin, Inc. for 'Chagrin in Three Parts' from *Collected Stories* by Graham Greene, copyright © Graham Greene 1967; the author and A. M. Heath and Company Limited for *The Well of Loneliness* by Radclyffe Hall (Hutchinson, 1986); Mrs Laura Huxley, Chatto & Windus Limited and Harper & Row, Inc., for extract from *Point Counter Point* by Aldous Huxley, copyright © 1928 by Aldous Huxley, André Deutsch Limited and Alfred A. Knopf, Inc., for extract from *Time After Time* by Molly Keane, copyright © 1983 by Molly Keane; The Marvell Press for 'Deceptions' from *The Less Deceived* by Philip Larkin (The Marvell Press, 1955); the author and The Hogarth Press for extract from *Cider With Rosie* by Laurie Lee (Hogarth, 1959); David Higham Associates Limited for extract from *In the Purely Pagan Sense* by John Lehmann (Blond and Briggs, 1976); Vision Press for 'Cantleman's Spring-Mate' from *Unlucky for Pringle: Unpublished and Other Stories* by Wyndham Lewis edited and introduced by C. J. Fox and Robert T. Chapman (Vision Press, 1973); Polygon for 'What the Pool Said, on Midsummer's Day' by Liz Lochhead from